Physiology
at a Glance

Physiology
at a Glance
Fourth Edition

Jeremy P.T. Ward

PhD
Professor of Respiratory Cell Physiology
Emeritus Professor of Physiology
Faculty of Life Sciences & Medicine
King's College London
London, UK

Roger W.A. Linden

BDS PhD MFDS RCS
Emeritus Professor of Craniofacial Biology
Faculty of Life Sciences & Medicine
King's College London
London, UK

WILEY Blackwell

This edition first published 2017 © 2017 by John Wiley & Sons, Ltd

Edition History
John Wiley & Sons, Ltd (3e 2013)

The right of Jeremy P.T. Ward and Roger W.A. Linden to be identified as the authors of this work has been asserted in accordance with law.

Registered Office(s)   John Wiley & Sons, Inc., 111 River Street, Hoboken, NJ 07030, USA
John Wiley & Sons Ltd, The Atrium, Southern Gate, Chichester, West Sussex, PO19 8SQ, UK

Editorial Office   9600 Garsington Road, Oxford, OX4 2DQ, UK

For details of our global editorial offices, customer services, and more information about Wiley products visit us at www.wiley.com.

Wiley also publishes its books in a variety of electronic formats and by print-on-demand. Some content that appears in standard print versions of this book may not be available in other formats.

Library of Congress Cataloging-in-Publication Data are available.

ISBN 9781119247272

Cover image: © SCIEPRO/ Gettyimages

Set in Minion Pro 9.5/11.5 by Aptara
Printed and bound by CPI Group (UK) Ltd, Croydon, CR0 4YY

C9781119247272_260724

Contents

Preface

Physiology is defined as 'the scientific study of the bodily function of living organisms and their parts'. There is a natural symbiosis between function (physiology) and structure (anatomy) from which physiology emerged as a separate discipline in the late 19th century. A good understanding of anatomy and physiology is an essential prerequisite for understanding what happens when things go wrong – the structural abnormalities and pathophysiology of disease – and as such underpins all biomedical studies and medicine itself. Following a century of reductionism, where the focus of research has progressively narrowed down to the function of individual proteins and genes, there is now a resurgence in integrative physiology, as it has been realized that to make sense of developments such as the Human Genome Project we have to understand body function as an integrated whole. This is considerably more complex than just the sum of its parts because of the multiplicity of interactions involved. True understanding of the role of a single gene, for example, can only be gained when placed in the context of the whole animal, as reflected by the often unexpected effects of knock-out of single genes on the phenotype of mice.

This volume is designed as a concise guide and revision aid to core topics in physiology, and should be useful to all students following a first-year physiology course, whether they are studying single honours, biomedical sciences, nursing, medicine or dentistry. It should also be useful to those studying system-based curricula. The layout of *Physiology at a Glance* follows that of the other volumes in the *At a Glance series*, with a two-page spread for each topic (loosely corresponding to a lecture), comprising a large diagram on one page and concise explanatory text on the other. For this fourth edition we have extensively revised the text and figures, there are three completely new chapters, on Cell signalling, Thermoregulation, and Altitude and aerospace physiology, and we have added a Glossary.

Physiology is a large subject, and in a book this size we cannot hope to cover anything but the core and basics. *Physiology at a Glance* should therefore be used primarily to assist basic understanding of key concepts and as an assistance to revision. Deeper knowledge should be gained by reference to full physiology and system textbooks, and in third-year honours programmes to original peer-reviewed papers. Students may find one or two sections of this book difficult, such as that on the physics of flow and diffusion, and detailed elements of cell signalling. Though such material may not be included in some introductory physiology courses, an understanding of these concepts can assist in learning how body systems behave in the way they do, and in understanding primary research papers.

In revising this fourth edition we have been helped immensely by constructive criticism and suggestions from our colleagues and students, and junior and senior reviewers of the last edition. We thank all those who have given us such advice; any errors are ours and not theirs. We would also like to thank the team at Wiley-Blackwell who provided great encouragement and support throughout the project.

Jeremy Ward
Roger Linden

Acknowledgements

Some figures in this book are taken or modified from:

Ward, J.P.T., Ward, J. and Leach, R.M. (2012) *The Respiratory System at a Glance* (4th edition). Wiley-Blackwell, Oxford.

Aaronson, P.I., Ward, J.P.T. and Connolly, M.J. (2012) *The Cardiovascular System at a Glance* (4th edition). Wiley-Blackwell, Oxford.

Mehta, A. and Hoffbrand, V. (2009) *Haematology at a Glance* (3rd edition). Wiley-Blackwell, Oxford.

Abbreviations

1,25-(OH)$_2$D	1,25-dihydroxycholecalciferol
2,3-DPG	2,3-diphosphoglycerate
5-HT	5-hydroxytryptamine; serotonin
μG	micro-gravity (weightlessness)
ACE	angiotensin-converting enzyme
ACh	acetylcholine
ACTH	adrenocorticotrophic hormone
ADH	antidiuretic hormone (also called vasopressin)
ADP	adenosine diphosphate
AIDS	acquired immune deficiency syndrome
AMH	anti-Müllerian hormone
AMS	acute mountain sickness
ANP	atrial natriuretic peptide
ANS	autonomic nervous system
AP	action potential
APC	active protein C *or* antigen presenting cell
ATP	adenosine triphosphate
ATPase	enzyme that splits ATP
AV node	atrioventricular node (heart)
AVAs	arteriovenous anastomoses
BAT	brown adipose tissue
BSA	body surface area
BTPS	body temperature and pressure, saturated with water
CaM	calmodulin
CaM-kinase	calcium–calmodulin kinase
cAMP	cyclic adenosine monophosphate
CaSR	calcium-sensing receptor (protein)
CCK	cholecystokinin
CDI	central diabetes insipidus
cGMP	cyclic guanosine monophosphate
CICR	Ca^{2+}-induced Ca^{2+} release
CNS	central nervous system
CO	cardiac output
COMT	catechol-*O*-methyl transferase
COX	cyclooxygenase
CRH	corticotrophin-releasing hormone
CSF	cerebrospinal fluid
CVP	central venous pressure
Da	Dalton (unit for molecular weight)
DAG	diacylglycerol
DHEA	dehydroepiandrosterone
D$_{L}$O$_2$	O_2 diffusing capacity in lung; transfer factor
DNA	deoxyribonucleic acid
DOPA	dihydroxyphenylalanine
E$_{(ion)}$	equilibrium potential for ion (e.g. K^+, Na^+, Ca^{2+} or Cl^-)
ECF	extracellular fluid
ECG (EKG)	electrocardiogram (or graph)
EDP	end diastolic pressure
EDV	end diastolic volume
EGF	epidermal growth factor
E$_m$	membrane potential
EMG	electromyogram
EPO	erythropoietin
EPP	end plate potential
ERV	expiratory reserve volume
ESV	end systolic volume
ETC	electron transport chain
F$_{ab}$	hypervariable region of antibody molecule
F$_c$	constant region of antibody molecule
FEV$_1$	forced expiratory volume in 1 s
FFA	free fatty acids
FGF	fibroblast growth factor
F$_{N_2}$ (F$_{O_2}$)	fractional concentration of nitrogen (oxygen) in a gas mixture
FRC	functional residual capacity
FSH	follicle-stimulating hormone
FVC	forced vital capacity
G-LOC	G-forces induced loss of consciousness
G-protein	GTP-binding protein
GDP	guanosine diphosphate
GFR	glomerular filtration rate
GH	growth hormone
GHRH	growth hormone-releasing hormone
GI	gastrointestinal
GIP	gastric inhibitory peptide
GLP-1	glucagon-like peptide 1
GLUT-1, 2 or 4	glucose transporters
GnRH	gonadotrophin-releasing hormone
GPCR	G-protein-coupled receptor
GRP	gastrin-releasing peptide
GTP	guanosine triphosphate
GTPase	enzyme that splits GTP
HACE	high-altitude cerebral oedema
HAPE	high-altitude pulmonary oedema
[Hb]	haemoglobin concentration

HbA	adult haemoglobin	**PLC**	phospholipase C
HbF	fetal haemoglobin	**PMCA**	plasma membrane Ca^{2+} ATPase
hCG	human chorionic gonadotrophin	**P_{O_2}**	partial pressure of oxygen
HIV	human immunodeficiency virus	**PRR**	pattern recognition receptor
HMWK	high molecular weight kininogen	**PTH**	parathyroid hormone
ICF	intracellular fluid	**Ras, Rho**	small monomeric GTPases
IgA, E, G, M	immunoglobulin A, E, G or M	**ROC**	receptor-operated channels
IGF-1 or 2	insulin-like growth factor (1 or 2)	**ROMK**	renal outer medullary potassium channel
IL-1b or 6	interleukin-1β or 6	**RPF**	renal plasma flow
IP_3	inositol trisphosphate	**RTK**	receptor tyrosine kinase
IRS-1	insulin receptor substrate 1	**RV**	residual volume *or* right ventricle
IRV	inspiratory reserve volume	**SA node**	sinoatrial node
ISF	interstitial fluid	**SERCA**	smooth endoplasmic reticulum Ca^{2+} ATPase
JAK	Janus kinase		
JGA	juxtaglomerular apparatus	**SH2**	Src-homology 2
LH	luteinizing hormone	**SMAD**	intracellular protein associated with streptokinases
MAO	monoamine oxidase		
MAP	mean arterial pressure	**SOC**	store-operated channels
MAPK(K)	mitogen-activated protein kinase (kinase)	**SP**	Substance P
		SR	sarcoplasmic reticulum
MEPP	miniature end plate potentials	**Src**	a non-receptor tyrosine kinase
MHC I, II	major histocompatibility complex I or II	**SST**	somatostatin
MIH	melanotrophin-inhibiting hormone	**STAT**	signal transduction and activation of transcription (protein)
MLC	myosin light chain		
MLCK	myosin light chain kinase	**STIM**	stromal interaction molecule
MLCP	myosin light chain phosphatase	**STPD**	standard temperature and pressure, dry gas
mRNA	messenger RNA		
MSH	melanotrophin-stimulating hormone	**SV**	stroke volume
Na^+ pump	Na^+-K^+ ATPase	**SWVP**	saturated water vapour pressure
NAD^+ or (NADH)	nicotinic adenine dinucleotide (oxidized and reduced forms)	**$T_{1 or 2}$**	mono- or di-iodotyrosine
		T_3	tri-iodothyronine
NCX	Na^+-Ca^{2+} exchanger	**T_4**	thyroxine
NDI	nephrogenic diabetes insipidus	**T_C**	Core temperature
NGF	nerve growth factor	**TF**	tissue factor
NK	natural killer (cells)	**TGFβ**	transforming growth factor β
NMJ	neuromuscular junction	**TH**	thyroid hormone
NO	nitric oxide	**TLC**	total lung capacity
NOS	nitric oxide synthase	**T_m**	tubular transport maximum (kidney)
P2Y or P2X	purinergic receptor type 2Y or 2X	**TNF**	tumour necrosis factor
PAH	*para*-aminohippuric acid	**TNZ**	thermoneutral zone
PAMP	pathogen-associated molecular pattern	**tPA**	tissue plasminogen activator
		TPR	total peripheral resistance
P_B	barometric pressure	**TRa**	thyroid hormone receptor
PDGF	platelet-derived growth factor	**TRE**	thyroid response element
PEFR	peak expiratory flow rate	**tRNA**	transfer RNA
PGE_2	prostaglandin E_2	**TSH**	thyroid-stimulating hormone
PGI_2	prostacyclin (prostaglandin I_2)	**TUC**	time of useful consciousness
PI-3 kinase	phosphatidylinositol-3 kinase	**TV**	tidal volume
pK	negative log of dissociation constant (buffers)	**TXA_2**	thromboxane A_2
		UCP-1, 2 or 3	uncoupling protein-1, 2 or 3
PKA	protein kinase A	**V_A/Q mismatch**	ventilation–perfusion mismatch (lungs)
PKC	protein kinase C	**VC**	vital capacity
PKG	protein kinase G	**VIP**	vasoactive intestinal polypeptide
PLA_2	phospholipase A2	**vWF**	von Willebrand factor

About the companion website

This book is accompanied by a companion website:

www.ataglanceseries.com/physiology

The website features:

- Interactive multiple choice questions
- Revision notes
- Interactive self-test flashcards

Introduction

Part 1

Chapters

1 Homeostasis and the physiology of proteins

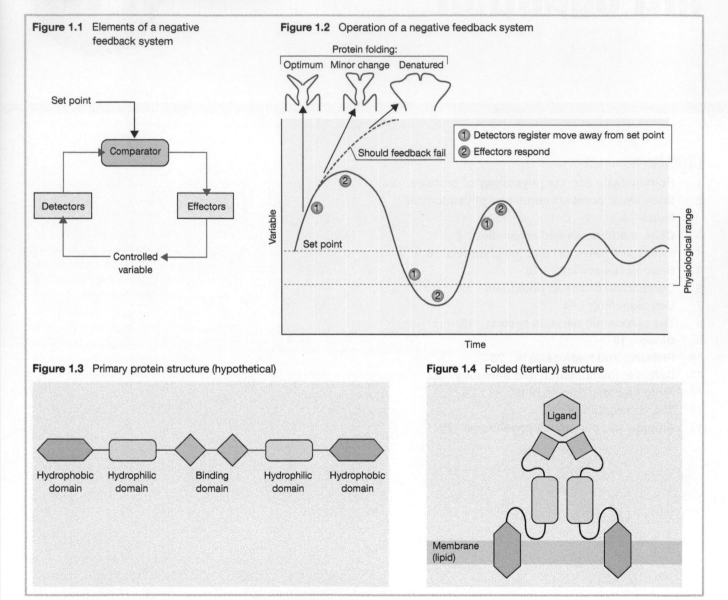

Figure 1.1 Elements of a negative feedback system

Set point

Comparator

Detectors

Effectors

Controlled variable

Figure 1.2 Operation of a negative feedback system

Protein folding:

Optimum Minor change Denatured

① Detectors register move away from set point
② Effectors respond

Should feedback fail

Variable

Set point

Time

Physiological range

Figure 1.3 Primary protein structure (hypothetical)

Hydrophobic domain Hydrophilic domain Binding domain Hydrophilic domain Hydrophobic domain

Figure 1.4 Folded (tertiary) structure

Ligand

Membrane (lipid)

Claude Bernard (1813–1878) first described 'le mileau intérieur' and observed that the internal environment of the body remained remarkably constant (or in equilibrium) despite the ever changing external environment. The term **homeostasis** was not used until 1929 when **Walter Cannon** first used it to describe this ability of physiological systems to maintain conditions within the body in a relatively constant state of equilibrium. It is arguably the most important concept in physiology.

Homeostasis is Greek for 'staying the same'. However, this so-called **equilibrium** is not an unchanging state but is a dynamic state of equilibrium causing a **dynamic constancy** of the internal environment. This **dynamic constancy** arises from the variable responses caused by changes in the external environment. Homeostasis maintains most physiological systems

and examples are seen throughout this book. The way in which the body maintains the H⁺ ion concentration of body fluids within narrow limits, the control of blood glucose by the release of insulin, and the control of body temperature, heart rate and blood pressure are all examples of homeostasis. The human body has literally thousands of control systems. The most intricate are genetic control systems that operate in all cells to control intracellular function as well as all extracellular functions. Many others operate within organs to control their function; others operate throughout the body to control interaction between organs. As long as conditions are maintained within the normal physiological range within the internal environment, the cells of the body continue to live and function properly. Each cell benefits from homeostasis and in turn, each cell contributes its share towards the maintenance of homeostasis. This reciprocal

Physiology at a Glance, Fourth Edition. Edited by Jeremy P.T. Ward and Roger W.A. Linden interplay provides continuity of life until one or more functional systems lose their ability to contribute their share. Moderate dysfunction of homeostasis leads to sickness and disease, and extreme dysfunction of homeostasis leads to death.

Negative feedback control

Most physiological control mechanisms have a common basic structure. The factor that is being controlled is called the **variable**. Homeostatic mechanisms provide the tight regulation of *all* physiological variables and the most common type of regulation is by *negative* feedback. A negative feedback system (Figure 1.1) comprises: **detectors** (often neural **receptor cells**) to measure the variable in question; a **comparator** (usually a neural assembly in the central nervous system) to receive input from the detectors and compare the size of the signal against the desired level of the variable (the **set point**); and **effectors** (muscular and/or glandular tissue) that are activated by the comparator to restore the variable to its set point. The term 'negative feedback' comes from the fact that the effectors always act to move the variable in the opposite direction to the change that was originally detected. Thus, when the partial pressure of CO_2 in blood increases above 5.3 kPa (40 mmHg), brain stem mechanisms increase the rate of ventilation to clear the excess gas, and *vice versa* when CO_2 levels fall below 5.3 kPa (Chapter 32). The term 'set point' implies that there is a single optimum value for each physiological variable; however, there is some tolerance in all physiological systems and the set point is actually a narrow *range* of values within which physiological processes will work normally (Figure 1.2). Not only is the set point not a point, but it can be reset in some systems according to physiological requirements. For instance, at high altitude, the low partial pressure of O_2 in inspired air causes the ventilation rate to increase. Initially, this effect is limited due to the loss of CO_2, but, after 2–3 days, the brain stem lowers the set point for CO_2 and allows ventilation to increase further, a process known as **acclimatization** (Chapter 14).

A common operational feature of all negative feedback systems is that they induce oscillations in the variable that they control (Figure 1.2). The reason for this is that it takes time for a system to detect and respond to a change in a variable. This delay means that feedback control always causes the variable to overshoot the set point slightly, activating the opposite restorative mechanism to induce a smaller overshoot in that direction, until the oscillations fall within the range of values that are optimal for physiological function. Normally, such oscillations have little visible effect. However, if unusually long delays are introduced into a system, the oscillations can become extreme. Patients with congestive heart failure sometimes show a condition known as **Cheyne–Stokes' breathing**, in which the patient undergoes periods of deep breathing interspersed with periods of no breathing at all (**apnoea**). This is partly due to the slow flow of blood from the lungs to the brain, which causes a large delay in the detection of blood levels of CO_2.

Some physiological responses use *positive* feedback, causing rapid amplification. Examples include initiation of an action potential, where sodium entry causes depolarization which further increases sodium entry and thus more depolarization

(Chapter 5), and certain hormonal changes, particularly in reproduction (Chapter 53). Positive feedback is inherently unstable, and requires some mechanism to break the feedback loop and stop the process (an off switch), such as time-dependent inactivation of sodium channels in the first example and the birth of the child in the second.

Protein form and function are protected by homeostatic mechanisms

The homeostatic mechanisms that are described in detail throughout this book have evolved to protect the integrity of the protein products of gene translation. Normal functioning of proteins is essential for life, and usually requires binding to other molecules, including other proteins. The specificity of this binding is determined by the three-dimensional shape of the protein. The **primary structure** of a protein is determined by the sequence of amino acids (Figure 1.3). Genetic mutations that alter this sequence can have profound effects on the functionality of the final molecule. Such gene **polymorphisms** are the basis of many genetically based disorders. The final shape of the molecule (the **tertiary structure**), however, results from a process of **folding** of the amino acid chain (Figure 1.4). Folding is a complex process by which a protein achieves its lowest energy conformation. It is determined by electrochemical interactions between amino acid side-chains (e.g. hydrogen bonds, van der Waals' forces), and is so vital that it is overseen by **molecular chaperones**, such as the **heat shock proteins**, which provide a quiet space within which the protein acquires its final shape. In healthy tissue, cells can detect and destroy misfolded proteins, the accumulation of which damages cells and is responsible for various pathological conditions, including **Alzheimer's disease** and **Creutzfeldt–Jakob disease**. Folding ensures that the functional sequences of amino acids (**domains**) that form, e.g. binding sites for other molecules or hydrophobic segments for insertion into a membrane, are properly orientated to allow the protein to serve its function.

The relatively weak nature of the forces that cause folding renders them sensitive to changes in the environment surrounding the protein. Thus, alterations in acidity, osmotic potential, concentrations of specific molecules/ions, temperature or even hydrostatic pressure can modify the tertiary shape of a protein and change its interactions with other molecules. These modifications are usually reversible and are exploited by some proteins to detect alterations in the internal or external environments. For instance, nerve cells that respond to changes in CO_2 (chemoreceptors; Chapter 32) possess **ion channel** proteins (Chapter 4) that open or close to generate electrical signals (Chapter 5) when the acidity of the medium surrounding the receptor (CO_2 forms an acid in solution) alters by more than a certain amount. However, there are limits to the degree of fluctuation in the internal environment that can be tolerated by proteins before their shape alters so much that they become non-functional or irreversibly damaged, a process known as **denaturation** (this is what happens to egg-white proteins in cooking). Homeostatic systems prevent such conditions from arising within the body, and thus preserve protein functionality.

2 Body water compartments and physiological fluids

Figure 2.1 Physiological fluid compartments

Interstitial fluid

Cell
(cytosol, ICF)

Diffusion
between
plasma and
cytosol

Capillary
(plasma)

ATP

Na+
pump

2K+   3Na+

Plasma membrane:
• Permeable to water
• Impermeant to ions
  except via ion channels
• Impermeant to proteins

Na+ pump (Na+–K+ ATPase):
• Maintains cytosolic ionic
  concentrations by pumping
  K+ into the cell and Na+ out

Capillary wall:
• Permeable to
  everything except
  plasma proteins

Constituents of physiological fluids (approximate values, intracellular varies between tissues)		Plasma	Interstitial	Intracellular	Unit
Water:	% total body water	13%	22%	65%	%
	(volume in a **70 kg** person)	(3.5)	(9.5)	(27)	L
Osmolality		290	290	290	mosmol/kg H_2O
Cations:	Na+	140	140	10	mmol/L
	K+	4	4	140	mmol/L
	Ca2+ (free)	1	1	0.0001	mmol/L
Anions:	Cl−	108	129	3–30	mmol/L
	HCO_3^-	26	26	9	mmol/L
	Proteins−	10	1	50	mmol/L
	Other anions (mainly PO_4^{3-}, SO_4^{3-})	3	0	60–88	mmol/L

Notes: Ca^{2+} (and Mg^{2+}) tend to bind to plasma proteins, and their free concentrations are about 50% of the total. Ionic concentrations are sometimes given in mEq/L to reflect the amount of charge, where an equivalent (Eq) is 1 mole of charge. So 1 Eq of a monovalent ion such as Na^+ = 1 mole, but 1 Eq of Ca^{2+} = 0.5 mole

Figure 2.2 Effects of ingesting fluids of differing osmotic potential

Hypertonic fluid

Plasma volume expands
Plasma becomes concentrated
Free movement of water and
ions from plasma leads to
expansion of interstitial fluid

Interstitial fluid becomes
concentrated
Osmotic potential draws water
out of cells

Cells lose water and shrink
Intracellular fluid concentrated

Water movement

Plasma

ISF

ICF

Isotonic fluid

Plasma volume expands
Free movement of water and
ions from plasma leads to
expansion of interstitial fluid

Fluid is isotonic so no osmotic
potential generated between
ISF and cells

Intracellular fluid unaffected

Water movement

Plasma

ISF

ICF

Hypotonic fluid

Plasma diluted
Oncotic pressure reduced
Water moves into interstitial
fluid

Interstitial fluid diluted
Osmotic potential generated
between ISF and cells
Water moves into cells

Intracellular fluid diluted
Cells swell

Water movement

Plasma

ISF

ICF

Physiology at a Glance, Fourth Edition. Edited by Jeremy P.T. Ward and Roger W.A. Linden.
© 2017 John Wiley & Sons, Ltd. Published 2017 by John Wiley & Sons, Ltd. Companion website: www.ataglanceseries.com/physiology

Osmosis

Osmosis is the passive movement of water across a **semi-permeable membrane** from regions of low solute concentration to those of higher solute concentration. Biological membranes are semi-permeable in that they usually allow the free movement of water but restrict the movement of solutes. The creation of **osmotic gradients** is the primary method for the movement of water in biological systems. This is why the osmotic potential (**osmolality**) of body fluids is closely regulated by a number of homeostatic mechanisms (Chapter 38). A fluid at the same osmotic potential as plasma is said to be **isotonic**; one at higher potential (i.e. more concentrated solutes) is **hypertonic** and one at lower potential is **hypotonic**. The osmotic potential depends on the number of osmotically active particles (molecules) per litre, irrespective of their identity. It is expressed in terms of osmoles, where 1 osmole equals 1 mole of particles, as **osmolarity** (osmol/L), or **osmolality** (osmol/kg H_2O). The latter is preferred by physiologists as it is independent of temperature, though in physiological fluids the values are very similar. The osmolality of plasma is ~290 mosmol/kg H_2O, mostly due to dissolved ions and small molecules (e.g. glucose and urea). These diffuse easily across capillaries, and the **crystalloid osmotic pressure** they exert is therefore the same either side of the capillary wall. Proteins do not easily pass through capillary walls, and are responsible for the **oncotic** (or colloidal osmotic) pressure. This is much smaller than crystalloid osmotic pressure, but is critical for fluid transfer across capillary walls because it differs between plasma and interstitial fluid (Chapter 26). Oncotic pressure is expressed in terms of pressure, and in plasma is normally ~25 mmHg. Maintenance of plasma osmolality is vital for regulation of blood volume (Chapter 25). Drinking fluids of differing osmotic potentials has distinct effects on the distribution of water between cells and extracellular fluid (Figure 2.2).

Body water compartments

Water is the solvent in which almost all biological reactions take place (the other being membrane lipid), and so it is fitting that it accounts for some 50–70% of the body mass (i.e. about 40 L in a 70 kg person). The nature of biological membranes means that water moves freely within the body, but the materials dissolved in it do not. There are two major 'fluid compartments': the water within cells (**intracellular fluid, ICF**), which accounts for about 65% of the body total, and the water outside cells (**extracellular fluid, ECF**). These compartments are separated by the plasma membranes of the cells, and differ markedly in terms of the concentrations of the ions that are dissolved in them (Figure 2.1; Chapter 4). Approximately 65% of the ECF comprises the tissue fluid found between cells (**interstitial fluid, ISF**), and the rest is made up of the liquid component of blood (**plasma**). The barrier between these two fluids consists of the walls of the capillaries (Figure 2.1; Chapter 26).

Intracellular versus extracellular fluid

Many critical biological events, including all bioelectrical signals (Chapter 5), depend on maintaining the composition of physiological fluids within narrow limits. Figure 2.1 shows the concentrations of ions in the three main fluid compartments. It should be noted that, *within* any one compartment, there *must* be electrical neutrality, i.e. the total number of positive charges must equal the total number of negative charges. The most important difference between ICF and ECF lies in the relative concentrations of cations. The K^+ ion concentration is much higher inside the cell than in ECF, while the opposite is true for the Na^+ ion concentration. Ca^{2+} and Cl^- ion concentrations are also higher in ECF. The question arises as to how these differences come about, and how they are maintained. Ion channel proteins allow the cell to determine the flow of ions across its own membrane (Chapter 4). In most circumstances, relatively few channels are open so that the leakage of ions is low. There is, however, always a steady movement of ions across the membrane, with Na^+ and K^+ following their concentration gradients into and out of the cell, respectively. Uncorrected, the leak would eventually lead to the equalization of the compositions of the two compartments, effectively eliminating all bioelectrical signalling (Chapter 5). This is prevented by the activity of the Na^+-K^+ ATPase, or Na^+ pump (Chapter 3). Of the other ions, most Ca^{2+} in the cell is transported actively either out of the cell or into the endoplasmic reticulum and mitochondria, leaving very low levels of free Ca^{2+} in ICF. Cl^- ions are differentially distributed across the membrane by virtue of their negative charge. Intracellular proteins are negatively charged at physiological pH. These and other large anions that cannot cross the plasma membrane (e.g. phosphate, PO_4^{3-}) are trapped within the cell and account for most of the anion content of ICF. Cl^- ions, which *can* diffuse across the membrane through channels, are forced out of the cell by the charge on the fixed anions. The electrical force driving Cl^- ions out of the cell is balanced by the chemical gradient driving them back in, a situation known as the **Gibbs–Donnan equilibrium**. Variations in the large anion content of cells mean that the concentration of Cl^- ions in ICF can vary by a factor of 10 between cell types, being as high as 30 mM in cardiac myocytes, although lower values (around 5 mM) are more common.

Interstitial fluid versus plasma

The main difference between these fluids is that plasma contains more protein than does ISF (Figure 2.1). The plasma proteins (Chapter 9) are the only constituents of plasma that do not cross into ISF, although they are allowed to escape from capillaries in very specific circumstances (Chapter 11). The presence of impermeant proteins in the plasma exerts an osmotic force relative to ISF (**plasma oncotic pressure**; see previously) that almost balances the hydrostatic pressure imposed on the plasma by the action of the heart, which tends to force water out of the capillaries, so that there is a small net water movement out of the plasma into the interstitial space. The leakage is absorbed by the **lymphatic system** (Chapter 26). **Transcellular fluid** is the name given to fluids that do not contribute to any of the main compartments, but which are derived from them. It includes cerebrospinal fluid and exocrine secretions, particularly gastrointestinal secretions (Chapters 40–44), and has a collective volume of approximately 2 L.

Cells, membranes and organelles

Figure 3.1 Main features of an eukaryotic cell

Golgi apparatus

Lysosomes

Microtubules
(part of cytoskeleton)

Smooth endoplasmic reticulum

Rough endoplasmic reticulum

Ribosomes

Nucleus

Nuclear envelope

Nuclear pore

Nucleolus

Plasma membrane

Mitochondria

(Organelles not to scale)

Figure 3.2 Fluid mosaic model of membrane

Membrane phospholipid

Phosphate and glycerol head (hydrophilic)

Fatty acid tails (hydrophobic)

Carbohydrate tails

Glycoprotein

Extracellular

Glycolipids

Ion channel protein

Integrins

Extracellular matrix

Glycocalyx

Membrane

Attachment to cytoskeleton and signalling proteins

Protein (e.g. receptor)

Cholesterol

Enzyme (e.g. phospholipase)

Cytosol

Figure 3.3 Energy production and mitochondria

Cell

Anaerobic respiration   Aerobic

O_2
CO_2

Lactate

Glucose → Glycolysis → Pyruvate NADH → ATP

Fatty acids

Mitochondria – oxidative phosphorylation

Outer membrane

Inner membrane

Matrix

Electron transport chain

H^+ H^+ H^+ H^+

I II III IV

Pyruvate Fatty acids + NAD^+

NADH, $FADH_2$

O_2

ADP+P

Citric acid (Krebs') cycle → CO_2

ATP synthase (driven by H^+ gradient)

ATP

Physiology at a Glance, Fourth Edition. Edited by Jeremy P.T. Ward and Roger W.A. Linden.
© 2017 John Wiley & Sons, Ltd. Published 2017 by John Wiley & Sons, Ltd. Companion website: www.ataglanceseries.com/physiology

The aqueous internal environment of the cell is separated from the aqueous external medium by an envelope of fat molecules (**lipids**) known as the **plasma membrane**. About half the cell is filled with **cytosol**, a viscous, protein-rich fluid between the internal structures. These consist of **organelles** which are themselves enclosed by lipid membranes, and components of the **cytoskeleton** such as microtubules and actin filaments which provide structural stability and the ability of the cell to change shape or move. The reticular appearance of the cell interior is due to organelles whose membranes are folded to maximize surface area. These include the **rough endoplasmic reticulum** and **Golgi apparatus**, which are involved in protein assembly, and the **smooth endoplasmic reticulum** which serves as a store for intracellular Ca^{2+} and is the major site of lipid production (Figure 3.1). The arrangement of structures within the cell is highly organized, but also dynamic; organelles and structures can be rearranged according to need and function (e.g. cell division or migration).

Protein-processing organelles

The **nucleus** (Figure 3.1) contains the chromosomes and **nucleolus**, a membrane-less structure responsible for production of **ribosomes**. Ribosomes translocate to the **rough endoplasmic reticulum** (giving it its appearance), where they are responsible for protein assembly. The endoplasmic reticulum and **Golgi apparatus** perform post-translational processing of new proteins. This includes trimming amino acid chains to the right length, protein folding, addition of polysaccharide chains (**glycosylation**) and identification of improperly folded proteins. These and other proteins for recycling are tagged with multiple **ubiquitin** molecules, allowing them to be recognized and destroyed by **proteasomes** (proteolytic protein complexes). Proteins are delivered from the Golgi apparatus to specific intracellular destinations. For example, receptor and structural proteins are sent to the membrane and digestive enzymes to lysosomes, and molecules for extracellular action are packaged into secretory vesicles. **Lysosomes** are small vesicles containing acid hydrolase enzymes which catabolize macromolecules. They work optimally at pH 5.0, and as cytosolic pH is ~7.2, any leaking into the cytosol cannot attack the cell inappropriately. Lysosomes digest endocytosed, unwanted and defective proteins, thereby recycling raw materials and preventing accumulation of rubbish.

Membranes and membrane proteins

Membrane lipids (mostly phospholipids) comprise a **hydrophilic** (water-loving) head, with two short **hydrophobic** (water-repelling) fatty acid tails (Figure 3.2). In an aqueous medium they self-organize into a **bilayer** with the heads facing outwards and the tails inwards (Figure 3.2). They diffuse freely within each layer (**lateral diffusion**) so the membrane is fluid. The hydrophobic interior and hydrophilic exterior of the membrane means that lipid-soluble (hydrophobic) substances such as **cholesterol** incorporate into the membrane, whilst molecules with both hydrophobic and hydrophilic domains such as proteins can be tethered part in and part out of the membrane (the **fluid mosaic model**; Figure 3.2). Many such molecules provide signalling, transport or structural functions. The latter are provided by proteins such as **spectrin**, which binds to the inner layer and forms an attachment framework for the **cytoskeleton**. Lipid-soluble molecules such as O_2 and CO_2, and small molecules such as water and urea readily pass through the lipid bilayer. However, larger molecules such as glucose and polar (charged) molecules such as ions cannot, and their transport is mediated by **transporter** and **ion channel** membrane proteins (Chapter 4). Proteins and large particles can also be engulfed by membrane segments to form intracellular vesicles (**endocytosis**). Membrane components can diffuse laterally and move around the membrane. However, the cell can control exactly which proteins insert into which portion of the membrane. For example, cells lining the kidney tubules are polarized so that **Na^+–K^+ ATPase** transporters (Chapters 4 and 36) are located only on one side of the cell. Most cells are covered by a thin gel-like layer called the **glycocalyx**, containing glycoproteins and carbohydrate chains extending from the membrane and secreted proteins (Figure 3.2). It protects the membrane and also plays a role in cell function and cell–cell interactions.

Numerous membrane proteins are associated with cell signalling (see Chapter 7). These include enzymes bound to the inner surface (e.g. phospholipase), and **transmembrane** proteins such as **receptors**, transporters and **ion channels** (Figure 3.2) which penetrate the entire thickness of the bilayer. The intramembrane segments of such proteins are composed of hydrophobic amino acid residues whilst the extra- and intracellular portions predominantly contain hydrophilic residues. Other transmembrane proteins such as **integrins** and **cadherins** provide structural and signalling links with other cells and the **extracellular matrix** (Figure 3.2). Their cytosolic ends bind to components of the cytoskeleton, including **protein kinases** which can initiate or modulate processes such as gene transcription, cell growth or changes in cell shape.

Mitochondria and energy production

Mitochondria use molecular oxygen to, in effect, burn sugar and small fatty acid molecules to produce **adenosine triphosphate (ATP)**, which is used by all energy-requiring cellular reactions. Glucose is first converted to pyruvate in the cytosol by glycolysis, producing in the process a small net amount of ATP and reduced nicotinic adenine dinucleotide (**NADH**). Glycolysis does not require O_2, so when O_2 is limited, this **anaerobic respiration** can supply some ATP, with NADH being reoxidized to **NAD^+** by metabolism of the pyruvate to lactate (Figure 3.3). However, under normal conditions where there is sufficient O_2, **oxidative phosphorylation** in the mitochondria produces ~15-fold more ATP for each glucose molecule than does glycolysis. Pyruvate and fatty acids transported into the **mitochondrial matrix** act as substrates for enzymes that drive the **citric acid (Krebs') cycle**, which generates **NADH** and the waste product CO_2. The **electron transport chain**, a series of enzymes in the inner mitochondrial membrane, then uses molecular O_2 to re-oxidize NADH to NAD^+. In doing so, it generates a H^+ ion gradient across the inner membrane which drives the **ATP synthase** (Figure 3.3). Note that mitochondria are not solely devoted to ATP production, as they are also involved in other cellular processes, including Ca^{2+} homeostasis and signalling. The mitochondria are also the major source of body heat production (see Chapter 13).

4 Membrane transport and ion channels

Figure 4.1 Transporters

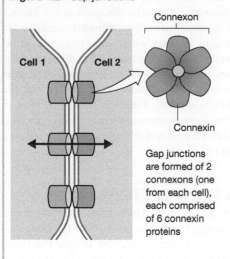

Primary active transport
Na⁺ pump

Secondary active transport
Na⁺–Ca²⁺ exchanger

K⁺ electrochemical gradient

Na⁺ electrochemical gradient

Ca²⁺ electrochemical gradient

Primary active transport uses energy from ATP to pump ions against their electrochemical gradients

Secondary active transport most often uses the Na⁺ electrochemical gradient to pump another ion (or molecule) against its electrochemical (or concentration) gradient

The Na⁺ electrochemical gradient is maintained by the activity of the Na⁺ pump

Figure 4.2 Gap junctions

Connexon

Cell 1   Cell 2

Connexin

Gap junctions are formed of 2 connexons (one from each cell), each comprised of 6 connexin proteins

Figure 4.3 Voltage-gated sodium channel

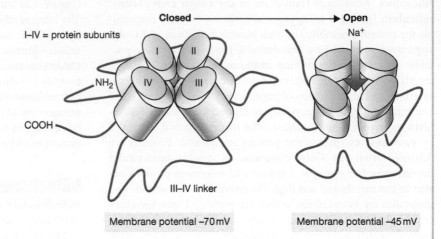

Closed ⟶ Open

I–IV = protein subunits

Na⁺

NH₂

COOH

III–IV linker

Membrane potential –70 mV

Membrane potential –45 mV

Figure 4.4 Gating of voltage-gated sodium channel

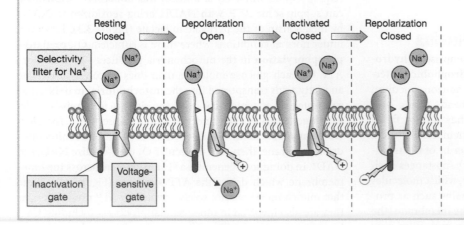

Resting
Closed

Depolarization
Open

Inactivated
Closed

Repolarization
Closed

Selectivity filter for Na⁺

Na⁺

Na⁺

Na⁺

Na⁺

Na⁺

Na⁺

Na⁺

Inactivation gate

Voltage-sensitive gate

Na⁺

Figure 4.5 Receptor-gated non-selective cation channel

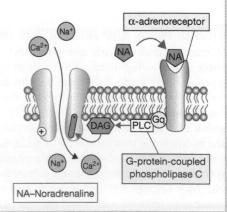

α-adrenoreceptor

Na⁺

Ca²⁺

NA

NA

DAG

PLC

Gq

Na⁺

Ca²⁺

G-protein-coupled phospholipase C

NA–Noradrenaline

Physiology at a Glance, Fourth Edition. Edited by Jeremy P.T. Ward and Roger W.A. Linden.
© 2017 John Wiley & Sons, Ltd. Published 2017 by John Wiley & Sons, Ltd. Companion website: www.ataglanceseries.com/physiology

Proteins provide several routes for the movement of materials across membranes: (i) pores or channels constructed of several protein subunits that allow bulk flow of water, ions or sometimes larger molecules, e.g. water channels (**aquaporins**, Chapter 37) and **gap junctions** connecting the cytosol of adjacent cells (Figure 4.2); (ii) transporter molecules, some of which use metabolic energy (either direct or indirect) to move molecules against chemical and/or electrical gradients; and (iii) ion channels, specialized to allow the passage of particular ion species across the membrane under defined conditions.

Carrier-mediated transport

Transporter (or carrier) proteins can move a single type of molecule in one direction across a membrane (a **uniporter**), several different molecules in one direction (a **symporter**) or different molecules in opposite directions (an **antiporter**) (Figure 4.1). Transporters can allow the movement of molecules down chemical concentration gradients (**facilitated diffusion**), when the energy required for conformational changes in the transporter protein is provided by the concentration gradient rather than by metabolic activity. Important transporters for glucose and amino acids, found in the kidney and the gut, are in fact driven by the Na^+ electrochemical gradient that exists across the cell membrane (Chapter 2). These symporters must bind Na^+ *and* the primary transported molecule at the external surface of the membrane before the conformational change will take place. Antiporters such as the Na^+–Ca^{2+} exchanger similarly use the Na^+ gradient, in this case to extrude one Ca^{2+} out of the cell in exchange for three Na^+ into the cell. These processes are known as **secondary active transport**, as the Na^+ gradient is set up by a process requiring metabolic energy. The uneven distribution of Na^+ ions across the cell membrane is produced by the best known of all transporters, the **Na^+–K^+ ATPase**, also known as the **Na^+ pump** (Figure 4.1). This protein is an antiporter that uses metabolic energy to move Na^+ ions out of the cell and K^+ ions in, *against their respective concentration gradients*. The ATPase binds extracellular K^+ and intracellular Na^+ ions, usually in the ratio of 2:3, and hydrolyses adenosine triphosphate (ATP) to provide the energy needed to change its conformation, leading to the ejection of Na^+ into the extracellular medium and K^+ into the cytosol; this allows the cell to maintain a high concentration of K^+ ions and a low concentration of Na^+ ions inside the cell (Chapter 2). The Na^+ pump works continuously, although its activity is stimulated by high intracellular levels of Na^+ ions and can be modulated by second messenger-mediated phosphorylation. The action of the Na^+-K^+ ATPase is the most important example of **primary active transport**.

Ion channels

Ions can *diffuse* across cell membranes down their electrochemical gradient through **ion channels**. These transmembrane proteins, which are invariably constructed of several subunits containing several membrane-spanning domains (e.g. Figure 4.3), provide a charged, hydrophilic pore through which ions can move across the lipid bilayer. They possess a number of important features that confer upon the cell the ability to control closely the movement of ions across the membrane. Ion channels are **selective** for particular ions, i.e. they allow the passage of only one type of ion or a few related ions. There are numerous specialized channels for Na^+, K^+, Cl^- and Ca^{2+} ions, as well as non-specific channels for monovalent, divalent or even all cations (positively charged ions) or anions (negatively charged ions). The charge on the transmembrane pore determines whether the channel is for cations or anions, and selection between different ion types depends on the size of the ion and its accompanying water of hydration. Different types of channel for the same ion can however allow greatly differing amounts of that ion to move through them per second for the same electrochemical gradient; this is called channel **conductance**, and is best understood in the following way. Ions carry charge and so their movement causes an **electrical current**. Ohm's law states that V (voltage) = I (current) × R (resistance). In terms of ion channels, V = membrane potential and I = ionic current, so one can calculate the resistance of the channel. The reciprocal of resistance is conductance, which has units called Siemens; 1 Siemens (S) = 1/Ohm. Single ion channels generally have conductances in the 2–300 pS (10^{-12} S) range.

The second key feature of ion channels is that their pores are either **open** or **closed**; the transition between these states is called **gating**. Gating is brought about by a change in the conformation of the protein subunits that opens or closes the ion-permeable pore (e.g. Figure 4.3). Many channels are opened or closed according to the potential difference (voltage) across the cell membrane (**voltage** gating; Chapter 5), whereas others are gated by the presence of a specific signal molecule (**ligand** or **receptor** gating). The function of some channels may additionally be modified by phosphorylation of channel proteins by enzymes such as protein kinase C or A (Chapter 7). The **voltage-gated fast inward Na^+ channel** responsible for the upstroke of the action potential (Chapter 5) has two gates, one that opens as the cell depolarizes beyond ~−55 mV (its **threshold**) and another that shuts (**inactivates**) the channel as the potential becomes positive (Figure 4.4). This latter gate can only be reset by repolarization almost to the resting potential (Chapter 5). Some ligand-gated channels are directly gated by extracellular molecules, such as neurotransmitters or hormones, whereas others respond indirectly via intracellular signals, such as diacylglycerol (DAG; Figure 4.5) or cyclic adenosine monophosphate (cAMP) (Chapter 7). Specialized cells that detect changes in the internal and external environments (receptor cells) possess ion channels that are gated by the particular signal that is detected by the receptor, e.g. pH or light. The characteristics of ion channels, in concert with the activities of ion pumps, give cells the ability to control precisely the movement of ions across the cell membrane. This is crucial for many important physiological processes, including electrical signalling (Chapters 5 and 6), initiation of muscle contraction (Chapters 15 and 16) and secretion of materials such as neurotransmitters, hormones and digestive enzymes.

5 Biological electricity

Figure 5.1 Nernst equation and K+ equilibrium potential

E = potential
z = valency (1 for K+)
F = Faraday (charge per mole)
 (96 485 Coulombs per mole)

R = gas constant
 (8.314 Joules/mole/degree K)
T = absolute temperature (Kelvin)

Extracellular   **Cytosol**

$[K^+] = 120\,mM$

Electrical gradient

Driving force:
EzF

Concentration gradient

Driving force:
$RT \times Ln\left(\frac{4}{120}\right)$

Fixed charge

$[K^+] = 4\,mM$

K+ channel

At equilibrium:

Electrical gradient   **Concentration gradient**

Driving force:
EzF   **=**   Driving force:
$RT \times Ln\left(\frac{4}{120}\right)$

Rearrange:

$$E = \frac{RT}{zF} \times Ln\left(\frac{4}{120}\right)$$

The Nernst equation

Solving for R, z and F, 37ºC, and log base 10:

$$E_k = 61 \times Log\left(\frac{4}{120}\right) = -90\ mV$$

Figure 5.2 Voltage and permeability changes in an action potential of a nerve

Voltage-gated K+ channels activate

Voltage-gated Na+ channels inactivate

Depolarization

Voltage-gated Na+ channels activate

Repolarization

Voltage-gated K+ channels inactivated

Ligand-gated Na+ channels activate

Threshold

Stimuli not reaching threshold

After hyperpolarization

Resting E_m

Stimulus e.g. neurotransmitter

— Voltage
- - - P_{Na}
- - - P_K

Membrane potential (mV)

Relative permeability

Time (ms)

Physiology at a Glance, Fourth Edition. Edited by Jeremy P.T. Ward and Roger W.A. Linden.
© 2017 John Wiley & Sons, Ltd. Published 2017 by John Wiley & Sons, Ltd. Companion website: www.ataglanceseries.com/physiology

lectrical events in biological tissues are caused by the movement of ions across the membrane. A potential difference exists across the membranes of all cells (**membrane potential**, E_m), but only **excitable tissues** can generate **action potentials** (transient depolarization of a cell as a result of ion channel activity). Action potentials transmit information in nerve cells (Chapter 6) and trigger contractions in muscle cells (Chapter 15). Cell membranes are electrically polarized so that the inside is negative relative to the outside. In excitable tissues, resting E_m is usually between –60 and –90 mV.

The resting membrane potential

The resting membrane is more permeable to K^+ and Cl^- than to other ions (Chapter 4). The cell contains negatively charged molecules (e.g. proteins) which cannot cross the membrane. This fixed negative charge attracts K^+, leading to accumulation of K^+ within the cell (Chapter 2). However, the consequent increase in the K^+ concentration gradient drives K^+ back out of the cell. This means fewer K^+ ions move into the cell than are required to achieve electrical neutrality with the fixed negative charges, and the inside of the cell therefore remains negatively charged compared to the outside, causing a potential difference across the membrane. Equilibrium is reached when the *electrical* forces exactly balance those due to *concentration* differences (**Gibbs–Donnan equilibrium**); the net force or **electrochemical gradient** for K^+ is then zero. If the membrane were *only* permeable to K^+, the voltage at which this would occur (K^+ **equilibrium potential**, E_K) is defined purely by the K^+ concentration gradient, and can be calculated from the **Nernst equation** (see Figure 5.1 for derivation). Thus, if intracellular $[K^+]$ were 120 mmol/L and extracellular $[K^+]$ 4 mmol/L, E_K = ~–90 mV. This applies to any ion, so if the membrane were *only* permeable to Na^+ (only Na^+ channels open) and intracellular and extracellular $[Na^+]$ were 10 and 140 mmol/L, respectively, the potential obtained at equilibrium (E_{Na}) would be +70 mV. To summarize, for any given intracellular and extracellular ionic concentrations, the equilibrium potential for that ion is the membrane potential required for the intracellular and extracellular concentrations to be in equilibrium, i.e. for the electrochemical gradient to be zero. The difference between the actual E_m and the equilibrium potential for any ion is therefore a measure of that ion's electrochemical gradient, the force driving it into or out of the cell.

Real cell membranes are permeable to other ions besides K^+, but at rest their K^+ permeability (P_K) is much greater than that for other ions. In particular, the ratio of P_K to Na^+ permeability (P_{Na}) ranges between 25:1 and 100:1 in nerve, skeletal and cardiac muscle cells. As a result E_m in such cells at rest (**resting membrane potential**) is close to E_K (–60 to –85 mV) and the electrochemical gradient for K^+ is small. E_m does not equal E_K because there is permeability to other ions, notably Na^+. As E_{Na} is much more positive than E_m, the Na^+ electrochemical gradient is strongly inwards, forcing Na^+ into the cell. However, as P_{Na} is relatively low, only a small amount of Na^+ can leak in, though this is sufficient to slightly depolarize the membrane from E_K. A consequence of the above is that if P_{Na} were suddenly increased to more than P_K, then E_m would shift towards E_{Na}. This is exactly what happens during an action potential, when Na^+ channels open so that P_{Na} becomes 10-fold greater than P_K, and the membrane depolarizes.

The action potential

Action potentials are initiated in nerve and skeletal muscle by activation of **ligand-gated Na^+ channels** by neurotransmitters (Chapter 4 and 15). This increases P_{Na} and causes E_m to move towards E_{Na} (i.e. become positive; Figure 5.2). This initial increase in P_{Na} is however relatively modest, so the depolarization is similarly small. However, if the stimulus is sufficiently strong, E_m depolarizes enough to reach the **threshold potential** (~–55 mV), at which point **voltage-gated Na^+ channels** (Chapter 4) activate, causing further depolarization. This activates more voltage-gated Na^+ channels so the process becomes explosively self-regenerating, leading to a large transient increase in P_{Na} so it is 10-fold greater than P_K. As a result, E_m rapidly approaches E_{Na} (~+65 mV; see previously), causing the sharp positive 'spike' or **depolarization** of the action potential, which lasts about 1 ms in nerve and skeletal muscle. The spike is transient because as E_m becomes positive, the voltage-gated Na^+ channels **inactivate** (Chapter 4) and P_{Na} plummets, whereas a type of voltage-gated K^+ channel (**delayed rectifier**) activates. Thus P_K is again much larger than P_{Na} and E_m returns towards E_K (**repolarization**); this takes about 1–2 ms. Delayed closure of the delayed rectifier K^+ channels means that the P_K:P_{Na} ratio remains transiently greater than normal after repolarization, causing a transient hyperpolarization (Figure 5.2).

Following depolarization the Na^+ channels remain **inactive** for about 1 ms until the cell is largely repolarized and, during this period, they cannot be opened by any amount of depolarization. This is known as the **absolute refractory period** during which it is impossible to generate another action potential. For the following 2–3 ms, the transient hyperpolarization renders the cell more difficult to depolarize, an interval known as the **relative refractory period**, when an action potential can be generated only in response to a larger than normal stimulus. The refractory period limits the frequency at which action potentials can be generated to <1000/s and ensures that, once initiated, an action potential can travel only in one direction. Once triggered, an action potential will travel over the entire surface of an excitable cell (it is **propagated**) and will always have the same amplitude (it is **all-or-nothing**). The minute changes in ion concentrations that occur during an action potential are restored by the action of the Na^+ pump; it is important to understand that the action potential is *not* due to changes in ionic concentrations, but to changes in **ionic permeability**. Note that action potentials in cardiac muscle differ somewhat from those in nerves and skeletal muscle (Chapter 22).

6 Conduction of action potentials

Figure 6.1 Unmyelinated nerve

Extracellular space

Movement of +ve charges (local current flow)

Na⁺

K⁺

Refractory area

Axon

Plasma membrane

Na⁺

Direction of propagation of action potential

Figure 6.3 Classification of fibres

Myelinated   Unmyelinated

20   15   10   5   1   2   0.5
Diameter (µm)

120   90   60   30   4   2   0.5
Conduction velocity (m/s)

Erlanger/Gasser classification

B   C

A

α

β

γ

δ

Lloyd/Hunt classification

I   II   III   IV

IA

IB

Examples of functions

Primary muscle spindles	Secondary muscle spindles	
Golgi tendon organs	Skin mechano-receptors	
		Deep pressure and touch
		Temperature
		Fast pain

Sensory function

Temperature
Slow pain

Motor function

Motor to skeletal muscles	Fusimotor	
		Preganglionic sympathetic

Postganglionic sympathetic

Figure 6.2 Myelinated nerve

Extracellular space

Myelin

Movement of +ve charges (local current flow)

Na⁺

K⁺

Axon

K⁺

Na⁺

Refractory node of Ranvier

Active node of Ranvier

Inactive node of Ranvier

Direction of propagation of action potential

Figure 6.4 Compound action potentials recorded at various distances from the initial stimulation point

Mixed nerve bundle

Stimulating electrodes   +ve   −ve

A (α, β, γ, δ)

Recording electrode 1

Recording electrode 2

A (α, β, γ, δ)

Recording electrode 3

Recording electrode 4

mm from stimulation point

0

20

40

90

150

B   C

B   C

A

α   β   γ   δ

B   C

10ms

A

α   β   γ   δ

B   C

Physiology at a Glance, Fourth Edition. Edited by Jeremy P.T. Ward and Roger W.A. Linden.
© 2017 John Wiley & Sons, Ltd. Published 2017 by John Wiley & Sons, Ltd. Companion website: www.ataglanceseries.com/physiology

The **action potential** described in Chapter 5 is a local event that can occur in all excitable cells. This local event is an **all-or-nothing** response, leading to reversal of the polarity from negative (−70 mV) to positive (+40 mV) on the inside of the cell with respect to the outside for a short time during the course of the action potential.

Local currents are set up around the action potential because the positive charges from the membrane ahead of the action potential are drawn towards the area of negativity surrounding the action potential (current sink or local current). This decreases the polarity of the membrane ahead of the action potential.

This electronic depolarization initiates a local response that causes the opening of the voltage-gated ion channels (Na^+ followed by K^+); when the threshold for firing of the action potential is reached, it **propagates** the action potential and this, in turn, leads to the local depolarization of the next area, and so on. Once initiated, an action potential does not depolarize the area behind it sufficiently to initiate another action potential because the area is **refractory** (Chapter 5).

This successive depolarization moves along each segment of an **unmyelinated** nerve until it reaches the end. It is all-or-nothing and does not decrease in size (Figure 6.1).

Saltatory conduction

Conduction in **myelinated** axons depends on a similar pattern of current flows. However, because **myelin** is an insulator and because the membrane below it cannot be depolarized, the only areas of the myelinated axon that can be depolarized are those that are devoid of any myelin, i.e. at the **nodes of Ranvier**. The depolarization jumps from one node to another and is called **saltatory**, from the Latin *saltare* (to jump) (Figure 6.2). Saltatory conduction is rapid and can be up to 50 times faster than in the fastest unmyelinated fibres.

Saltatory conduction not only increases the velocity of impulse transmission by causing the depolarization process to jump from one node to the next, but also **conserves energy** for the axon because depolarization only occurs at the nodes and not along the whole length of the nerve fibre, as in unmyelinated fibres. This leads to up to 100 times less movement of ions than would otherwise be necessary, therefore conserving the energy required to re-establish the Na^+ and K^+ concentration differences across the membranes following a series of action potentials being propagated along the fibre.

All nerve fibres are capable of conducting impulses in either direction if stimulated in the middle of their axon; however, normally they conduct impulses in one direction only (**orthodromically**), from either the receptor to the axon terminal or from the synaptic junction to the axon terminal. **Antidromic** conduction does not normally occur.

Fibre diameters and conduction velocities

Some information needs to be transmitted to and from the central nervous system very rapidly, whereas other information does not. Nerve fibres are able to cover both of these extremes and any in between by virtue of their size, and therefore conduction velocity, and whether or not they are myelinated. Nerve fibres come in all sizes, from 0.5 to 20 μm in diameter, with the smallest diameter unmyelinated fibres being the slowest conducting and the largest myelinated fibres the fastest conducting.

Classification of nerve fibres

Unfortunately, there are two classifications of nerve fibres. One, originally described by Erlanger and Gasser, and often referred to as the **general** classification, uses the letters **A, B and C, with A further subdivided into α, β, γ and δ**. The second, originally described by Lloyd and Hunt, and often referred to as the **sensory** or **afferent** classification, uses the Roman numerals **I, II, III and IV, with I further subdivided into A and B**. The groups are subdivided differently in the two classifications and so, unfortunately, it is not possible to rely on only one of the classifications for the description of nerve fibres. **The fibres of groups A and B and also of groups I, II and III are all myelinated, and those of group C and IV are unmyelinated**. These classifications, conduction velocities, fibre diameters and examples of their functions are shown in Figure 6.3. A word of caution is necessary concerning the average conduction velocities of the larger myelinated fibres: in reality, although there may be a few larger diameter fibres in the human body that do indeed conduct impulses as fast as 120 m/s, a more common observation is that the fastest proprioceptive (sensory) fibres conduct at below 100 m/s, with the average being closer to 80 m/s. The same applies to the α-motor neurones in that the conduction velocities rarely exceed 90 m/s, with the average being closer to 60 m/s.

Compound action potentials

Peripheral nerves in most animals comprise a number of axons bound together by a fibrous tissue called the **epineurium**. When extracellular recording electrodes are placed close to a peripheral nerve, the recorded voltage signal, when an action potential is initiated in the bundle, is much smaller (microvolts) than that recorded by an electrode inserted directly into the axon (millivolts). The extracellular recorded signal is made up of the electrical events occurring in all of the active fibres within the nerve bundle. If all the nerve fibres in a nerve bundle are synchronously stimulated at one end of a nerve, and recording electrodes are placed at a number of locations along the length of the bundle, a **compound action potential** is recorded at each electrode. The waveform recorded from each of the electrodes will differ due to the different conduction velocities of each group of fibres that makes up the bundle. Theoretically, if the nerve bundle were to contain examples of all classifications of nerve fibres (i.e. Aα, Aβ, Aγ, Aδ, B and C), the recorded compound action potential would be seen as a **multi-peaked** display, as the action potentials in the fastest conducting fibres (Aα) would reach the electrode before those in the slowest conducting fibres (C). Action potentials in the fibres with conduction velocities between these two extremes would arrive between these two times (Figure 6.4).

7 Cell signalling

Notes: Cell signalling differs between tissues because the cells express different receptors, protein kinases and enzymes. In this diagram pathways and interactions are often simplified for clarity; e.g. in some cases it is actually an ancillary protein that is phosphorylated, not the target protein itself, but the end effect is the same.

Figure 7.1 G-protein coupled receptor

Figure 7.2 Receptor tyrosine kinase
NB Indicative only, RTKs differ in details of structure and operation

PI3 kinase: phosphatidylinositol-3-kinase; Akt: protein kinase B; Ras: monomeric G-protein like Rho; MAP kinase: mitogen-activated kinase; JAK: Janus kinase; RTK: receptor tyrosine kinase; STAT: signal transduction and activation of transcription

Figure 7.3 G-protein coupled receptor associated signalling pathways

Ryanodine receptors (RyR) and Ca^{2+}-induced Ca^{2+} release (CICR) are described in Chapters 22 and 24. CREB, cAMP response element-binding protein (transcription factor); CaM, calmodulin; PMCA, plasma membrane Ca^{2+} ATPase; SERCA, sarcoendoplasmic reticulum Ca^{2+} ATPase; NCX, Na^+-Ca^{2+} exchanger; MLC, myosin light chain; MLCP, MLC phosphatase

Physiology at a Glance, Fourth Edition. Edited by Jeremy P.T. Ward and Roger W.A. Linden.
© 2017 John Wiley & Sons, Ltd. Published 2017 by John Wiley & Sons, Ltd. Companion website: www.ataglanceseries.com/physiology

Cells respond to stimuli through numerous signalling mechanisms. Membrane-spanning proteins including **ion channels** (Chapter 4) and **receptors** allow signals to be transferred across the membrane. Binding of a molecule (**ligand**) to its receptor initiates intracellular signalling pathways. These include activation of enzymes attached to the membrane inner surface that generate **second messengers** to promulgate the signal. Second messengers can be substrates for other enzymes, activate **protein kinases** which **phosphorylate** proteins to alter their function, or trigger a rise in cytosolic Ca^{2+} (itself a key second messenger). Ca^{2+} may act directly (e.g. on troponin; Chapter 15), or via the Ca^{2+} binding protein **calmodulin** (CaM), which on binding 4 Ca^{2+} activates Ca^{2+}-dependent protein kinases (e.g. myosin light chain kinase, **MLCK**; Chapter 24). Cell signalling can be highly compartmentalized, with clusters of interacting receptors, channels, enzymes and/or kinases forming **micro-signalling domains** within the cell.

Membrane-bound enzymes generating second messengers include **phospholipases** and **adenylate cyclase** (Figure 7.3). Phospholipase A_2 (**PLA$_2$**) cleaves membrane phospholipids to release **arachidonic acid**, which is converted by cyclooxygenase (COX) into the substrate for synthesis of **eicosanoids** (prostaglandins and leukotrienes). Phospholipase C (**PLC**) cleaves PIP2 (phosphatidylinositol-bisphosphate) into inositol-trisphosphate (**IP$_3$**) and diacylglycerol (**DAG**), which evoke Ca^{2+} mobilization and activation of **protein kinase C** (PKC). Adenylate cyclase generates cyclic adenosine monophosphate (**cAMP**) which activates **protein kinase A** (PKA), and **guanylate cyclase** generates **cGMP** (cyclic guanosine monophosphate), activating **protein kinase G** (PKG). Both cyclases also have soluble (cytosolic) isoforms. cAMP and cGMP also have kinase-independent effects, including activation of cyclic nucleotide-gated ion channels.

To terminate signalling, cytosolic Ca^{2+} is pumped back into the endoplasmic reticulum by **SERCA** (sarco/endoplasmic reticulum Ca^{2+}-ATPase) and out of the cell by **PMCA** (plasmamembrane Ca^{2+}-ATPase) and **NCX** (Na^+-Ca^{2+} exchanger) (Chapter 4), cAMP and cGMP are broken down by **phosphodiesterases**, and proteins are dephosphorylated by **phosphatases** (though this *activates* some kinases).

Receptor types

Many receptors are members of the **G-protein coupled receptor** (**GPCR**) superfamily with seven membrane-spanning domains (Figure 7.1). When *inactive* (no ligand), GPCRs attach to **heterotrimeric G-proteins** (*guanine nucleotide-binding*) consisting of a GTPase-containing **α-subunit** (G_α), and **β** and **γ** subunits (as a dimer, $G_{\beta\gamma}$). At this point G_α is bound to **GDP** (guanosine diphosphate). On GPCR activation by a ligand (e.g. neurotransmitter, hormone) or light for rhodopsin receptor (Chapter 60), G_α exchanges GDP for **GTP** (guanosine triphosphate) and G_α-GTP and $G_{\beta\gamma}$ dissociate from the GPCR and each other, though remaining tethered to the membrane. Classical pathways activated by G_α-GTP are discussed in the next paragraph; $G_{\beta\gamma}$ signals to some phospholipases, ion channels and lipid kinases.

Four types of G_α are associated with three GPCR-coupled signalling pathways (Figure 7.3). $G_{\alpha i}$ *inhibits* and $G_{\alpha s}$ *stimulates* adenylate cyclase; **β-adrenergic receptors** are archetypical examples of $G_{\alpha s}$-coupled GPCRs, the **muscarinic M$_2$ receptor** (acetylcholine) an example for $G_{\alpha i}$. $G_{\alpha q}$ activates **phospholipase C-β** (PLCβ) so generating IP$_3$ and DAG; IP$_3$ initiates Ca^{2+} release from the endoplasmic reticulum and DAG activates receptor-operated channels (ROC) and PKC (Chapters 4, 24). The **α$_1$-adrenergic receptor** is a typical $G_{\alpha q}$-coupled GPCR. $G_{\alpha 12/13}$ activates **Rho** (a *small monomeric* G-protein) and the **Rho/Rho kinase** pathway, which is involved in cytoskeletal regulation, cell migration and smooth muscle contraction (Chapter 24). Most $G_{\alpha 12/13}$-coupled GPCRs also couple to $G_{\alpha q}$, so one receptor activates both pathways; the α$_1$-adrenergic receptor is an example.

Receptor tyrosine kinases (**RTKs**; Figure 7.2) are high affinity receptors for polypeptide growth factors, cytokines and insulin. Ligand binding causes receptor dimerization and transphosphorylation of tyrosine residues in their cytoplasmic tails, creating a binding site for **SH2** (Src-homology 2) and **PTB** (phosphotyrosine binding) domain proteins. These initiate diverse signalling pathways, many affecting gene transcription, and regulate cell growth, proliferation, differentiation, survival and responses to stress and inflammatory cytokines. Some RTKs also activate **PLCγ**, which like PLCβ generates IP$_3$ and DAG.

Ionotropic receptors are ion channels directly activated by ligand binding, the classic example being the cholinergic **nicotinic receptor** (Chapters 8 and 16); cholinergic *muscarinic* receptors are GPCRs. Cytosolic **nuclear receptors** bind membrane-permeable signalling molecules including steroids and thyroid hormones, before translocating to the nucleus to alter gene expression.

Protein kinases

Protein kinases recognize target proteins by specific amino acid sequences (motifs) surrounding the residue (amino acid) that will be phosphorylated. The same motif can occur in different proteins, so a protein kinase can potentially phosphorylate multiple targets. The same protein kinase can therefore elicit different responses in different cell types (or even sub-cellular locations) depending on which targets are expressed there. Conversely two protein kinases may phosphorylate a single protein, but at different motifs which affect its function in different ways. **Threonine/serine kinases** phosphorylate threonine or serine residues (e.g. PKA, PKG, PKC, MLCK, Rho kinase). **Tyrosine kinases** include RTKs (see previous section) and **non-receptor tyrosine kinases**, which regulate and integrate the actions of other kinases and small monomeric G-proteins.

PKA is the primary effector for $G_{\alpha s}$-coupled GPCRs such as β-adrenergic, prostacyclin and glucagon receptors, and key functions include smooth muscle relaxation (Chapter 24), glucose mobilization (Chapter 46), and renal water reabsorption (Chapter 38). Its targets include channels, transporters, metabolic enzymes and the transcription factor CREB. **PKG** is highly expressed in smooth muscle and platelets. It mediates the effects of nitric oxide (which activates *soluble* guanylate cyclase) (Chapters 10 and 24) by inhibiting Ca^{2+} release from stores and activating Ca^{2+}-dependent K^+ channels (causing hyperpolarization), thus reducing cytosolic $[Ca^{2+}]$. **PKCs** target a vast range of proteins, including ion channels, transporters (e.g. Na^+-K^+ ATPase) and many enzymes. **Conventional** PKCs are activated by both DAG and Ca^{2+}, **novel** isoforms only by DAG, **atypical** by neither. The depolarization elicited by agonists of $G_{\alpha q}$-coupled GPCRs is thought to be due to inhibition of K^+ channels by conventional PKCs activated by DAG and the rise in $[Ca^{2+}]$ (Figure 7.3).

The *yin-yang* relationship between protein kinases and phosphatases is typified by the regulation of smooth muscle contraction (Chapter 24), which also exemplifies **convergence** of signalling pathways (Figure 7.3). Activation of α$_1$-adrenergic receptors leads to elevation of $[Ca^{2+}]$ and Ca^{2+}-calmodulin-induced activation of MLCK. MLCK phosphorylates myosin light chain (MLC), promoting force development. This would be impeded by myosin light chain phosphatase (MLCP) which *dephosphorylates* MLC, but MLCP is inhibited by Rho kinase and PKC, also activated by α$_1$-adrenergic receptors. The effect of the elevation in $[Ca^{2+}]$ on force development is thus potentiated (Ca^{2+} sensitization).

8 The autonomic nervous system

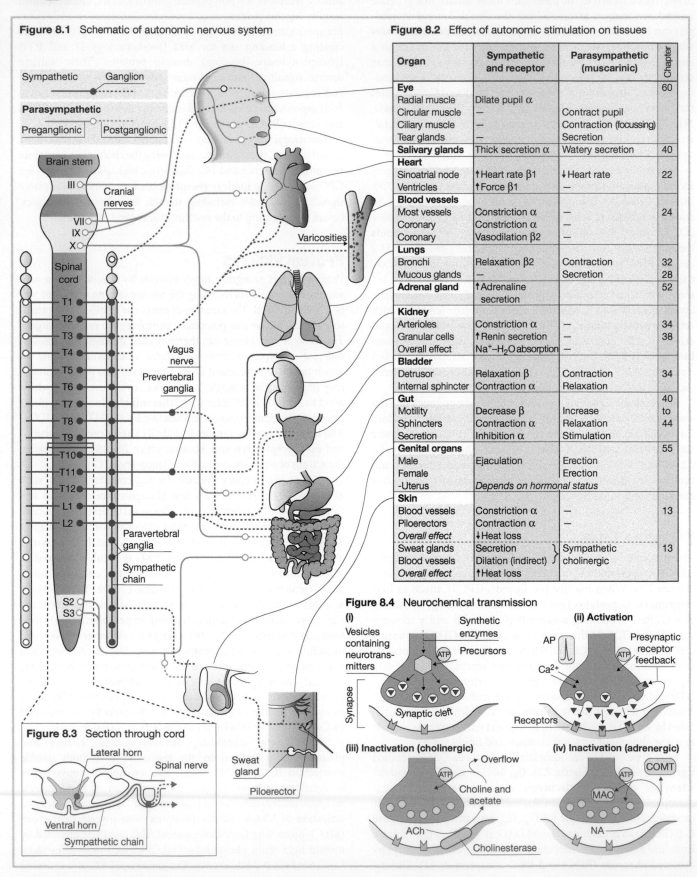

Figure 8.1 Schematic of autonomic nervous system

Sympathetic ——— Ganglion
Parasympathetic
Preganglionic ——— Postganglionic

Brain stem
III
Cranial nerves
VII
IX
X
Spinal cord
T1
T2
T3
T4
T5
T6
T7
T8
T9
T10
T11
T12
L1
L2
S2
S3

Vagus nerve
Prevertebral ganglia
Paravertebral ganglia
Sympathetic chain
Varicosities

Figure 8.3 Section through cord

Lateral horn
Spinal nerve
Ventral horn
Sympathetic chain
Sweat gland
Piloerector

Figure 8.2 Effect of autonomic stimulation on tissues

Organ	Sympathetic and receptor	Parasympathetic (muscarinic)	Chapter
Eye			60
Radial muscle	Dilate pupil α		
Circular muscle	—	Contract pupil	
Ciliary muscle	—	Contraction (focussing)	
Tear glands	—	Secretion	
Salivary glands	Thick secretion α	Watery secretion	40
Heart			
Sinoatrial node	↑Heart rate β1	↓Heart rate	22
Ventricles	↑Force β1	—	
Blood vessels			
Most vessels	Constriction α	—	24
Coronary	Constriction α	—	
Coronary	Vasodilation β2	—	
Lungs			
Bronchi	Relaxation β2	Contraction	32
Mucous glands	—	Secretion	28
Adrenal gland	↑Adrenaline secretion		52
Kidney			
Arterioles	Constriction α		34
Granular cells	↑Renin secretion	—	38
Overall effect	Na⁺–H₂O absorption	—	
Bladder			
Detrusor	Relaxation β	Contraction	34
Internal sphincter	Contraction α	Relaxation	
Gut			40
Motility	Decrease β	Increase	to
Sphincters	Contraction α	Relaxation	44
Secretion	Inhibition α	Stimulation	
Genital organs			55
Male	Ejaculation	Erection	
Female		Erection	
-Uterus	*Depends on hormonal status*		
Skin			
Blood vessels	Constriction α	—	13
Piloerectors	Contraction α	—	
Overall effect	↓Heat loss		
Sweat glands	Secretion	} Sympathetic cholinergic	13
Blood vessels	Dilation (indirect)		
Overall effect	↑Heat loss		

Figure 8.4 Neurochemical transmission

(i)
Vesicles containing neurotransmitters
Synthetic enzymes
Precursors
ATP
Synapse
Synaptic cleft

(ii) **Activation**
AP
Ca²⁺
Presynaptic receptor feedback
ATP
Receptors

(iii) Inactivation (cholinergic)
Overflow
ATP
Choline and acetate
ACh
Cholinesterase

(iv) Inactivation (adrenergic)
COMT
ATP
MAO
NA

Physiology at a Glance, Fourth Edition. Edited by Jeremy P.T. Ward and Roger W.A. Linden.
© 2017 John Wiley & Sons, Ltd. Published 2017 by John Wiley & Sons, Ltd. Companion website: www.ataglanceseries.com/physiology

The **autonomic nervous system** (ANS) provides the **efferent** pathway for the **involuntary** control of most organs, excluding the motor control of skeletal muscle (Chapters 15 and 16). The ANS provides the effector arm for **homeostatic reflexes** (e.g. control of blood pressure), and allows the integration and modulation of function by central mechanisms in the brain in response to *environmental* and *emotional* stimuli (e.g. exercise, thermoregulation, 'fight or flight'). Figure 8.1 shows a simplified schematic diagram of the ANS, and Figure 8.2 its actions on major organs.

The ANS is divided into **sympathetic** and **parasympathetic** systems. Both contain **preganglionic neurones** originating in the central nervous system that synapse with non-myelinated **postganglionic neurones** in the **peripheral ganglia**; postganglionic neurones innervate the target organ or tissue (Figures 8.1 and 8.2). Preganglionic neurones of both sympathetic and parasympathetic systems release **acetylcholine** in the synapse, which acts on **cholinergic nicotinic** receptors on the postganglionic fibre. The postganglionic neurotransmitters and receptors depend on the system and organ (see below). Parasympathetic peripheral ganglia are generally found close to or in the target organ, whereas sympathetic ganglia are largely located in two **sympathetic chains** either side of the vertebral column (*paravertebral ganglia*), or in diffuse *prevertebral ganglia* of the visceral plexuses of the abdomen and pelvis (Figure 8.1). Sympathetic postganglionic neurones are therefore generally long, whereas parasympathetic neurones are generally short. An exception is the sympathetic innervation of the **adrenal gland**, where preganglionic neurones directly innervate the adrenal medulla.

The sympathetic system is more pervasive than the parasympathetic; where an organ is innervated by both systems, they often act antagonistically (Figure 8.2). However, there is a high degree of central coordination, so that an increase in sympathetic activity to an organ is commonly accompanied by a decrease in parasympathetic activity. Sympathetic and parasympathetic activity may modulate different functions in the same organ (e.g. genital organs). In loose terms, the sympathetic system might be said to coordinate '*flight or fight*' responses, and the parasympathetic system '*rest and digest*' responses.

Sympathetic system

Sympathetic preganglionic neurones originate in the *lateral horn* of segments T1–L2 of the spinal cord, and exit the cord via the *ventral horn* (Figure 8.3) on their way to the paravertebral or prevertebral ganglia. Sympathetic postganglionic neurones terminate in the effector organs, where they release **noradrenaline** (NA; **norepinephrine**). Noradrenaline and **adrenaline** (**epinephrine**), which is released by the adrenal medulla, are catecholamines, and activate **adrenergic** receptors, which are linked via G-proteins to cellular effector mechanisms (Chapter 7). There are two main classes of adrenergic receptor, α and β, and these are further subdivided into several subtypes (e.g. α_1, α_2, β_1, β_2, β_3). Noradrenaline and adrenaline are equally potent on α_1-receptors, which are linked to G_q-proteins and are commonly associated with smooth muscle contraction (e.g. blood vessels). The α_2-receptors are $G_{i/o}$-protein linked and are often inhibitory. All β-receptors are linked to G_s-protein and activate adenylyl cyclase to make cyclic adenosine monophosphate (cAMP). Noradrenaline is more potent at β_1-receptors and adrenaline is more potent at β_2-receptors. The

activation of β-receptors is associated with the relaxation of smooth muscle (e.g. blood vessels, airways), but it increases heart rate and force (Figure 8.2).

A few sympathetic neurones release acetylcholine at the effector (e.g. sweat glands), and are thus known as **sympathetic cholinergic** neurones.

Parasympathetic system

Parasympathetic preganglionic neurones originate in the brain stem, from which they run in cranial nerves III, VII, IX and X (**vagus**), and also from the second and third sacral segments of the spinal cord (Figure 8.1). Parasympathetic postganglionic neurones release acetylcholine (ACh), which acts on **cholinergic muscarinic** receptors. Parasympathetic activation causes secretion in many glands (e.g. bronchial mucous glands), and either contraction (e.g. bladder detrusor) or relaxation (e.g. bladder internal sphincter) of smooth muscle, although it has little effect on blood vessels. Notable exceptions, however, include vasodilatation in the penis and clitoris with subsequent erection (Chapter 54).

Neurochemical transmission

Action potentials (APs) in incoming neurones are transmitted by the release of neurotransmitters that bind to receptors on the postganglionic neurone or effector tissue. Between neurones (e.g. in ganglia), this occurs within a classical **synapse**, where the axon terminates in a bulbous swelling or **bouton** separated from the target by a narrow (10–20 nm) synaptic cleft (Figure 8.4i). Postganglionic neurones branch repeatedly and have numerous boutons along their length, forming **varicosities** (e.g. see blood vessel in Figure 8.1). The boutons may either be close (~20 nm) to the effector membrane, allowing fast and specific delivery of the signal, or at some distance (100–200 nm), allowing a more distributed but slower effect. The mechanisms of neurochemical transmission are similar, and although the next paragraph and Figure 8.4i–iv refer to synapses, the same principles apply.

Synthetic enzymes are transported down the axon into the bouton, where they synthesize neurotransmitter (acetylcholine, noradrenaline) from precursors transported into the bouton. The neurotransmitter is stored in 50-nm **vesicles** (Figure 8.4i). The arrival of an AP at the nerve ending causes an influx of Ca^{2+}, the fusion of vesicles with the membrane and the release of neurotransmitter; this binds to postsynaptic receptors and activates the response. Neurotransmitter release can be suppressed by feedback onto **presynaptic inhibitory receptors** (α_2-*receptors* for adrenergic synapses) (Figure 8.4ii). Neurotransmitters must be removed at the end of activation. In *cholinergic* synapses, **cholinesterase** rapidly breaks down acetylcholine into *choline* and *acetate*, which are recycled; some may escape into interstitial fluid (*overflow*) (Figure 8.4iii). In adrenergic synapses, most noradrenaline is rapidly taken up again by the nerve ending via an adenosine triphosphate (ATP)-dependent transporter called **uptake-1**; recovered noradrenaline is recycled. Some facilitated diffusion (**uptake-2**) also occurs into smooth muscle. Excess noradrenaline and sympathomimetic amines, such as tyramine (found in some foodstuffs), are metabolized in the neurone by mitochondrial **monoamine oxidase** (MAO). Noradrenaline and other catecholamines that enter the circulation are metabolized sequentially by **catechol-*O*-methyl transferase** (COMT) and MAO (Figure 8.4iv).

9 Blood

Figure 9.1 Blood cell counts and haematocrit

Erythrocytes	male	4.7–6.1	$\times 10^{12}$/L
	female	4.2–5.4	
Packed cell volume (PCV)	male	0.41–0.52	(no unit)
(haematocrit)	female	0.36–0.48	
Haemoglobin (Hb)	male	130–180	g/L
	female	120–160	
Leucocytes (total)		4–11	$\times 10^9$/L
(white blood cell count, WBCC)			
Platelets		150–400	$\times 10^9$/L

Figure 9.2 Plasma proteins

	Content (g/L)	Typical functions
Albumin	48	Oncotic pressure
		Binds hormones and drugs
α-globulins	5.5	Copper transport
		Antiproteases
β-globulins:		
Transferrin	3	Iron transport
Prothrombin	1	Haemostasis
Plasminogen	0.7	Haemostasis
Complement	1.6	Immune system
Fibrinogen	3	Haemostasis
γ-globulins	13	Immune system

Figure 9.3 Erythropoiesis and the life cycle of the erythrocyte

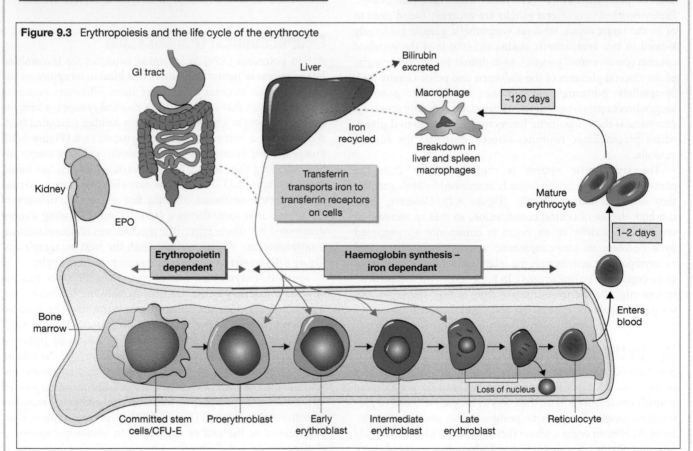

GI tract
Liver
Bilirubin excreted
Macrophage
~120 days
Iron recycled
Breakdown in liver and spleen macrophages
Transferrin transports iron to transferrin receptors on cells
Mature erythrocyte
Kidney
EPO
1–2 days
Erythropoietin dependent
Haemoglobin synthesis – iron dependant
Enters blood
Bone marrow
Loss of nucleus
Committed stem cells/CFU-E | Proerythroblast | Early erythroblast | Intermediate erythroblast | Late erythroblast | Reticulocyte

Figure 9.4 White blood cells (numbers and proportions change greatly in disease)

Granulocytes

Lymphocytes
20–40% total
1500–3000 $\times 10^6$/L

Monocytes
2–8% total
300–600 $\times 10^6$/L

Basophils
~0.5% total
0–100 $\times 10^6$/L

Eosinophils
1–4% total
150–300 $\times 10^6$/L

Neutrophils
50–70% total
3000–6000 $\times 10^6$/L

Physiology at a Glance, Fourth Edition. Edited by Jeremy P.T. Ward and Roger W.A. Linden.
© 2017 John Wiley & Sons, Ltd. Published 2017 by John Wiley & Sons, Ltd. Companion website: www.ataglanceseries.com/physiology

The primary function of blood is to deliver O_2 and energy to the tissues, and remove CO_2 and waste products. It is also important for the defence and immune systems, regulation of temperature, and transport of hormones and signalling molecules between tissues. Blood consists of **plasma** (Chapter 2) and blood cells. **Red blood cells** contain haemoglobin and transport respiratory gases (Chapter 31), whereas **white cells** form part of the defence system (Chapter 11). In adults, all blood cells are produced in the red bone marrow. Normal values for cell counts, haemoglobin and proportion of blood volume due to red cells (**haematocrit** or **packed cell volume**; estimated by centrifuging a blood sample) are shown in Figure 9.1. **Platelets** are discussed in Chapter 10.

Plasma proteins

Plasma contains several important proteins (Figure 9.2), with a total concentration of 65–83 g/L. Most, other than γ-globulins (see later), are synthesized in the liver. Proteins can ionize as either acids or bases because of the presence of both NH_2 and COOH groups. At pH 7.4 they are mostly in the anionic (acidic) form. Their ability to accept or donate H^+ means they can act as **buffers** (Chapter 39). Plasma proteins have important **transport functions**, as they bind many hormones (e.g. cortisol and thyroxine) and metals (e.g. iron). They are classified into **albumin**, **globulin** and **fibrinogen** fractions. Globulins are further classified as **α-, β- and γ-globulins**. Examples and their major functions are shown in Figure 9.2.

Red blood cells

Red blood cells (**erythrocytes**) are biconcave discs ~8 μm wide, and uniquely have no nucleus. They therefore cannot repair themselves and have a lifespan of only 100–120 days. The shape and flexibility of red cells allows them to deform easily and pass through capillaries. Importantly, they contain **haemoglobin** which is responsible for carriage of O_2, and also plays a role in acid–base buffering (Chapter 31 and 39).

Red cells are formed by a process called **erythropoiesis** (Figure 9.3). They originate from **committed stem cells** (CFU-E; colony forming unit-erythroid) in the bone marrow of the adult, and liver and spleen of the fetus. The glycoprotein hormone **erythropoietin** (EPO) increases the number of committed stem cells and promotes production of red cells. Erythropoietin is produced mainly by the kidneys in adults, and liver in the fetus. The key stimulus for increased erythropoietin is low O_2 (**hypoxia**). Stem cells differentiate into **erythroblasts** (**early normoblasts**), which are relatively large (~15 μm) and nucleated. As differentiation proceeds, the cells shrink and **haemoglobin** is synthesized, which requires **iron**, **folate** and **vitamin B_{12}**. In the **late normoblast** the nucleus breaks up and disappears. The young red cell shows a reticulum on staining, and is called a **reticulocyte**. As it ages, the reticulum disappears and the characteristic biconcave shape develops. Normally 1–2% of circulating red cells are reticulocytes. This increases when erythropoiesis is enhanced (e.g. by hypoxia). About 2×10^{11} red cells are produced from the marrow each day. The spleen holds a reserve of red cells that can be released following blood loss.

Red cells are destroyed by **macrophages** in the liver and spleen after ~120 days. The haem group is split from haemoglobin and converted to **biliverdin** and then **bilirubin**. The iron is conserved and recycled via **transferrin**, an iron transport protein, or stored in **ferritin**. Bilirubin is a brown–yellow compound which is excreted in the bile. An increased rate of haemoglobin breakdown results in excess bilirubin, which stains the tissues (**jaundice**).

An inadequate amount of red cells and/or haemoglobin is called **anaemia**. This is commonly a result of **haemorrhage** (e.g. heavy menstruation), but also occurs when the diet contains insufficient iron, folate or vitamin B_{12}, or they are poorly absorbed in the gut (Chapter 42). Anaemia is also caused by abnormalities of haemoglobin (**thalassaemia**), the **sickle cell** mutation and **leukaemia** (white cell cancers).

Red cells have surface **antigens** that can react with specific antibodies in the plasma. The antigens and antibodies present are determined genetically, forming the basis of **blood groups**. The most important systems are **ABO** (A, B, both or neither antigens present) and **Rh** (Rhesus; D or no D antigen). Matching of blood groups is essential during blood transfusions, because red cells with a different antigen to the recipient will react with antibodies in the plasma, stick together (**agglutinate**) and **haemolyse** (break apart). The Rh system is important in pregnancy, because an Rh- mother can be sensitized (produce antibodies) to red cells from a Rh+ fetus during birth. This can be a problem for a second pregnancy with another Rh+ fetus, as antibodies cross the placenta.

White blood cells

White blood cells (**leucocytes**) defend the body against infection by foreign material, and the white cell count (Figure 9.1) increases greatly in disease. Three main types are present in blood: granulocytes, lymphocytes and monocytes.

Granulocytes are further classified as **neutrophils** (neutral-staining granules), **eosinophils** (acid-staining granules) and **basophils** (basic-staining granules) (Figure 9.4). All contribute to inflammation by releasing mediators. **Neutrophils** have a key role in the **innate immune system**, and migrate to areas of infection (**chemotaxis**) within minutes, where they destroy bacteria by **phagocytosis** (engulfing them). They are a major component of pus. Neutrophils live for ~6 h in blood, longer in tissues. **Eosinophils** are less motile but longer lived, and phagocytose larger parasites. They are increased in allergic disease, to which they contribute by releasing inflammatory mediators. **Basophils** release histamine and heparin as part of the inflammatory response and are similar to tissue **mast cells**.

Lymphocytes originate in the bone marrow but mature in the lymph nodes, thymus and spleen before returning to the circulation. Most remain in the lymphatic system. Lymphocytes are critical components of the **immune system** and are of three main forms: **B cells** which produce γ-globulins (*immunoglobulins*, antibodies), **T cells** which coordinate the immune response, and **natural killer** (NK) cells which kill infected or cancerous cells (Chapter 11).

Monocytes are phagocytes but larger and longer lived than granulocytes. After formation in the marrow they circulate in the blood for ~72 h before entering tissues to become **macrophages**, which unlike granulocytes can also dispose of dead cell debris. Macrophages form the **reticuloendothelial system** in liver, spleen and lymph nodes.

10 Platelets and haemostasis

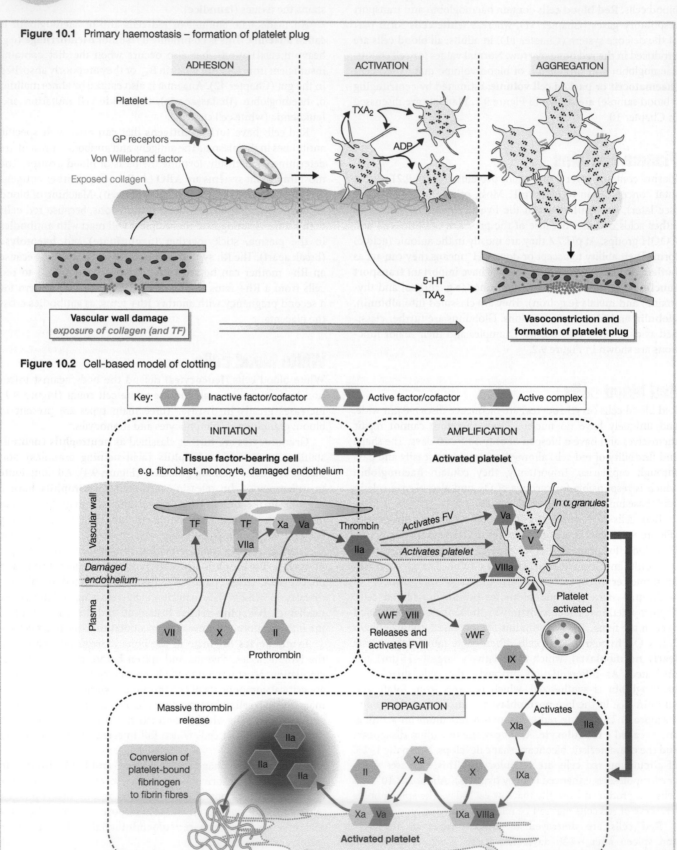

Figure 10.1 Primary haemostasis – formation of platelet plug

| ADHESION | ACTIVATION | AGGREGATION |

Platelet
GP receptors
Von Willebrand factor
Exposed collagen

TXA_2
ADP

5-HT
TXA_2

Vascular wall damage
exposure of collagen (and TF)

Vasoconstriction and formation of platelet plug

Figure 10.2 Cell-based model of clotting

Key: Inactive factor/cofactor Active factor/cofactor Active complex

INITIATION

Tissue factor-bearing cell
e.g. fibroblast, monocyte, damaged endothelium

AMPLIFICATION

Activated platelet

In α granules

Vascular wall

TF   TF   Xa   Va   Thrombin   Activates FV   Va
      VIIa   IIa   *Activates platelet*   V

Damaged endothelium   VIIIa

Plasma

VII   X   II   vWF VIII   vWF   Platelet activated

Prothrombin   Releases and
                         activates FVIII

                                            IX

PROPAGATION

Massive thrombin release   Activates

                        IIa   XIa   ◄ IIa

Conversion of   IIa   IIa
platelet-bound
fibrinogen   IIa
to fibrin fibres
                              II   Xa   X   IXa

                        Xa Va   IXa VIIIa

Activated platelet

Physiology at a Glance, Fourth Edition. Edited by Jeremy P.T. Ward and Roger W.A. Linden.

Leaks in the cardiovascular system can lead to loss of blood and must be rapidly plugged. This is the purpose of **haemostasis**, a complex process that includes formation of the blood clot, a tough mesh of **fibrin** entrapping platelets and blood cells. Its complexity is in part due to the precarious balance that must be maintained between providing a rapid and effective means of stopping leaks, and inappropriate formation of clots in blood vessels (**thrombosis**). Thrombosis is associated with many serious conditions such as coronary artery disease.

Platelets play a critical role in haemostasis. They circulate in the blood but are not true cells, being small (~3 μm) vesicle-like structures formed from megakaryocytes in the bone marrow. They have a lifespan of ~4 days. Platelets have multiple surface receptors and clearly visible dense granules. These contain mediators such as serotonin and adenosine diphosphate (ADP), which are released on activation.

Primary haemostasis

The immediate response to damage of a blood vessel wall is **vasoconstriction**, which reduces blood flow and thus loss; it is an intrinsic property of the blood vessel. This is followed by a sequence of events that eventually leads to sealing of the wound by a clot (Figure 10.1). Damage to the vessel wall exposes collagen, to which a plasma protein called **von Willebrand factor** (vWF) binds. Tissue factor (TF) is also exposed (see below). **Platelets** have **glycoprotein** (GP) receptors which avidly bind to vWF, tethering the platelet. Further receptors including **integrins** (Chapter 3) bind directly to collagen. Together these cause **adhesion** of the platelet to the damaged area. Binding to these receptors also initiates **platelet activation**, partly by increasing intracellular Ca^{2+}. Platelets change shape, put out pseudopodia and make **thromboxane A_2** (TXA_2) via **cyclooxygenase** (COX). TXA_2 stimulates release of **serotonin (5-HT**; 5-hydroxytryptamine), **ADP** and other compounds from the platelet granules. TXA_2 and serotonin also enhance the vasoconstriction. The process propagates because **ADP** directly activates more platelets via purinergic (**P2Y**) receptors. It also causes activation of fibrinogen receptors (**GPIIb/IIIa**) on their surface, which bind to **fibrinogen** in the plasma causing the platelets to become sticky and **aggregate**, forming a soft platelet plug (Figure 10.1). This is stabilized during clotting by conversion of the fibrinogen to **fibrin**. Note that **thrombin** (see later) is also a potent platelet activator.

Formation of the blood clot (coagulation)

The process leading to formation of the blood clot involves sequential conversion of **proenzymes** to active enzymes (**clotting factors**; e.g. factor X → Xa) in an amplifying cascade. Most clotting factors are produced in the liver, which requires **vitamin K**, and many (e.g. thrombin, factor X) require Ca^{2+} to act. The ultimate purpose is to produce a massive burst of **thrombin** (factor IIa; a protease which cleaves fibrinogen to fibrin), and thus rapid formation of the clot. The **cell-based model of clotting** (Figure 10.2) has replaced the older extrinsic and intrinsic pathways. Most of the action in this model only occurs on cell or platelet surfaces (hence its name).

The **initial phase** of clotting occurs when cells that express a protein called **tissue factor** (TF; thromboplastin) become exposed to plasma as a result of vascular damage. Such cells include fibroblasts, monocytes and damaged endothelial cells. **Factor VIIa** from the plasma is then able to bind to TF (**TF:VIIa**), and this complex consequently activates a key protein in the clotting process, **factor X**. It is this, when combined with **cofactor Va** to form **prothrombinase**, that converts **prothrombin** to **thrombin**; importantly, it can only do so when tethered to the cell by phospholipids. However, insufficient thrombin is produced at this stage for clot formation, and the signal has to be amplified.

The **amplification phase** takes place on the surface of **platelets** (Figure 10.2). The small amount of thrombin produced above activates nearby platelets, and also cofactor V on their surface. **Cofactor VIII** is normally bound to plasma vWF, which protects it from degradation. Thrombin cleaves factor VIII from vWF and activates it, when it also binds to the platelet surface. The end product is a large number of activated platelets, each with a large surface area (due to pseudopodia) covered with the active cofactors, all stuck together by fibrinogen (see previously).

The scene is now set for the **propagation phase**. Thrombin activates a short cascade that leads to activation of **factor IX** (also activated by TF:VIIa). Factor IXa forms a complex with cofactor VIIIa on the platelet surface to form **tenase**, a much more powerful activator of factor X than TF:VIIa. The large amount of factor Xa thus generated binds to cofactor Va also on the platelet surface to form a similarly large amount of **prothrombinase**. There is consequently a massive burst of thrombin production, 1000-fold greater than in the initial phase. Thrombin cleaves the **fibrinogen** bound around the platelets to form **fibrin monomers**, which spontaneously polymerize to a fibrous mesh of fibrin, entrapping the platelets and other blood cells. The fibrin polymer is finally cross-linked by **factor XIIIa** (also activated by thrombin) to create a tough network of fibrin fibres and a stable clot. Retraction of entrapped platelets contracts the clot by ~60%, making it tougher and assisting repair by drawing the edges of the wound together.

Inhibitors of haemostasis and fibrinolysis

Because thrombin both activates and is produced by the mechanisms described above, there is an element of **positive feedback**, and the whole process is intrinsically unstable. Multiple inhibitory mechanisms counteract this to prevent inappropriate clotting. Undamaged endothelium produces **prostacyclin** and **nitric oxide** (Chapter 27), which impede platelet adhesion and activation and so limit them to damaged areas. Plasma **antithrombin** inhibits thrombin, factor Xa and tenase, and is strongly potentiated by **heparin** and **heparans** on endothelial cells. **Thrombomodulin** (also on endothelial cells) binds thrombin and converts it so it no longer cleaves fibrinogen but instead activates **protein C** (APC; activated protein C), which with **protein S** inactivates factors Va and VIIIa, and hence tenase and prothrombinase. Finally, the clot is broken down by **plasmin**, a process called **fibrinolysis**. This occurs when plasma **plasminogen** binds to fibrin, and is converted to plasmin by **tissue plasminogen activator** (tPA). Plasmin is itself inactivated by α_2-antiplasmin.

11 Defence: inflammation and immunity

Figure 11.1 Innate immune response and inflammation
– See text for details. Note that phagocytes release powerful cytotoxins including reactive oxygen species and lysozymes, which also damage the tissue, a serious problem in chronic inflammation. NK cells not shown for clarity.

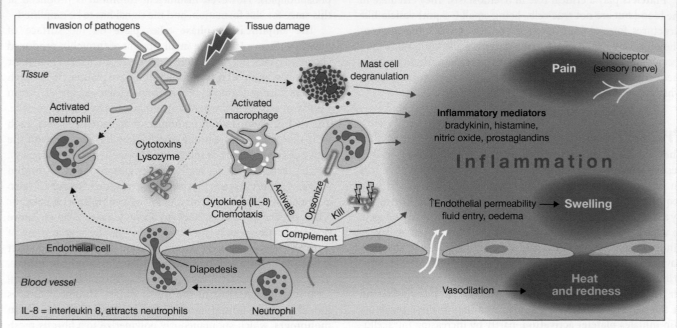

Invasion of pathogens

Tissue damage

Tissue

Mast cell degranulation

Pain

Nociceptor (sensory nerve)

Activated neutrophil

Activated macrophage

Inflammatory mediators
bradykinin, histamine, nitric oxide, prostaglandins

Cytotoxins Lysozyme

I n f l a m m a t i o n

Activate

Opsonize

Kill

Cytokines (IL-8) Chemotaxis

Complement

↑Endothelial permeability fluid entry, oedema → **Swelling**

Endothelial cell

Diapedesis

Blood vessel

Vasodilation → **Heat and redness**

IL-8 = interleukin 8, attracts neutrophils

Neutrophil

Figure 11.2 Antibodies

Antigen binding sites
Hypervariable regions

F_{ab}

Light chain

F_c

Heavy chain

F_c differs between classes, and binds to class-specific F_c receptors on immune cells, and also complement

Classes: mostly **monomers**
IgG Most common (80%)
IgE Antihelminth, binds to and activates mast cells in allergy
IgD Naïve B cell antigen receptor
IgA Mucosal immunity in gut and airways, dimer
IgM Naïve B cell antigen receptor Secreted as a **pentamer**, a strong activator of complement, in T cell independent humoral responses

Class switching:
Activated B cells can switch the class of antibody they make, e.g. from IgM to IgG or IgE. This is regulated by T_H cytokines. Plasma cells cannot class switch, being pre-programmed

Figure 11.3 Humoral immunity

Figure 11.4 Cell-mediated immunity

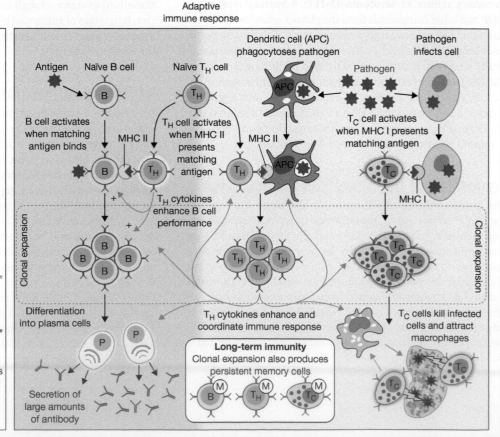

Adaptive immune response

Dendritic cell (APC) phagocytoses pathogen

Pathogen infects cell

Antigen   Naïve B cell

Naïve T_H cell

APC

Pathogen

B cell activates when matching antigen binds

T_H cell activates when MHC II presents matching antigen

MHC II

MHC II

APC

T_C cell activates when MHC I presents matching antigen

T_C

MHC I

Clonal expansion

T_H cytokines enhance B cell performance

Clonal expansion

Differentiation into plasma cells

T_H cytokines enhance and coordinate immune response

T_C cells kill infected cells and attract macrophages

Long-term immunity
Clonal expansion also produces persistent memory cells

Secretion of large amounts of antibody

Physiology at a Glance, Fourth Edition. Edited by Jeremy P.T. Ward and Roger W.A. Linden.
© 2017 John Wiley & Sons, Ltd. Published 2017 by John Wiley & Sons, Ltd. Companion website: www.ataglanceseries.com/physiology

Physical defence against infection by **bacteria**, **viruses**, **fungi**, and **parasites** is provided by the skin, and epithelia lining the airways and gut. The latter secrete **antimicrobial** chemicals and **mucus**, which traps microorganisms and is removed by cilia (Chapter 28) or peristalsis. Haemostasis quickly seals breaches (Chapter 10). Organisms evading these defences are targeted by the **immune system**, where **leucocytes** play a central role (Chapter 9). The **innate** immune response is fast but *non-specific* and causes **inflammation**, characterized by **heat**, **redness**, **swelling** and **pain**. The **adaptive** response is slower, *highly specific*, and more potent.

Innate immune response

Tissue damage and invasion of pathogens activate **mast cells** (similar to *basophils*) and resident **phagocytes**, primarily **macrophages** and **dendritic cells**, which release **inflammatory mediators**, signalling molecules (**cytokines**) and **cytotoxic agents** (Figure 11.1). Inflammatory mediators cause **vasodilation** (*heat and redness*), stimulate **nociceptors** (*pain*) and increase **endothelial permeability**, leading to *extravasation* of protein and fluids and thus **oedema** (*swelling*) (Chapters 2 and 26). Cytokines (e.g. interleukin 8, IL-8) attract many more phagocytes, chiefly **neutrophils** (**chemotaxis**); these leave the blood by squeezing between endothelial cells (**diapedesis**). Phagocytes ingest (**phagocytose**) microorganisms, and in the case of macrophages also damaged cells and debris. Pathogens can be detected because they express **pathogen-associated molecular patterns** (**PAMPs**) not found in mammals (e.g. bacterial mannose residues, viral RNA and fungal glucans). PAMPs are recognized by phagocyte **pattern recognition receptors** (**PRRs**); relatively few different PRRs are required (<1000) because PAMPs are common across wide groups of pathogen. On binding a PAMP, PRRs initiate phagocytosis and release of cytokines and cytotoxins. Injured, infected or cancerous cells express PAMP-like molecules recognized by **natural killer** (**NK**) lymphocytes, which kill the cells and activate macrophages to remove the debris. In major infections cytokines such as IL-1 cause *fever* (Chapter 13); high temperatures may assist the immune response.

Complement is an important *non-cellular* mechanism comprised of a cascade of plasma proteins. On activation it coats and **opsonizes** (*facilitates phagocytosis*) pathogens, kills by membrane rupture, recruits phagocytes and induces inflammation. It is activated by some surface molecules (e.g. bacterial mannose) and by *antibodies* (e.g. IgM; Figure 11.2) that have 'tagged' a pathogen or material as foreign.

Antibodies (immunoglobulins)

Adaptive immunity depends on **antibodies**, which are made by **lymphocytes** and recognize highly specific molecular sequences (**epitopes**) on proteins, polysaccharides, lipids and small chemicals. Molecules that react with antibodies are called **antigens**. There are five antibody classes (Figure 11.2). All have a constant region (F_C) attached to two *hyper-variable* branches (F_{ab}) which recognize the epitope. The hypervariability is due to random mutations in antibody genes during lymphocyte maturation, so each cell can end up with one of ~10^9 different antibodies. Although *individual cells express just one variant*, the large number of lymphocytes and random nature of production means that every variant will be expressed somewhere, if only in a small group of cells. Such groups of lymphocytes with identical antibodies are called **clones**. Any lymphocytes with antibodies directed against *self* are (normally) destroyed during maturation. Antibodies *neutralize* toxins and prevent attachment of pathogens; *target, opsonize* or *agglutinate* (clump together) antigens for phagocytosis; *target* pathogens and foreign material for complement; and, crucially, act as **antigen receptors** on lymphocytes.

Adaptive immune response

The adaptive response takes ~5 days to become effective, and peaks after 1–2 weeks. It has two intertwined branches: **humoral immunity**, mediated by **B lymphocytes** (B cells) which mature in **bone marrow**, and **cell-mediated immunity**, mediated by **T lymphocytes** (T cells) which mature in the **thymus**. **Naïve** (not yet activated) lymphocytes continually **recirculate** between **lymphoid tissues** (e.g. lymph nodes, tonsils and spleen) until they encounter a matching antigen.

Humoral immunity (Figure 11.3) is particularly effective against extracellular pathogens, as it involves secretion of antibodies into extracellular fluid. Only B cells can do this, or have antigen receptors that can recognize *all* types of antigen (e.g. protein, polysaccharide, lipid, etc.). When an antigen binds to its matching receptor on naïve B cells, the latter activate and undergo **clonal expansion** – rapid proliferation resulting in a large number of identical cells expressing the same antibody. These differentiate into **plasma cells**, which secrete the antibody in massive amounts. For non-protein antigens the whole process is *T cell independent*. However, if the antigen is a protein, **T helper** (T_H, CD4+) cells substantially enhance the response. T cells only recognize protein (or peptide) antigens, and then only when they are *presented* to them by **major histocompatibility complex** (**MHC II**) on **antigen presenting cells** (**APC**), which include dendritic cells, macrophages and B cells. B cells activated by protein antigen attract and attach to T_H cells, to which they present the antigen via MHC II. If a T_H cell's receptors identify the antigen, the cell proliferates and releases cytokines which strongly potentiate B cell proliferation and performance; this is often essential for an effective response. T_H cytokines also induce B cell **class switching**, e.g. from production of IgM to IgE (Figure 11.2).

Memory cells which persist for years are also produced during clonal expansion. These respond much more rapidly and powerfully to subsequent exposures to the same pathogen, and provide **long term immunity**. This is the basis of immunization.

Cell-mediated immunity (Figure 11.4) is directed towards antigens *within* cells, which are made visible by MHC. **MHC I** is found on the surface of all cells and displays *cytosolic* antigens (e.g. viral proteins), but only to **cytotoxic T_C** (CD8+) cells, which proliferate on recognizing the antigen and destroy any similarly infected cells. In contrast, MHC II displays antigens *retained within vesicles*, i.e. that have been phagocytosed, and is found *only* in APCs which activate T_H cells. **Dendritic cells**, and to a lesser extent macrophages, are the most important phagocytic APCs. After phagocytosing a pathogen they migrate to lymphoid tissues and present the antigen (via MHC II) to naïve T_H cells. T_H cells that recognize the antigen activate, proliferate and stimulate B cells (and thus a *humoral* response) as described above. Importantly, they also release cytokines that regulate the activity of other immune cells, including macrophages, T_H, T_C, NK, plasma and mast cells. T_H cells therefore play a critical coordinating role in the immune response.

12 Principles of diffusion and flow

Figure 12.8 Wall tension

$$\text{Wall tension} = P_t\left(\frac{r}{w}\right)$$
(Laplace's law)

r = radius
w = wall thickness
P_t = pressure

Figure 12.5
Axial flow of red blood cells

Figure 12.6
Narrowing increases velocity, and can cause turbulent flow

Figure 12.2
Flow through whole circuit
= $(P_1 - P_2)$/total resistance
(Darcy's law)

Figure 12.7
Resistance of parallel circuits =
$$1/(1/R_a + 1/R_b + 1/R_c + 1/R_d)$$

Figure 12.3
For individual small vessels, non-pulsatile flow is described by the Poiseuille equation:

$$\text{Flow} = \Delta P \left(\frac{\pi r^4}{8VL}\right)$$

Flow very dependent on radius

Resistance term

P = pressure, r = radius
V = viscosity, L = length

Figure 12.4
Laminar flow

Laminar flow
Fastest in centre of vessel

Flow velocity

Velocity = zero at vessel wall

Circulations to organs in parallel

Constriction of thick-walled arterioles controls perfusion of vascular beds

Capillaries

Figure 12.1 Diffusion across a membrane (application of Fick's Law)

Rate of diffusion $(J_S) = -pA(C_1 - C_2)$
where p is permeability, A is area, and C_1, C_2 are concentration

Membrane

Area

C_1 C_2

Diffusion and bulk flow

Materials are carried around the body by a combination of bulk flow and diffusion. **Bulk flow** simply means transport *with* the carrying medium (blood, air). **Passive diffusion** refers to movement down a *concentration gradient*, and accounts for transport across small distances, e.g. within the cytosol and across membranes. The rate of **diffusion in a solution** is described by **Fick's law**:

$$J_s = -DA(\Delta C/\Delta x) \qquad \text{(Eqn 12.1)}$$

where J_s is the amount of substance transferred per unit time, ΔC is the difference in concentration, Δx is the diffusion distance and A is the surface area over which diffusion occurs. The negative sign reflects movement *down* the concentration gradient. D is the **diffusion coefficient**, a measure of how easy it is for the substance to diffuse. D is related to temperature, solvent viscosity and the size of the molecule, and is normally *inversely proportional to the cube root of the molecular weight*. **Diffusion across a membrane** is affected by the **permeability** of the membrane. The permeability (p) is related to the membrane thickness and composition, and the diffusion coefficient of the substance. Fick's equation can be rewritten as:

$$J_s = -pA\Delta C \qquad \text{(Eqn 12.2)}$$

where A is the membrane area and ΔC is the concentration difference across the membrane. The rate of diffusion across a capillary wall is therefore related to the *concentration difference* across the wall and the *permeability* of the wall to that substance (Figure 12.1).

Flow through a tube

Flow through a tube is dependent on the pressure difference across the ends of the tube ($P_1 - P_2$) and the resistance to flow provided by the tube (R):

$$\text{Flow} = (P_1 - P_2)/R \qquad \text{(Eqn 12.3)}$$

This is **Darcy's law** (analogous to *Ohm's law* in electronics; Figure 12.2).

Resistance is due to frictional forces, and is determined by the **diameter** of the tube and the **viscosity** of the fluid:

$$R = (8VL)/(\pi r^4) \qquad \text{(Eqn 12.4)}$$

This is **Poiseuille's law**, where V is the viscosity, L is the length of the tube and r is the radius of the tube. Combining equations (12.3) and (12.4) shows an important principle, namely that **flow $\propto$ (radius)^4**:

$$\text{Flow} = [(P_1 - P_2)\pi r^4]/(8VL) \qquad \text{(Eqn 12.5)}$$

Therefore, small changes in radius have a large effect on flow (Figure 12.3). Thus, the constriction of an artery by 20% will decrease the flow by ~60%.

Viscosity. Treacle flows more slowly than water because it has a higher viscosity. Plasma has a similar viscosity to water, but blood contains cells (mostly erythrocytes) which effectively increase the viscosity by three- to fourfold. Changes in cell number, e.g. *polycythaemia* (increased erythrocytes), therefore affect the blood flow.

Laminar and turbulent flow. Frictional forces at the sides of a tube cause drag on the fluid touching them. This creates a *velocity gradient* (Figure 12.4) in which the flow is greatest at the centre. This is termed **laminar flow**, and describes the flow in the majority of cardiovascular and respiratory systems at rest. A consequence of the velocity gradient is that blood cells tend to move away from the sides of the vessel and accumulate towards the centre (**axial streaming**; Figure 12.5); they also tend to align themselves to the flow. In small vessels, this *effectively reduces the blood viscosity* and minimizes the resistance (the **Fåhraeus–Lindqvist effect**).

At high velocities, especially in large arteries and airways, and at the edges or branches where the velocity increases sharply, flow may become **turbulent**, and laminar flow is disrupted (Figure 12.6). This significantly increases the resistance. The narrowing of airways and large arteries (or valve orifices), which increases the fluid velocity, can therefore cause turbulence, which is heard as **lung sounds** (e.g. wheezing in asthma) and **cardiac murmurs** (Chapter 21).

Turbulent flow is also responsible for the sounds heard when measuring blood pressure using a **sphygmomanometer** and stethoscope (**Korotkoff sounds**). A rubber cuff round the arm is inflated to a pressure well above predicted arterial pressure and then slowly deflated. When the pressure in the cuff approaches systolic pressure, the blood is able to force its way through the constricted artery in the arm for part of the pulse. The high velocity of the blood through the narrowed artery causes turbulence and therefore a sound; the first appearance of this is taken as systolic pressure. As the pressure in the cuff falls further and so below diastolic pressure, flow is continuous because the pressure is greater than that in the cuff throughout the pulse. As a result the sound fades and disappears, and the cuff pressure at this point is taken as diastolic pressure.

Resistances in parallel and in series. The cardiovascular and respiratory systems contain a mixture of *series* (e.g. arteries $\Rightarrow$ arterioles $\Rightarrow$ capillaries $\Rightarrow$ venules $\Rightarrow$ veins) and *parallel* (e.g. lots of capillaries) components (Figure 12.7). Flow through a *series* of tubes is restricted by the resistance of each tube in turn, and the total resistance is the **sum** of the resistances:

$$R_T = R_1 + R_2 + R_3 + \ldots \qquad \text{(Eqn 12.6)}$$

In a parallel circuit, the addition of extra paths reduces the total resistance, and so:

$$R_T = 1/(1/R_a + 1/R_b \ldots) \qquad \text{(Eqn 12.7)}$$

Although the resistance of individual capillaries or terminal bronchioles is high (small radius, *Poiseuille's law*), the huge number of them in parallel means that their contribution to the total resistance of the cardiovascular and respiratory systems is comparatively small.

Wall tension and pressure in spherical or cylindrical containers

Pressure across the wall of a flexible tube (*transmural pressure*) tends to extend it, and increases wall tension. This can be described by **Laplace's law**:

$$P_t = (Tw)/r \qquad \text{(Eqn 12.8)}$$

where P_t is the transmural pressure, T is the wall tension, w is the wall thickness and r is the radius (Figure 12.8). Thus, a small bubble with the same wall tension as a larger bubble will contain a greater pressure, and will collapse into the larger bubble if they are joined. In the lung, small alveoli would collapse into larger ones were it not for *surfactant* which reduces the surface tension more strongly as the size of the alveolus decreases (Chapter 29). Laplace's law also means that a large dilated heart (e.g. heart failure) has to develop more wall tension (contractile force) in order to obtain the same ventricular pressure, making it less efficient.

13 Thermoregulation

Figure 13.1 Thermoregulation: Concept of core and shell

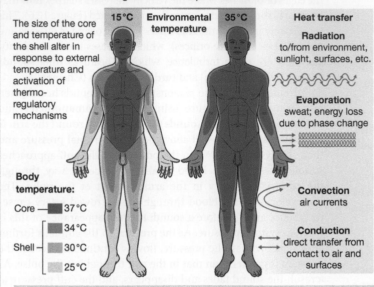

The size of the core and temperature of the shell alter in response to external temperature and activation of thermo-regulatory mechanisms

Environmental temperature

15°C   35°C

Body temperature:

Core — 37°C

Shell —
34°C
30°C
25°C

Heat transfer

Radiation
to/from environment, sunlight, surfaces, etc.

Evaporation
sweat; energy loss due to phase change

Convection
air currents

Conduction
direct transfer from contact to air and surfaces

Figure 13.2 Thermoregulatory centres in the hypothalamus
(lines reflect signalling routes not neural tracts)

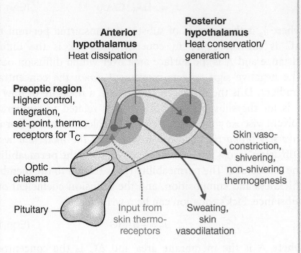

Anterior hypothalamus
Heat dissipation

Posterior hypothalamus
Heat conservation/generation

Preoptic region
Higher control, integration, set-point, thermo-receptors for T_C

Optic chiasma

Pituitary

Input from skin thermo-receptors

Skin vaso-constriction, shivering, non-shivering thermogenesis

Sweating, skin vasodilatation

Figure 13.3 Cartoon of cutaneous circulation (simplified)

When cool, vasoconstriction limits blood flow and heat loss.
When warm, vasodilatation increases blood flow (particularly in AVAs, only present in hair-less skin), greatly increasing heat loss.

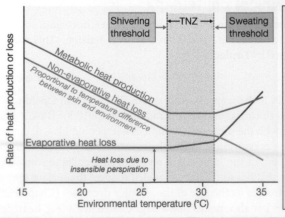

Epidermis

Dermis

Artery
Vein

Capillary loops

Heat Heat Heat

Subpapillary plexus

Dermal venous plexus

Arteriovenous anastomoses

Sympathetic adrenergic nerves *(noradrenaline)*

Figure 13.4 Sweat gland

Activated by sympathetic cholinergic nerves, sweat composition depends on flow rate

Evaporative loss of heat

Sweat

Sweat gland duct *(salt and water reabsorbed)*

Bradykinin NO, SP

Vasodilatation

Sweat gland

Sympathetic cholinergic nerves *(acetylcholine, + co-transmitters nitric oxide [NO] and substance P [SP])*

Figure 13.5 Piloerection

Activated by sympathetic adrenergic nerves; arrector pili muscle erects hair

Sebaceous gland

Arrector pili *(smooth muscle)*

Sympathetic adrenergic nerves

Hair follicle

Figure 13.6 Thermoneutral zone (TNZ) – for naked 70 kg man. Within the TNZ metabolic rate is constant, and thermoregulation occurs by regulation of vasomotor tone alone

Shivering threshold ← TNZ → Sweating threshold

Metabolic heat production

Non-evaporative heat loss
Proportional to temperature difference between skin and environment

Evaporative heat loss

Heat loss due to insensible perspiration

Rate of heat production or loss

Environmental temperature (°C)
15   20   25   30   35

Notes:
Shivering and sweating thresholds are modified by skin temperature: e.g. T_C does not need to fall so much to initiate shivering when skin is cool, and sweating starts at a lower T_C when skin is hot. These responses 'anticipate' the effect that changes in external temperature would have on T_C.

Shivering greatly increases heat production; sweating also has a metabolic cost and generates heat, but much less than it causes to be lost.

Figure 13.7 Acclimatization to the heat and consequences of inadequate thermoregulation

Hot (45°C) and dry

Cool

Core temperature (°C)
39.5
39.0
38.5
38.0
37.5

Sweat production

Days in heat
0   2   4   6   8

Heat exhaustion: $T_C > 39.5°C$, profuse sweating, ↓extracellular fluid volume, ↓blood pressure, ↑HR

Heat stroke: $T_C > 41°C$, failure of thermo-regulatory effectors, decreased sweating, BP variable, ↑↑HR

Physiology at a Glance, Fourth Edition. Edited by Jeremy P.T. Ward and Roger W.A. Linden.
© 2017 John Wiley & Sons, Ltd. Published 2017 by John Wiley & Sons Ltd. Companion website: www.ataglanceseries.com/physiology

Thermoregulation maintains **core temperature** (T_C) around the major organs (e.g. brain, heart, liver) close to a **set point** (Chapter 1). The extent of the core and temperature of the shell around it varies with conditions (Figure 13.1). T_C fluctuates with exercise, sleep, feeding and hormonal status (e.g. ovulation elevates T_C), and exhibits a circadian rhythm with minimum temperatures at night. Metabolic heat is transferred by blood to the skin, where it is lost by **radiation** (infrared), **conduction** (to objects and air), **convection** (air currents) and **evaporation**; skin is thus the **major thermoregulatory organ**. Heat production depends on body mass ($\propto$ metres^3), whereas heat loss depends on surface area (metres^2). As size increases, the **body surface area** (BSA) to mass ratio therefore decreases, so large animals (e.g. elephants) have problems losing heat, whilst small ones (e.g. shrews) have problems retaining it. Neonates, with a BSA/volume ratio about twice that of adults, are thus more susceptible to **hypothermia**.

Nearly all thermoregulatory mechanisms are controlled by the **hypothalamus** (Figure 13.2). T_C is sensed by **thermoreceptors** in the **preoptic region**, 75% of which are heat-sensitive. Conversely **skin** has more cold- than heat-sensitive thermoreceptors (Chapter 58). Deep body thermoreceptors in spinal cord and abdomen are also mostly cold sensitive, and protect against hypothermia. The **preoptic region** provides higher control; it integrates signals from all thermoreceptors, acts as comparator for the T_C set point (Chapter 1), and modulates activity of the hypothalamic effector areas. A **heat dissipation** effector area in the **anterior hypothalamus** controls sweating, skin vasodilatation and behaviour (e.g. shade-seeking), and a **heat conservation** area in the **posterior hypothalamus** controls skin vasoconstriction, piloerection (raising of skin hair, 'goosebumps'), shivering, non-shivering thermogenesis and heat-conserving behaviour.

Fever (elevated T_C) reflects resetting of the thermoregulatory set point by trauma, exercise or **pyrogens** (fever-inducing substances), particularly **interleukin-1** released during infection and inflammation (Chapter 11). Their effect on the set point is probably mediated by prostaglandin-E_2 (PGE_2); common **anti-pyretics** (paracetamol, aspirin, ibuprofen) inhibit cyclooxygenase (COX) so reducing substrate for PGE_2 synthesis (Chapter 4), and thus fever.

Thermoregulatory mechanisms

The skin contains **venous plexuses** which facilitate heat transfer from blood to the surface (Figure 13.3). In **glabrous** (hairless) skin of hands, feet and areas of the face, coiled, thick-walled **arteriovenous anastomoses** (AVAs) directly link arterial and venous vessels, bypassing capillaries and enabling high blood flows through the venous plexus and increased radiation of heat. Within the **thermoneutral zone** (TNZ; Figure 13.6) T_C is maintained solely by adjusting skin blood flow via vasoconstriction induced by sympathetic **adrenergic** nerves (*noradrenaline-releasing*) (Chapters 8, 24). Cooler temperatures detected by peripheral or central thermoreceptors increase sympathetic vasoconstrictor activity, AVAs being particularly strongly affected, and skin blood flow can fall as much as 90% (pale skin). Sympathetic stimulation also causes **piloerection** to trap an insulating layer of air; this is marginally effective in humans (Figure 13.5). Skin temperature can also directly affect blood flow, probably via local sensory reflexes and/or altered sensitivity to noradrenaline. **Prolonged cold** causes transient **paradoxical vasodilatations** in hands and feet, maintaining manual dexterity at the cost of some heat loss.

An elevated T_C **reduces** sympathetic-mediated vasoconstriction and increases blood flow, particularly through AVAs, and heat loss. If T_C exceeds the **sweating threshold** (Figure 13.6) sympathetic **cholinergic** (*acetylcholine-releasing*) nerves activate **sweat glands**, causing **sweating** and release of **bradykinin**, a powerful vasodilator (Figure 13.4). Neural co-transmitters (*nitric oxide, substance P*) contribute to the consequent increase in blood flow (also required to form sweat). In very hot conditions skin blood flow can increase 30-fold. Skin temperature affects the sweating threshold, an 'anticipatory' effect (Figure 13.6). Sweat glands produce a primary secretion similar to protein-free plasma. At low sweat rates most salt and water is subsequently reabsorbed in the duct, leaving a sweat rich in urea, lactate and K^+. At high sweat rates more salt than water is reabsorbed, creating a **hypotonic** sweat. Sweating greatly increases evaporative cooling, the only way heat can be lost to an environment hotter than T_C, but is highly dependent on humidity. We can tolerate 45 °C in a dry environment indefinitely after acclimatization (see next section), but with a humidity >40% we would be in extreme danger of heat stroke (Figure 13.7).

Shivering is initiated when T_C falls below the **shivering threshold**, and can increase heat production fivefold. Cool skin raises the temperature at which shivering starts, warm skin reduces it (Figure 13.6). Neurones from the shivering motor centre in the posterior hypothalamus increase voluntary muscle tone sufficiently to activate the muscle stretch reflex (Chapter 63), initiating asynchronous cycles of rapid contractions and reflex relaxations; motor neurone activity is not cyclic. Severe shivering causes and is limited by glycogen depletion and hypoglycaemia, a serious problem in severe cold.

Neonates have a poorly developed or absent shivering response, and generate heat by **non-shivering thermogenesis** in **brown adipose tissue** (BAT; brown fat). Activation of mitochondrial **uncoupling proteins** (UCP1) short-circuit the electron transport chain (ETC) (Chapter 3) to divert energy to heat rather than ATP production. The hypothalamus regulates non-shivering thermogenesis via sympathetic stimulation (noradrenaline) and circulating adrenaline, which act on β_3-**adrenergic receptors** to cause breakdown of triglyceride to free fatty acids (FFA). FFAs activate UCP1 and provide substrate for increased ETC activity. Cold environments and **thyroxine** (Chapter 48) increase UCP1 expression. Some non-shivering thermogenesis occurs in adults. An illegal and dangerous weight-loss drug (DNP) acts by uncoupling the ETC and mimicking the above, but in all tissues not just BAT; it can cause severe hyperthermia, convulsions, blindness and death.

Acclimatization

After several days in a hot climate sweating capacity increases by two- to threefold, with larger volumes of sweat over a greater area and a lower sweating threshold. Evaporative heat loss consequently increases as much as 10-fold (Figure 13.7), but loss of water and salt can reduce blood volume and Na^+ content. These stimulate a reduced urine output and increased production of aldosterone (Chapter 38), which potentiates salt reabsorption in sweat gland ducts (and kidney). There remains a risk of **dehydration** and **hyponatraemia** (low plasma $[Na^+]$), leading to heat cramps and heat exhaustion, common causes of collapse, e.g. in marathon runners. There is little evidence in humans for significant acclimatization to cold, though metabolic rate and non-shivering thermogenesis may increase.

14 Altitude and aerospace physiology

Figure 14.1 Change in barometric pressure with altitude and time of useful consciousness

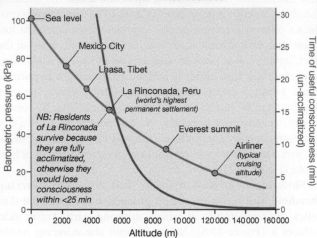

NB: Residents of La Rinconada survive because they are fully acclimatized, otherwise they would lose consciousness within <25 min

Labels on graph: Sea level; Mexico City; Lhasa, Tibet; La Rinconada, Peru (world's highest permanent settlement); Everest summit; Airliner (typical cruising altitude)

X-axis: Altitude (m); Y-axis left: Barometric pressure (kPa); Y-axis right: Time of useful consciousness (un-acclimatized) (min)

Figure 14.2 Effect of ascent to altitude and acclimatization

Acute response	Ascent to altitude	After acclimatization
	↓PO₂ →	↑Haematocrit (weeks)

Carotid body — Inhibits
Central chemoreceptors — Inhibits
↑Ventilation — No inhibition — Central chemoreceptors
pH of CSF normalized
↓PCO₂
Alkalosis
Renal compensation: no alkalosis

Outcome: ↓P_aCO_2, ↑blood pH; ↓P_aO_2, ↓O_2 content

Final outcome: ↓P_aCO_2, **normal** pH; ↑P_aO_2, ↑O_2 content

Figure 14.3 Factors affecting tolerance to +Gz forces and risk of G-LOC

Tissue energy reserves still adequate, venous pooling just starting

Maximum venous pooling, baroreceptor reflex not yet effective

Baroreceptors restore BP, venoconstriction increases CVP

Rapid onset then sustained

G-LOC region
G-LOC lasts ~12 sec after +Gz falls, followed by 15 sec of confusion

Moderate onset

Visual region
greyout, blackout

Gradual onset

Safe region

Rapid onset, rapid fall

X-axis: Seconds; Y-axis: Acceleration (+Gz)

Short periods of very high +Gz may evoke no effects, but if sustained G-LOC can occur without visual warning (e.g. greyout). Actual limits vary with individuals and counter-measures; an inexperienced, ill-prepared person could suffer G-LOC below +3 Gz.

Improves tolerance to +Gz:	Decreases tolerance to +Gz:
• Recent experience (e.g. on centrifuge)	• Alcohol or smoking beforehand
• Trained	• Untrained
• Well hydrated (↑blood volume)	• Dehydrated (↓blood volume)
• Well rested and fit	• Tired or unfit
• Exercise conditioning (resistance weights and aerobic)	• Aerobic exercise only (as this reduces heart rate)

Figure 14.4 Consequences of prolonged micro-gravity or bed rest

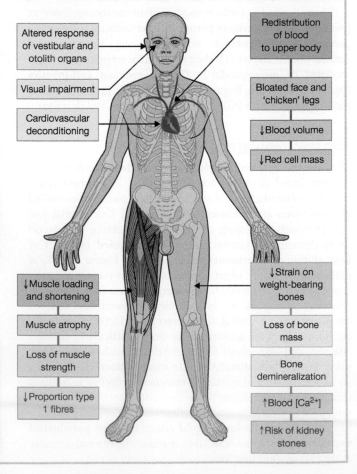

Altered response of vestibular and otolith organs

Visual impairment

Cardiovascular deconditioning

Redistribution of blood to upper body

Bloated face and 'chicken' legs

↓Blood volume

↓Red cell mass

↓Muscle loading and shortening

Muscle atrophy

Loss of muscle strength

↓Proportion type 1 fibres

↓Strain on weight-bearing bones

Loss of bone mass

Bone demineralization

↑Blood [Ca²⁺]

↑Risk of kidney stones

Physiology at a Glance, Fourth Edition. Edited by Jeremy P.T. Ward and Roger W.A. Linden.
© 2017 John Wiley & Sons, Ltd. Published 2017 by John Wiley & Sons, Ltd. Companion website: www.ataglanceseries.com/physiology

The way physiological systems respond to extreme conditions helps us understand the way they work in health and disease. These examples should be read in conjunction with the chapters referenced in the text.

Altitude

As altitude increases barometric pressure (P_B) falls from the sea level value of 101 kPa; at the summit of Everest (8850 m) it is 32 kPa (Figure 14.1). As the oxygen fraction (F_{O_2}) remains constant (0.21), P_{O_2} falls from 21 kPa to 6.7 kPa at the summit ($P_B \times 0.21$). If ventilation remained unchanged, this would inevitably lead to a reduction in arterial P_{O_2} (P_aO_2) but P_aCO_2 ($\propto$ to CO_2 production/alveolar ventilation) would be unaltered. At altitudes above 2500 m the consequent fall in P_aO_2 would be sufficient to stimulate the carotid body chemoreceptors and increase ventilation (Chapter 32). However, the latter would *reduce* P_aCO_2 below normal (hypocapnia), causing the central chemoreceptors to *depress* ventilation. This means that both P_aO_2 and P_aCO_2 end up too low, the latter causing respiratory alkalosis (Chapter 39). These effects contribute to **acute mountain sickness** (AMS), which commonly develops some hours after rapid ascent to altitudes above 3600 m with symptoms of fatigue, nausea, anorexia, dizziness, headache and sleep disturbance. Hypoxic pulmonary vasoconstriction (Chapter 33) may also cause pulmonary hypertension. AMS can progress to life-threatening high-altitude pulmonary oedema (**HAPE**) or cerebral oedema (**HACE**), which require immediate descent.

High altitude acclimatization (Figure 14.2): A more leisurely ascent over several days allows the body to acclimatize, with an increase in ventilation and P_aO_2 and reduced risk of AMS. Although hypocapnia is still present, renal bicarbonate excretion corrects the respiratory alkalosis (Chapter 39) and transport of bicarbonate out of the cerebrospinal fluid (CSF) normalizes CSF pH, the signal detected by the central chemoreceptor to control ventilation (Chapter 32). Thus although P_aCO_2 is low, it no longer impedes the effects of hypoxia on the carotid body (which may also increase sensitivity to hypoxia). In addition, hypoxia stimulates erythropoietin production (Chapter 9), increasing haemoglobin to >200 g/L and thus arterial O_2 content after a few weeks. Sudden exposure to the summit of Everest would cause an unacclimatized person to lose consciousness within 2 min (Figure 14.1), but some fit, fully acclimatized climbers have reached it without supplementary O_2.

Aerospace

Time of useful consciousness (TUC; Figure 14.1) is also an important consideration for sudden decompression of high altitude aircraft. Pilots of commercial airliners flying at 11–12 000 m may have a TUC of less than 30 s during which they must don O_2 masks before descending to a safe altitude (<2400 m). Military craft operate at higher altitudes; as TUC is only 4 s even at 15 000 m, pilots wear O_2 masks at all times. However, P_B at this altitude is 12 kPa, so even 100% O_2 cannot provide a sufficient P_{O_2} ($P_{O_2} = P_B$). All pilots flying above 12 500 m therefore wear *pressurized* O_2 masks to maintain the inspired P_{O_2} >19 kPa; **countermeasure suits** constrict the chest to aid expiration against the high inspired pressure.

G-forces are caused by acceleration, and described by a standard nomenclature. Thus +4 Gz denotes a force 4 × gravity acting from head to foot, such as when a pilot turns at speed with head towards the centre of the turn; −Gz is from foot to head, and Gy and Gx refer to lateral and horizontal forces. +9 Gz is not uncommon during rapid manoeuvring in fighters, and +4 Gx and +4 Gz during launch and return of space vehicles. The most critical physiological effects are those caused by +Gz on the cardiovascular system, which are akin to postural hypertension (Chapters 23 and 25). Venous pooling causes a fall in central venous pressure (CVP) and thus cardiac output due to Starling's Law, though the baroreceptor reflex rapidly restores blood pressure. However, as the head is above the heart, cerebral and retinal blood pressures fall, and above +3 Gz their perfusion may fall sufficiently to cause impaired (**greyout**) then complete loss (**blackout**) of vision (particularly sensitive to perfusion), followed by cerebral hypoxia and *G-induced loss of consciousness* (**G-LOC**). These effects are exacerbated by a fall in P_aO_2 due to ventilation/perfusion mismatch and right to left shunts caused by alveolar collapse (Chapter 33). Various factors including rate of +Gz onset affect the risk of G-LOC (Figure 14.3). G-LOC remains a significant cause of military and acrobatic aircraft losses, though countermeasures markedly improve tolerance. **Inflatable G-suits** compress the body during acceleration to reduce venous pooling, and **anti-G straining manoeuvres** including forced breathing and isometric muscle contraction assist cardiac filling and mobilization of blood from the limbs respectively.

Prolonged microgravity (μG; weightlessness) has similar consequences to extended bed rest (e.g. critically ill and immobile patients) (Figure 14.4). μG dramatically reduces mechanical loading of weight-bearing bones and muscles and most movement in μG is initiated by the upper body. The calf and thigh muscles thus atrophy and lose strength despite rigorous exercise routines, though impaired neuromuscular function may contribute. Interestingly the strength of upper body muscles also declines but to a lesser extent. The proportion of slow type 1 fibres (Chapter 17) also decreases, with potential for muscle damage and altered fatigability. Reduced strain on bone is detected by osteocytes and leads to demineralization, reduced bone formation and loss of matrix (akin to osteoporosis; Chapter 50). The consequent increase in plasma $[Ca^{2+}]$ can lead to kidney stones. Loss of gravity causes redistribution of blood to the upper body, which is interpreted as an increase in blood volume (Chapters 25 and 38); plasma volume and red blood cell mass consequently decline, though largely due to reduced fluid intake rather than urinary excretion. These changes contribute to cardiovascular deconditioning, which also includes reductions in muscle size and force, cardiac output and maximum O_2 uptake (VO_2 max, a measure of fitness). Extended μG also impairs orthostatic tolerance (ability to respond to changes in posture) (Chapter 25); this is sustained for days after return to Earth. Function of the vestibular and otolith organs (Chapter 61) is seriously compromised by μG, leading to disorientation and contributing to space motion sickness in the first few days until position sensing switches to visual cues.

Muscles

Part 2

Chapters

15 Skeletal muscle and its contraction

Figure 15.1 A reductionist's approach to skeletal muscle morphology, from gross anatomy (top) to the molecular level (bottom)

Tendon

Epimysium

Perimysium

Fasciculi

Muscle *in situ*

Fasciculus

Cisternae

T-tubules

Endomysium

Myofibre

A-band

I-band

H-zone

M-line

Z

Sarcomere

Z-line

M-line

I-band

A-band

I-band

A B C D

Cross-section through sarcomere at:

A Thin filament only

B M-line of thick filament

C Thick filament only

D Thick and thin filament

Actin

Troponin

Tropomyosin

Thin filament

Thick filament

Heavy chain

Myosin head

Myosin tail

Figure 15.2 Sliding filament theory

Tropomyosin   Troponin   Actin

Thin filament

Myosin head

Myosin tail

Thick filament

Binding of ATP to myosin head

ATP

ATP

Dissociation of myosin head from actin

ADP   P$_i$

Hydrolysis of ATP and tilt of myosin head

ADP   P$_i$

Binding of myosin head to actin

P$_i$

ADP

Power stroke of the cross-bridge. The thin filament moves relative to the thick filament. Followed by the release of ADP and cycle restarts as long as Ca^{2+} concentration is high

Physiology at a Glance, Fourth Edition. Edited by Jeremy P.T. Ward and Roger W.A. Linden.

Muscles make up about 50% of the adult body mass. There are three types of muscle: **skeletal** (muscle attached to the skeleton); **cardiac** (muscle in the heart; Chapter 18) (both of these are morphologically striated or striped and are commonly called **striated muscles**); and **smooth** (muscle involved in many involuntary processes in blood vessels, airways and gut; this type is not striated, hence its name; Chapter 18). A comparison of the properties of the three muscle types is shown in Appendix I.

Skeletal muscle

The **skeletal muscles** and the **skeleton** function together as the musculoskeletal system. Skeletal muscle is sometimes referred to as **voluntary muscle** because it is under conscious control. It uses about 25% of our oxygen consumption at rest and this can increase up to 20-fold during exercise.

General mechanisms of skeletal muscle contraction

The functions of muscle tissue are the development of tension and shortening of the muscle. Muscle fibres have the ability to shorten a considerable amount, which is brought about by the molecules sliding over each other. Muscle activity is transferred to the skeleton by the tendons, and the tension developed by the muscles is graded and adjusted to the load.

Fine structure of skeletal muscle (Figure 15.1)

The connective tissue surrounding the whole muscle is called the **epimysium**. The connective tissue that extends beyond the body of the muscle eventually blends into a **tendon**, which is attached to bone or cartilage. Skeletal muscle is composed of numerous parallel, elongated, multinucleated (up to 100) cells, referred to as **muscle fibres** or **myofibres**, which are between 10 and 100 μm in diameter and vary in length, and are grouped together to form **fasciculi**. Each fasciculus is surrounded by the **perimysium**. Each myofibre is encased by connective tissue called the **endomysium**. Beneath the endomysium is the **sarcolemma** (excitable plasma membrane). This has infoldings that invaginate the fibre interior, particularly at the motor end plate of the neuromuscular junction (Chapter 16). Each myofibre is made up of **myofibrils** 1 μm in diameter separated by cytoplasm and arranged in a parallel fashion along the long axis of the cell. Each myofibril is further subdivided into **thick** and **thin myofilaments** (thick, 10–14 nm in width, 1.6 μm in length; **thin**, 7 nm in width, 1 μm in length). These are responsible for the cross-striations. **Thin filaments** consist primarily of three proteins, **actin**, **tropomyosin** and **troponin**, in the ratio 7:1:1, and **thick filaments** consist primarily of **myosin**. The cytoplasm surrounding the **myofilaments** is called the **sarcoplasm**. Each myofibre is divided at regular intervals along its length into **sarcomeres** separated by **Z-discs** (in longitudinal sections, these are **Z-lines**). To the Z-lines are attached the thin filaments held in a hexagonal array. The **I-band** extends from either side of the Z-line to the beginning of the thick filament (myosin). The myosin filaments make up the **A-band**.

The **H-zone** is at the centre of the sarcomere, and the **M-line** is a disc of delicate filaments in the middle of the H-zone that holds the myosin filaments in position so that each one is surrounded by six actin filaments.

The thin filaments consist of two intertwining strands of actin with smaller strands of tropomyosin and troponin between them. Each strand of actin is made up of ~200 units of globular or G-actin containing binding sites for myosin. At rest, these sites are covered by tropomyosin preventing myosin binding.

The thick filaments are made up of about 100 myosin molecules; each molecule is club shaped, with a thin tail (shaft) comprising two coiled peptide chains and a head made up of two heavy peptide chains and four light peptide chains that have a regulatory function. The ATPase activity of the myosin molecule is concentrated in the head.

The thin tails of the myosin molecules form the bulk of the thick filaments, whereas the heads are 'hinged' and project outward to form cross-bridges between the thick filaments and their neighbouring thin filaments. Six thin filaments surround each thick filament.

Between the myofibrils are a large number of mitochondria and glycogen granules, as found in other cells, but muscle cells have regular invaginations which project from outside the cell and wrap around the sarcomeres, particularly where the thin and thick filaments overlap. These invaginations are called transverse or **T-tubules** and contain extracellular fluid. The specialized smooth endoplasmic reticulum, the **sarcoplasmic reticulum (SR)**, is enlarged to form **terminal cisternae** close to the T-tubules. Ca^{2+} is transported from the cytosol into the SR by the sarco/endoplasmic reticulum Ca^{2+}-ATPase (SERCA).

Like fingers of the hands sliding over one another, actin and myosin molecules slide past each other. The myosin heads bind to the actin chain and tilt. There is a constant process of binding, tilting, releasing and rebinding of cross-bridges, as well as rotation of the myosin filaments as they interact with the actin filaments and bind with the alternate myofibril in the hexagonal structure. This results in the contraction of the whole muscle. The cross-bridges are formed asynchronously so that some are active, whilst others are resting.

The interaction of actin (thin filaments) and myosin (thick filaments) brings about contraction of the muscle, which is caused by the cross-bridges, a result of the interaction of troponin and Ca^{2+}. This mechanism is called the **sliding filament theory**. The contraction of muscle is triggered by release of Ca^{2+} from the SR (Chapter 16). Ca^{2+} floods out of the cisternae, where it is stored by binding reversibly with a protein, **calsequestrin**. This raises the concentration of calcium from 0.1 μmol/L to more than 10 μmol/L, saturating the binding sites on troponin. This results in a shift of tropomyosin, thus allowing myosin cross-bridges to bind with actin and begin the contraction cycle (Figure 15.2). The heads tilt after attachment by hydrolysing the adenosine triphosphate (ATP) energy stores, releasing adenosine diphosphate (ADP) and inorganic phosphate (P_i), which leads to a greater binding of the cross-bridges. ADP and P_i escape from the head, freeing the head for another molecule of ATP. This releases the binding of the head and, if Ca^{2+} is still present, the cycle continues. Otherwise, the binding is inhibited. Contraction is maintained as long as Ca^{2+} is high. The duration of the contraction is dependent on the rate at which SERCA pumps the Ca^{2+} back into the SR.

16 Neuromuscular junction and whole muscle contraction

Figure 16.1 Diagram of the structure of part of the neuromuscular junction

Motoneurone

Myelin

Axon

Mitochondria

Schwann cell sheath

Thin layer of AChE (in cleft)

Synaptic cleft

Na^+
K^+

Ca^{2+}

Vesicles containing ACh

Ca^{2+}

Muscle cell nucleus

End plate

Na^+

ACh receptors

Junctional folds (containing voltage-dependent Na^+ and K^+ channels)

Myofibril

Figure 16.2 Neuromuscular junction transmitter release and recycling

ACh

Empty vesicle

Choline acetyl transferase

ACh

Prejunctional membrane

Choline + acetate

Synaptic cleft

K^+

AChE

ACh

ACh

Postjunctional membrane

Na^+

ACh receptor

Figure 16.3 Diagram of potentials at the end plate

Voltage (mV)

Action potential

Threshold

−50

EPP

MEPP

−70

0   2   4   6   8

Time (ms)

Figure 16.4 Relationship between initiating action potential and fast and slow twitch muscle types

+40

mV

Action potential

−70

Muscle tension

Fast twitch

Slow twitch

0   0.1   0.2   0.3

Time (s)

Figure 16.5 Mechanical components of muscle

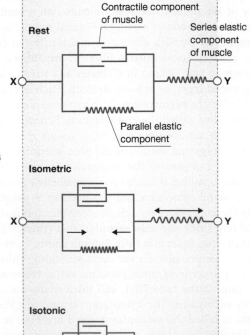

Rest

Contractile component of muscle

Series elastic component of muscle

X   Y

Parallel elastic component

Isometric

X   Y

Isotonic

X   Y

Figure 16.6 Length–tension relationship of muscle during active tension and passive stretch

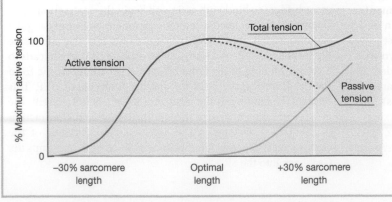

% Maximum active tension

100

Total tension

Active tension

Passive tension

0

−30% sarcomere length

Optimal length

+30% sarcomere length

Physiology at a Glance, Fourth Edition. Edited by Jeremy P.T. Ward and Roger W.A. Linden.
© 2017 John Wiley & Sons, Ltd. Published 2017 by John Wiley & Sons, Ltd. Companion website: www.ataglanceseries.com/physiology

Neuromuscular junction

For **skeletal (voluntary) muscle** to contract, there must be neuronal activation to the muscle fibres themselves from either higher centres in the brain or via reflex pathways involving either the spinal cord or the brain stem. The neurones that innervate skeletal muscles are called **α-motor neurones**. Each motor axon splits into a number of branches that make contact with the surface of individual muscle fibres in the form of bulb-shaped endings. These endings make connections with a specialized structure on the surface of the muscle fibre, called the **motor end plate**, and together form the **neuromuscular junction (NMJ)** (Figure 16.1).

The role of the NMJ is the one-to-one transmission of excitatory impulses from the α-motor neurone to the muscle fibres it innervates. It allows a reliable transmission of the impulses from nerve to muscle and produces a predictable response in the muscle. In other words, an action potential in the motor neurone must produce an action potential in the muscle fibres it innervates; this, in turn, must produce a contraction of the muscle fibres. The process by which the **NMJ** produces this one-to-one response is shown in Figures 16.1 and 16.2.

The motor neurone axon terminal has a large number of vesicles containing the transmitter substance **acetylcholine (ACh)**. At rest, when not stimulated, a small number of these vesicles release their contents, by a process called **exocytosis**, into the synaptic cleft between the neurones and the muscle fibres. ACh diffuses across the cleft and reacts with specific ACh receptor proteins (**nicotinic receptors**) in the postsynaptic membrane (motor end plate). These receptors contain an integral ion channel, which opens and allows the movement inwards (influx) of small cations, mainly Na^+. There are more than 10^7 receptors on each end plate (**postjunctional membrane**); each of these can open for about 1 ms and allow small positively charged ions to enter the cell. This movement of positively charged ions generates an **end plate potential** (EPP). This is a depolarization of the cell with a rise-time of approximately 1–2 ms and may vary in amplitude (unlike the all-or-nothing response seen in the action potential; Chapter 6). The random release of ACh from the vesicles at rest gives rise to small, 0–4-mV depolarizations of the end plate, called **miniature end plate potentials (MEPP)** (Figure 16.3).

However, when an **action potential** reaches the **prejunctional nerve terminal**, there is an enhanced permeability of the membrane to Ca^{2+} ions due to opening of voltage-gated Ca^{2+} channels. This causes an increase in the exocytotic release of ACh from several hundred vesicles at the same time. This sudden volume of ACh diffuses across the cleft and stimulates a large number of receptors on the postsynaptic membrane, and thus produces an EPP that is above the threshold for triggering an action potential in the muscle fibre. It triggers a **self-propagating muscle action potential**. The depolarizing current (the **generator potential**) generated by the numbers of quanta of ACh is more than sufficient to cause the initiation of an action potential in the muscle membrane surrounding the postsynaptic junction. The typical summed **EPP** is usually four times the potential necessary to trigger an action potential in the muscle fibre, and so there is a large inherent safety factor.

The effect of ACh is rapidly abolished by the activity of the enzyme **acetylcholinesterase (AChE)**. ACh is hydrolysed to **choline** and **acetic acid**. About one-half of the choline is recaptured by the presynaptic nerve terminal and used to make more ACh. Some ACh diffuses out of the cleft, but the enzyme destroys most of it. The number of vesicles available in the nerve ending is said to be sufficient for only about 2000 nerve–muscle impulses, and therefore the vesicles reform very rapidly within about 30 s (Figure 16.2).

Whole muscle contraction

As the action potential spreads over the muscle fibre, it invades the T-tubules and releases Ca^{2+} from the **sarcoplasmic reticulum** into the **sarcoplasm**, and the muscle fibres that are excited contract. This contraction will be maintained as long as the levels of Ca^{2+} are high. The single contraction of a muscle due to a single action potential is called a **muscle twitch**. Fibres are divided into **fast** and **slow twitch fibres** depending on the time course of their twitch contraction. This is determined by the type of myosin in the muscles and the amount of sarcoplasmic reticulum. Different muscles are made up of different proportions of these two types of fibre, leading to a huge variation in overall muscle contraction times (Figure 16.4).

At rest, muscles exert tension when stretched. Muscles have a passive elastic property and act both in series and parallel to the contractile element (Figure 16.5).

Isometric contraction occurs when the two ends of a muscle are held at a fixed distance apart, and stimulation of the muscle causes the development of tension within the muscle without a change in muscle length. **Isotonic contraction** occurs when one end of the muscle is free to move and the muscle shortens whilst exerting a constant force. In practice, most contractions are made up of both elements.

The relationships between resting, active and total tensions developed in skeletal muscle are shown in Figure 16.6. The **passive curve** is due to the stretching of the elastic components, the **active curve** is due to contraction of the sarcomeres alone (contractile component), and the **total curve** is due to the sum of the passive and active tensions developed. It can be seen that the active tension developed is dependent on the length of the muscle. The optimum length occurs where the thick and thin filaments are thought to provide a maximum number of active cross-bridge sites for interaction (this length is very close to that of the resting length of a particular muscle). As the muscle length is increased, the thick and thin filaments overlap less, providing fewer cross-bridge sites for interaction; as the muscle shortens below the optimal length, the thin filaments overlap one another and, in so doing, reduce the number of active sites available for interaction with the thick filaments.

17 Motor units, recruitment and summation

Figure 17.1 Diagram of spinal cord, and a motor unit incorporating an α-motor neurone and the muscle fibres it innervates

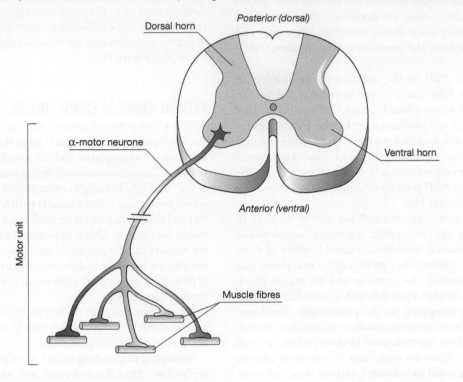

Figure 17.2 Diagram of time course of tension during twitches and tetanus

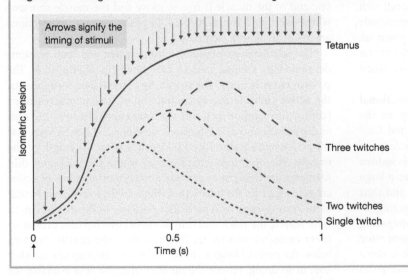

Figure 17.3 Electromyograms recorded at four different levels

In normal skeletal muscle, fibres never contract as isolated individuals. Several contract at almost the same time, as they are all supplied by the same α-motor neurone. The single motor neurone and all the fibres it innervates is called the **motor unit** (Figure 17.1). This is the smallest part of a muscle that can be made to contract independently of other parts of the muscle. The number of muscle fibres innervated by one motor unit can be as low as five or as high as 2000. The number is correlated with the precision with which the tension developed by the muscle is graded.

Within the muscle, the muscle fibres of each motor unit are widely distributed amongst the fibres of many other units. This, in effect, distributes the demands made on the muscle's circulatory support. The ratio between the number of α-motor neurones and the total number of skeletal muscle fibres is small in muscles such as the extraocular muscles that provide fine smooth movements (1 : 5), but large in muscles such as the gluteus maximus that need to generate powerful but coarse movements (1 : >1000).

Fibres have been classified into three types, on the basis of various structural and functional properties of motor units and their integral muscles. Table 17.1 outlines the relationship between the properties of the motor units (with their defining characteristics of conduction speed, resistance to fatigue and also size of activity pattern) and the properties of the muscle fibres they contain (the type of myosin which determines the speed of contraction, and the type of metabolism, which is highly correlated with the resistance to fatigue), and also the names given to these types in human muscles. Most muscles contain all three types (I, IIA, IIB), but differ in the proportions of each according to the function of the muscle as a whole. Posture muscles, such as the soleus, have mostly slow, fatigue-resistant, oxidative-type units, whereas movement muscles, such as the gastrocnemius, have a high proportion of the other two types. Training and exercising can alter these proportions.

The cell bodies of α-motor neurones also vary in size according to the type of motor unit: **motor neurones innervating type I fibres have the smallest cell bodies, and those innervating type IIB fibres have the largest**.

During graded contraction, there is a recruitment order of the units, such that the smallest cells discharge first and the largest last (the so-called **size principle**). **Force** is controlled not only by **varying the unit recruitment**, but also by **varying the firing rate of the units**. A single action potential in a single motor unit produces a delayed rise in tension in all the muscle fibres that make up that motor unit. A second and third action potential that occur soon after the first produce a summed contraction, or a series of twitches. The tension developed by the first action potential has not completely decayed when the second contraction is grafted on to the first, and so on for the third action potential and contraction. This is called **summation** (Figure 17.2). If the muscle fibres are stimulated repeatedly at a faster frequency, a sustained contraction results in which individual twitches cannot be detected. This is called **tetanus**. The tension of tetanus is much greater than the maximum tension of a single, double or triple twitch (Figure 17.2). For most units, the firing rate for a steady contraction is between 5 and 8 Hz. It can rise to 40 Hz or more, but only for very brief periods. During a gradual increase in contraction of a muscle, the first units start to discharge and increase their firing rate and, as the force needs to increase, new units are recruited and, in turn, also increase their firing rate. When there is a need to gradually decrease the force output, the pattern is reversed, so that those units that were recruited last will be the first to decrease their firing and then stop, and the last units to fire will be the smallest units. Because the unitary firing rates for each motor unit are different and not synchronized, the overall effect is a smooth force profile from the muscle. The greater the desynchronized firing, the smoother the movements observed. When synchronized firing does occur, such as in fatigued states and Parkinson's disease, marked muscle tremors are seen.

The summed excitatory impulses (action potentials) of the motor units can be recorded in an **electromyogram** (EMG). The EMG is an extracellular recording made from either the skin surface overlying a muscle or from electrodes inserted extracellularly within the body of the muscle. The increase in recruitment of individual motor units (**motor unit recruitment**), as well as the increased rate of firing of the units (**rate or frequency recruitment**), can sometimes be seen in the EMG during increased force of contraction (Figure 17.3).

Table 17.1 Properties of motor units and muscle fibres

Motor unit properties			
Contraction speed	Slow	Fast	Fast
Resistance to fatigue	Resistant	Resistant	Fatigable
Motor unit force	Small	Larger	Largest
Motor unit activity pattern	Long-lasting low frequency, e.g. postural	Frequent short bursts of moderate force	Rare, very short bursts for high forces
Motor unit name	SR (slow resistant)	FR (fast resistant)	FF (fast fatigable)
Muscle fibre properties			
Myosin isoform	I	IIA	IIX
Contraction speed	Slow	Fast	Fast
Metabolic process	Oxidative	Oxidative and glycolytic	Glycolytic
Capillary density	High	Medium	Low
Fibre type name			
Physiological	SO (slow oxidative)	FOG (fast oxidative and glycolytic)	FG (fast glycolytic)
Diagnostic	Type I	Type IIA	Type IIB/X

18 Cardiac and smooth muscle

Figure 18.1 Gross anatomy and histology of the heart

See Chapter 20 for more detail

Myocardium

50 μm

Capillary

Nucleus

Intercalated disc

Desmosome

Connexons

Gap junction (nexus)

Figure 18.2 The sarcomere (the contractile element)

Sarcomere

I A H A I

Myosin

Actin

Z M Z

2.2 μm

Sarcoplasmic reticulum

Sarcolemma

Mitochondria

T-tubule

Figure 18.3 Smooth muscle cell ultrastructure

Dense bodies

Actin filaments

Myosin filaments

Dense bands

Nucleus

Intermediate filaments

Sarcoplasmic reticulum

Cardiac muscle

The muscles of the heart, the **myocardium**, generate the force of contraction of the atrial and ventricular muscles. The myocardium is composed of cardiac muscle cells called **myocytes**. These cells are striated due to the orderly arrangement of the thick and thin filaments which, as in skeletal muscle, make up the bulk of the muscle. However, they are less organized than in skeletal muscle (Figures 18.1 and 18.2). The **myocytes** have dimensions of $100 \times 20\,\mu m$, are branched, with a **single nucleus**, and are also **rich in mitochondria**. The normal pumping action of the heart is dependent on the synchronized contraction of all cardiac cells. Their contraction is not dependent on an external nerve supply, as in skeletal muscle, but instead the heart generates its own rhythm (**inherent rhythmicity**). The nerves innervating the heart only speed up or slow down the rhythm and can modify the force of contraction (termed **chronotropic** and **inotropic** effects respectively; Chapter 22).

The synchronicity between myocytes occurs because all adjacent cells are linked to one another at their ends by specialized **gap junctions** (formed of **connexons**, Chapter 4) within the **intercalated discs** (Figure 18.1), which essentially provide low-resistance electrical pathways between cells. These allow action potentials to spread rapidly from one cell to another and enable the cardiac muscle to act as a **functional syncytium** (i.e. it acts as a single unit although comprising individual cells). The intercalated discs also provide structural attachments (**desmosomes**) between myocytes to distribute force. Although a rise in intracellular Ca^{2+} initiates contraction in the same way as in skeletal muscle (Chapter 15), the mechanisms leading to this rise in intracellular Ca^{2+} are fundamentally different, and are discussed in Chapter 22.

Smooth muscle

The **absence of striations** within the cells and the poorer organization of the fibres give this type of muscle its name. Each cell contains only **one nucleus** situated near the centre. Smooth muscle is involved in many involuntary processes in blood vessels, airways, gut and elsewhere. The smooth muscle of each organ is distinctive from that of most other organs, and there is considerable variation in the structure and function of smooth muscle in different parts of the body. However, it can essentially be divided into **unitary** (or **visceral**) and **multiunit** smooth muscle types.

Smooth muscle cells are spindle-shaped with dimensions of 50–$400\,\mu m$ in length by 2–$10\,\mu m$ thick. They are joined, like cardiac muscle, by special intercellular connections called **desmosomes**. Because the actin and myosin filaments are not regularly arranged, they lack striations. Smooth muscle cells shorten by sliding of the myofilaments towards and over one another, but at a much slower rate than in other muscle types. For this reason, they are capable of prolonged, maintained contraction, without fatigue and with little energy consumption (Figure 18.3).

The **unitary muscle type** or **visceral smooth muscle** exhibits many gap junctions between cells, and a steady wave of contraction can pass through a whole sheet of muscle as if it were a single unit. It is commonly found in the stomach, intestines, urinary bladder, urethra and blood vessels, and is capable of bringing about **autorhythmical activity** (seen particularly in the digestive tract where it is modulated by neuronal activity).

Tonic activity causes smooth muscle to remain in a constant state of contraction or tonus. It is commonly found in sphincters that control the movement of digestive products through the gastrointestinal tract.

Multiunit smooth muscle is made up of individual fibres not connected by gap junctions, but separately stimulated by autonomic motor neurones. Each smooth muscle fibre can contract independently from the others. Examples include the ciliary muscles of the eye, the iris of the eye and piloerector muscles that cause erection of hairs when stimulated by the sympathetic system.

The factors that influence the neural control of smooth muscle are:

1 The type of innervation and the transmitter released.
2 The receptor of the neurotransmitter on the muscle cell itself.
3 The anatomical arrangement of the nerve in relation to the muscle fibres.

There are three types of innervation: **extrinsic** – from the autonomic part of the nervous system, mainly sympathetic (arteries), parasympathetic (ciliary muscles) and both sympathetic and parasympathetic (gut); **intrinsic** – a plexus of nerves within the smooth muscle itself (seen in the gut); and **afferent sensory neurones** – these indirectly lead to the reflex activation of motor neurones.

Smooth muscle cells also respond to local tissue factors and hormones, i.e. changes in the fluids that surround them (interstitial fluids). In addition, many hormones that circulate in the bloodstream also cause smooth muscle contraction (hormones such as adrenaline [epinephrine], angiotensin, oxytocin, antidiuretic hormone [ADH], noradrenaline [norepinephrine] and serotonin). Also, a lack of oxygen in the tissues causes smooth muscle cells to relax and vasodilate; an increase in CO_2 or H^+ also causes vasodilatation (Chapter 24).

Contractile mechanisms of smooth muscle

Smooth muscle contains no troponin, but has twice as much actin and tropomyosin as striated muscle. Myosin is also present, but only in about one-quarter of the amount found in striated muscle fibres. The rate at which cross-bridges are formed and released is slower (some 300 times) than that in striated muscle fibres, in part due to the different mechanisms involved.

Although contraction of smooth muscle is initiated by an increase in Ca^{2+}, unlike striated muscle this is not mediated via the interaction of Ca^{2+} with troponin (there is none). Instead, cross-bridge formation is controlled from the myosin side in a rather more complex fashion. Ca^{2+} binds to the protein **calmodulin**, which activates **myosin light chain kinase**. This phosphorylates myosin which allows it to form cross-bridges with actin, using energy from adenosine triphosphate (ATP). It follows that there must be a means by which myosin is dephosphorylated. This is provided by **myosin light chain phosphatase**. Many factors that contract smooth muscle do so by inhibiting myosin phosphatase at the same time as raising Ca^{2+}, so maximizing the degree of myosin phosphorylation (Chapters 7 and 24).

A comparison of the properties of skeletal, cardiac and smooth muscle is shown in the Appendix I.

The cardiovascular system

Chapters

19 Introduction to the cardiovascular system

Figure 19.1 Schematic of cardiovascular system

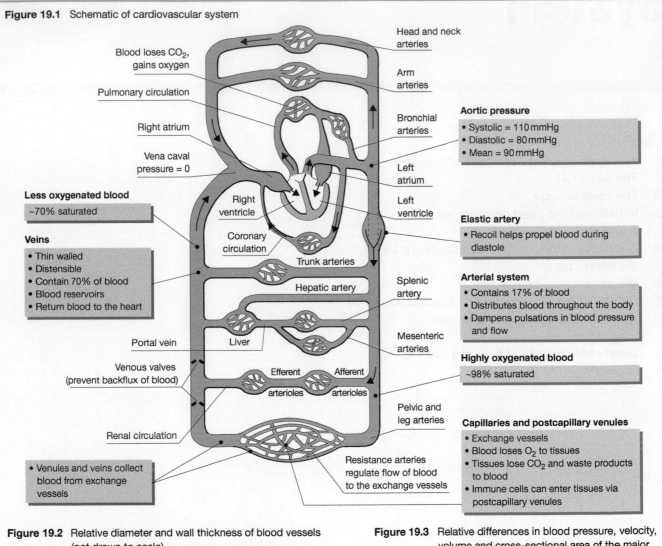

Blood loses CO_2, gains oxygen

Pulmonary circulation

Right atrium

Vena caval pressure = 0

Less oxygenated blood
~70% saturated

Veins
• Thin walled
• Distensible
• Contain 70% of blood
• Blood reservoirs
• Return blood to the heart

Portal vein   Liver

Venous valves (prevent backflux of blood)

Renal circulation

• Venules and veins collect blood from exchange vessels

Head and neck arteries

Arm arteries

Bronchial arteries

Left atrium

Left ventricle

Right ventricle

Coronary circulation

Trunk arteries

Hepatic artery   Splenic artery

Mesenteric arteries

Efferent arterioles   Afferent arterioles

Pelvic and leg arteries

Resistance arteries regulate flow of blood to the exchange vessels

Aortic pressure
• Systolic = 110 mmHg
• Diastolic = 80 mmHg
• Mean = 90 mmHg

Elastic artery
• Recoil helps propel blood during diastole

Arterial system
• Contains 17% of blood
• Distributes blood throughout the body
• Dampens pulsations in blood pressure and flow

Highly oxygenated blood
~98% saturated

Capillaries and postcapillary venules
• Exchange vessels
• Blood loses O_2 to tissues
• Tissues lose CO_2 and waste products to blood
• Immune cells can enter tissues via postcapillary venules

Figure 19.2 Relative diameter and wall thickness of blood vessels (not drawn to scale)

	Lumen diameter	Wall thickness
Ascending aorta	25 mm	2 mm
Muscular artery	4 mm	1 mm
Arteriole	20 m	15 m
Capillary	5 m	1 m
Venule	20 m	2 m
Vein	5 mm	0.5 mm
Vena cava	30 mm	1.5 mm

Figure 19.3 Relative differences in blood pressure, velocity, volume and cross-sectional area of the major components of the vascular system

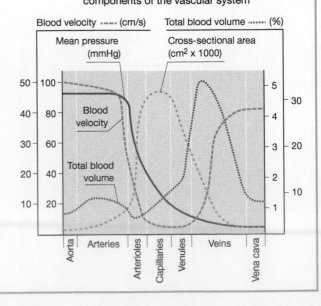

Blood velocity ---- (cm/s)   Total blood volume ...... (%)

Mean pressure (mmHg)   Cross-sectional area (cm² x 1000)

Blood velocity

Total blood volume

Aorta | Arteries | Arterioles | Capillaries | Venules | Veins | Vena cava

Physiology at a Glance, Fourth Edition. Edited by Jeremy P.T. Ward and Roger W.A. Linden.
© 2017 John Wiley & Sons, Ltd. Published 2017 by John Wiley & Sons, Ltd. Companion website: www.ataglanceseries.com/physiology

The cardiovascular system comprises the heart and blood vessels, and contains ~5.5 L of blood in a 70 kg man. Its main functions are to distribute O_2 and nutrients to tissues, transfer metabolites and CO_2 to excretory organs and the lungs, and transport hormones and components of the immune system. It is also important for thermoregulation (Chapter 13). The cardiovascular system is arranged mostly in **parallel**, i.e. each tissue derives blood directly from the aorta (Figure 19.1). This allows all tissues to receive fully oxygenated blood, and flow can be controlled independently in each tissue against a constant pressure head by altering the resistance of small arteries (i.e. arteriolar constriction or dilatation). The right heart, lungs and left heart are arranged in **series**. **Portal systems** are also arranged in series, where blood is used to transport materials directly from one tissue to another, such as the **hepatic portal system** between digestive organs and the liver. The function of the cardiovascular system is modulated by the autonomic nervous system (Chapter 8).

Blood vessels

The vascular system consists of **arteries** and **arterioles** that take blood from the heart to the tissues, thin-walled **capillaries** that allow the diffusion of gases and metabolites, and **venules** and **veins** that return blood to the heart. The blood pressure, vessel diameter and wall thickness vary throughout the circulation (Figures 19.2 and 19.3). Varying amounts of **smooth muscle** are contained within the vessel walls, allowing them to constrict and alter their resistance to flow (Chapters 12 and 24). Capillaries contain no smooth muscle. The inner surface of all blood vessels is lined with a thin monolayer of **endothelial cells**, important for vascular function (Chapter 24). Large arteries are **elastic** and partially damp out oscillations in pressure produced by the pumping of the heart; stiff arteries (age, atherosclerosis) result in larger oscillations. Small arteries contain relatively more muscle and are responsible for controlling tissue blood flow. Veins have a larger diameter than equivalent arteries, and provide less resistance. They have thin, distensible walls and contain ~70% of the total blood volume (Figure 19.3). Large veins are known as **capacitance vessels** and act as a *blood volume reservoir*; when required, they can constrict and increase the effective blood volume (Chapter 24). Large veins in the limbs contain **one-way valves**, so that when muscle activity (e.g. walking) intermittently compresses these veins they act as a pump, and assist the return of blood to the heart (the **muscle pump**).

The heart

The **heart** is a four-chambered muscular pump which propels blood around the circulation. It has an intrinsic pacemaker and requires no nervous input to beat normally, although it is modulated by the **autonomic nervous system** (Chapter 8). The volume of blood pumped per minute (**cardiac output**) is ~5 L at rest in humans, although this can increase to above 20 L during exercise. The volume ejected per beat (**stroke volume**) is ~70 mL at rest. The **ventricles** perform the work of pumping; **atria** assist ventricular filling. Unidirectional flow through the heart is maintained by **valves** between the chambers and outflow tracts. Contraction of the heart is called **systole** (pronounced *sis'-toley*); the period between each systole, when the heart refills with blood, is called **diastole** (*di-as'-to-ley*).

The systemic circulation

During systole, the pressure in the left ventricle increases to ~120 mmHg, and blood is ejected into the **aorta**. The rise in pressure stretches the elastic walls of the aorta and large arteries, and drives blood flow. **Systolic pressure** is the maximum arterial pressure during systole (~110 mmHg). During diastole, arterial blood flow is partly maintained by elastic recoil of the walls of large arteries. The minimum pressure reached before the next systole is the **diastolic pressure** (~80 mmHg). The difference between the systolic and diastolic pressures is the **pulse pressure**. Blood pressure is expressed as the systolic/diastolic arterial pressure, e.g. 110/80 mmHg. The **mean blood pressure** (mean arterial pressure, MAP) cannot be calculated by averaging these pressures, because for ~60% of the time the heart is in diastole. It is instead estimated as the *diastolic pressure plus one-third of the pulse pressure*, e.g. $80 + 1/3(110 - 80) \approx 90$ mmHg.

The **major arteries** divide repeatedly into smaller **muscular arteries**, the smallest of which (diameter <100 μm) are called **arterioles**. Tissue blood flow is regulated by the constriction of these small arteries, referred to as **resistance vessels**. The mean blood pressure at the start of the arterioles is ~65 mmHg. The arterioles divide into dense networks of **capillaries** in the tissues, and these rejoin into small and then larger **venules**, the smallest veins. Capillaries and small venules provide the exchange surface between blood and tissues, contain no smooth muscle and are called **exchange vessels**; some gas exchange also occurs across the walls of small arterioles. The pressure on the arterial side of capillaries is ~25 mmHg and, on the venous side, ~15 mmHg. Venules converge into veins and finally the **vena cava**. This returns the partially deoxygenated and CO_2-loaded blood to the right atrium. The pressure in the vena cava at the level of the heart is called the **central venous pressure** (CVP), and is close to 0 mmHg.

The pulmonary circulation

The right atrium helps to fill the right ventricle, which pumps blood into the **pulmonary artery** and lungs. The pulmonary circulation is shorter than the systemic, and has a lower resistance to flow. Less pressure is therefore required to drive blood through the lungs; the pulmonary artery pressure is ~20/15 mmHg. Gas exchange occurs in capillaries surrounding the alveoli (small air sacs) of the lungs. These rejoin to form pulmonary venules and veins, and oxygenated blood is returned through the pulmonary vein to the left atrium, and hence to the left ventricle. The metabolic requirements of the lungs are not met by the pulmonary circulation, but by the separate **bronchial circulation**, the venous outflow of which returns to the left side of the heart (Figure 19.1).

20 The heart

Figure 20.1 Anatomy of the heart

- Carotids
- Aortic arch
- Superior vena cava
- Pulmonary artery
- Right atrium
- Left atrium
- Mitral valve
- Inferior vena cava
- Pulmonary valve
- Tricuspid valve
- Left ventricle
- Right ventricle
- Septum
- Papillary muscles

Myocardium

- Cardiac muscle cell
- 50 μm
- Capillary
- Nucleus

Figure 20.2 Cardiac muscle microstructure

Intercalated disc

- Gap junction (nexus)
- Desmosome
- Connexons

Figure 20.3 Conduction pathways

1. Stimulus initiated in SAN
2. Conduction via atrial muscle and internodal tracts (1 m/s)
3. Conduction via AVN (0.05 m/s)
4. Dispersion via bundle of His, left and right bundles, and Purkinje fibres to ventricular mass (4 m/s)
5. Finally from endocardium to epicardium (0.3 m/s)

- Aorta

Figure 20.4 The electrocardiogram

- Einthoven's triangle
- Lead I: RA–LA
- Lead II: RA–LL
- Lead III: LA–LL

Figure 20.5 Coronary circulation

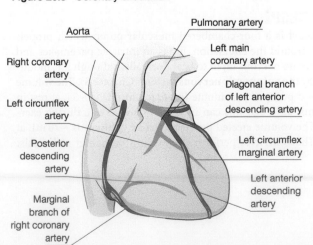

- Aorta
- Pulmonary artery
- Right coronary artery
- Left main coronary artery
- Left circumflex artery
- Diagonal branch of left anterior descending artery
- Posterior descending artery
- Left circumflex marginal artery
- Marginal branch of right coronary artery
- Left anterior descending artery

The heart consists of four chambers – two thin-walled **atria** and two muscular **ventricles**. The atria are separated from the ventricles by a band of fibrous connective tissue (**annulus fibrosus**), which provides a skeleton for the attachment of muscle and the insertion of cardiac valves. It also prevents electrical conduction between the atria and ventricles, except at the **atrioventricular node** (AVN). The walls of the heart are formed from **cardiac muscle** (**myocardium**). As the systemic circulation has a 10–15-fold greater resistance to flow than the pulmonary circulation, the left ventricle needs to develop more force and has more muscle than the right ventricle. The inner surface of the heart is covered by a thin layer of cells called the **endocardium**, similar to vascular **endothelial** cells (Chapter 24). This provides an antithrombogenic surface (inhibits clotting). The outer surface is covered by the **epicardium**, a layer of mesothelial cells. The whole heart is enclosed in a thin fibrous sheath (the **pericardium**), containing interstitial fluid as a lubricant, which protects the heart from damage caused by friction and prevents excessive enlargement.

Cardiac valves

Blood flows from the right atrium into the right ventricle via the **tricuspid** (three cusps or leaflets) atrioventricular (AV) valve, and from the left atrium to the left ventricle via the **mitral** (two cusps) AV valve. The AV valves are prevented from being everted into the atria by the high pressures developed in the ventricles by fine cords (**chordae tendinae** or *trabeculae*) attached between the edge of the valve cusps and **papillary muscles** in the ventricles (Figure 20.1). Blood is ejected from the right ventricle through the **pulmonary semilunar** valve into the pulmonary artery, and from the left ventricle via the **aortic semilunar** valve into the aorta; both semilunar valves have three cusps. The cusps are formed from connective tissue covered in a thin layer of **endocardial** or **endothelial** cells. When closed, the cusps form a tight seal at the **commissure** (line at which the edges meet). Both sets of valves open and close *passively* according to the pressure difference across them. Disease or the malformation of valves can have serious consequences. **Stenosis** describes narrowed valves; stenotic AV valves impair ventricular filling, and stenotic outflow valves increase **afterload** and thus ventricular work. **Incompetent** valves do not close properly and leak (**regurgitate**).

Cardiac pacemaker, conduction of the impulse and electrocardiogram

Cardiac muscle is described in Chapter 18. The heart beat is initiated in the **sinoatrial node** (SAN), a region of specialized myocytes in the right atrium, close to the coronary sinus. Spontaneous depolarization of the SAN (Chapter 22) provides the impulse for the heart to contract. Its rate is modulated by **autonomic nerves**. Action potentials (Chapter 22) in the SAN activate adjacent atrial myocytes via **gap junctions** contained within the **intercalated discs**; **desmosomes** provide a physical link (Figure 20.2; Chapters 18 and 22). A wave of depolarization and contraction therefore sweeps through the atrial muscle. This is prevented from reaching the ventricles directly by the **annulus fibrosus** (see above), and the impulse is channelled through the **AVN**, located between the right atrium and ventricle near the atrial septum.

The AVN contains small cells and conducts slowly; it therefore delays the impulse for ~120 ms, allowing time for atrial contraction to complete ventricular filling. Once complete, effective pumping requires rapid activation throughout the ventricles, and the impulse is transmitted from the AVN by specialized, wide and thus fast conducting myocytes in the **bundle of His** and **Purkinje fibres**, by which it is distributed over the inner surface of both ventricles (Figure 20.3). From here, a wave of depolarization and contraction moves from myocyte to myocyte across the endocardium until the whole ventricular mass is activated.

Electrocardiogram (Figure 20.4). The waves of depolarization through the heart cause *local currents* in surrounding fluid, which are detected at the body surface as small changes in voltage. This forms the basis of the **electrocardiogram** (**ECG**). The classical ECG records the voltage between the left and right arm (**lead I**), the right arm and left leg (**lead II**), and the left arm and left leg (**lead III**). This is represented by **Einthoven's triangle** (Figure 20.4). The size of voltage at any time depends on the quantity of muscle depolarizing (more cells generate more current), and the **direction** in which the wave of depolarization is travelling (i.e. it is a **vector** quantity). Thus, lead II normally shows the largest deflection during ventricular depolarization, as the muscle mass is greatest and depolarization travels from apex to base, more or less parallel to a line from the left hip to the right shoulder. The basic interpretation of the ECG is described in Chapter 21.

Coronary circulation

The heart requires a rich blood supply, which is derived from the **left** and **right coronary arteries** arising from the aortic sinus (Figure 20.5). Cardiac muscle has an extensive system of capillaries. Most of the blood returns to the right atrium via the **coronary sinus**. The **large** and **small** coronary veins run parallel to the right coronary arteries, and empty into the coronary sinus. Small vessels, such as the **thebesian veins**, empty into the cardiac chambers directly. The left ventricle is mostly supplied by the left coronary artery; occlusion in coronary artery disease can lead to serious damage. The coronary circulation is, however, capable of developing a good collateral system over time, where new arteries by-pass occlusions and improve perfusion. During systole, contraction of the ventricles compresses the coronary arteries and suppresses blood flow; this is of greatest effect in the left ventricle, where during systole the ventricular pressure is the same as or greater than that in the arteries. As a result, *more than 85% of left ventricular perfusion occurs during diastole*. This is problematic in disease if the heart rate is increased (e.g. exercise), as the diastolic interval is shorter.

21 The cardiac cycle

Figure 21.1 Pressures, volumes and key events during the cardiac cycle

A Atrial systole

B Isovolumetric contraction

C Rapid ventricular ejection
D Reduced ventricular ejection

E Isovolumetric relaxation

F Rapid ventricular filling
G Reduced ventricular filling

Aortic valve closes

Aorta

Aortic valve opens

Dicrotic notch

Left ventricle pressure

Mitral valve closes

Left atrium pressure

Mitral valve opens

Heart sounds

Ventricular volume (mL)

Aortic flow (L/min)

Jugular venous pulse

ECG (mV)

200ms

Figure 21.2 Ventricular pressure–volume loop

↑Contractility

Normal

↑EDV

Left ventricular volume (mL)

Physiology at a Glance, Fourth Edition. Edited by Jeremy P.T. Ward and Roger W.A. Linden.
© 2017 John Wiley & Sons, Ltd. Published 2017 by John Wiley & Sons, Ltd. Companion website: www.ataglanceseries.com/physiology

The cardiac cycle (Figure 21.1) describes the events that occur during one beat of the heart. These are shown in the figure for the left side of the heart, together with the pressures and volumes in the chambers and main vessels. At the start of the cycle, towards the end of **diastole**, the whole of the heart is relaxed. The atrioventricular (AV) valves are open (right, **tricuspid**; left, **mitral**), because the atrial pressure is still slightly greater than the ventricular pressure. The **pulmonary** and **aortic valves** are closed, as the pulmonary artery and aortic pressures are greater than that in the ventricles. The cycle starts when the **sinoatrial node** (SA node) initiates atrial systole (Chapter 22).

Atrial systole (**A**). At rest, atrial contraction only contributes the last ~15–20% of the final ventricular volume, as most of the filling has already occurred due to venous pressure. The atrial contribution increases with heart rate, as diastole shortens and there is less time for ventricular filling. There are no valves between the veins and atria, and atrial systole causes a small pressure rise in the great veins (**a wave**). The ventricular volume after filling is complete (**end-diastolic volume**, EDV) is ~120–140 mL in humans. The **end-diastolic pressure** (EDP) is less than 10 mmHg, and is higher in the left ventricle than in the right due to the thicker and therefore stiffer left ventricular wall. EDV strongly affects the strength of ventricular contraction (see **Starling's law**; Chapter 23). Atrial depolarization causes the **P wave** of the electrocardiogram (**ECG**); it should be noted that atrial *repolarization* is too diffuse to be seen on the ECG.

Ventricular systole (**B, C**). The ventricular pressure rises sharply during contraction, and the AV valves close as soon as this is greater than the atrial pressure. This causes a vibration which is heard as the **first heart sound** (S_1). Ventricular depolarization is associated with the **QRS** complex of the ECG. For a short period, while force is developing, both the AV and outflow (semilunar) valves are closed and there is no ejection, as the ventricular pressure is still less than that in the pulmonary artery and aorta. This is called **isovolumetric contraction** (**B**), as the ventricular volume does not change. The increasing pressure makes the AV valves bulge into the atria, causing a small atrial pressure wave (**c wave**), followed by a fall (**x descent**).

Ejection. Eventually, the ventricular pressure exceeds that in the aorta or pulmonary artery, the outflow valves open and blood is ejected. The flow is initially very rapid (**rapid ejection phase, C**) but, as contraction wanes, ejection is reduced (**reduced ejection phase, D**). During the second half of ejection, the ventricles stop actively contracting, and the muscle starts to repolarize; this is associated with the **T wave** of the ECG. The ventricular pressure during the reduced ejection phase is slightly less than that in the artery, but initially blood continues to flow out of the ventricle because of momentum. Eventually, the flow briefly reverses, causing the closure of the outflow valve, a small increase in aortic pressure (**dicrotic notch**) and the **second heart sound** (S_2). The amount of blood ejected in one beat is the **stroke volume**, ~70 mL. About 50 mL of blood is therefore left in the ventricle at the end of systole (**end-systolic volume, ESV**). The proportion of EDV that is ejected (stroke volume/EDV) is the **ejection fraction**; this is normally ~0.6, but is reduced below 0.5 in heart failure.

Diastole. Immediately after the closure of the outflow valves, the ventricles rapidly relax. The AV valves remain closed, however, because the ventricular pressure is initially still greater than that in the atria (**isovolumetric relaxation, E**). This is called isometric relaxation because again the ventricular volume does not change. Meanwhile, the atrial pressure has been increasing due to filling from the veins (**v wave**). When the ventricular pressure falls sufficiently, the AV valves open and the atrial pressure falls (**y descent**) as the ventricles rapidly refill (**rapid filling phase, F**). This is assisted by elastic recoil of the ventricular walls, essentially sucking blood into the ventricle. Filling during the last two-thirds of diastole is slower and due to venous flow alone (**reduced filling phase, G**). Diastole is twice the length of systole at rest, but decreases as the heart rate increases.

Ventricular pressure–volume loop

The ventricular pressure plotted against volume generates a loop (Figure 21.2), the area of which represents the work performed. Its shape is affected by the force of ventricular contraction (contractility), factors that alter refilling (EDV) and the pressure against which the ventricle has to pump (e.g. aortic pressure, **afterload**). An estimate of **stroke work** is calculated from the mean arterial pressure × stroke volume.

The pulse

The **peripheral arterial pulse** reflects the pressure waves travelling down through the blood from the heart; these move much faster than the blood itself. The shape of the pulse is affected by the compliance (stretchiness) and diameter of the artery; stiff (e.g. atherosclerosis) or small arteries have sharper pulses because they cannot absorb the energy so easily. Secondary peaks are due to reflections of the pressure wave at bifurcations of the artery. The **jugular venous pulse** reflects the right atrial pressure, as there is no valve between the jugular vein and right atria, and has corresponding **a**, **c** and **v waves**.

Heart sounds

Heart sounds are caused by vibrations in the blood due, for example, to closure of the cardiac valves (see earlier). Normally, only the **first** and **second** heart sounds are detectable (S_1, S_2), although a third sound (S_3) can occasionally be heard in fit young people. When the atrial pressure is raised (e.g. in heart failure), both a third and fourth sound may be heard, associated with rapid filling and atrial systole, respectively; this sounds like a galloping horse (**gallop rhythm**). Cardiac **murmurs** are caused by turbulent blood, and a benign murmur is sometimes heard in young people during the ejection phase. Pathological murmurs are associated with the narrowing of valves (**stenosis**), or **regurgitation** of blood backwards through valves that do not close properly (**incompetence**).

22

Initiation of the heart beat and excitation–contraction coupling

Figure 22.1 Cardiac ventricular muscle action potential

Figure 22.2 Relationship between tension and AP

Figure 22.5 Action potentials in other regions of the heart

Atria

Purkinje fibres

Phase 1

Figure 22.3 Sinoatrial node action potential

Decay of pacemaker potential determines heart rate

Figure 22.4 Control of heart rate: chronotropic agents

Normal

Sympathetic (noradrenaline)

Vagal (acetylcholine)

Threshold

Faster decay

Slowed decay + hyperpolarization

Figure 22.6 Cardiac muscle excitation–contraction coupling and relaxation mechanisms

Physiology at a Glance, Fourth Edition. Edited by Jeremy P.T. Ward and Roger W.A. Linden.
© 2017 John Wiley & Sons, Ltd. Published 2017 by John Wiley & Sons, Ltd. Companion website: www.ataglanceseries.com/physiology

The process linking depolarization to contraction is called **excitation–contraction coupling**. The basics of action potentials (**APs**) are described in Chapter 5.

Cardiac muscle electrophysiology

Ventricular muscle action potential (Figure 22.1). The resting potential of ventricular myocytes is approximately −90 mV (close to E_K) and stable (phase 4; Figure 22.1). An AP is initiated when the myocyte is depolarized to a **threshold potential** of approximately −65 mV, as a result of transmission from an adjacent myocyte via **gap junctions** (Chapters 4 and 20). Fast, voltage-gated Na$^+$ channels are activated, leading to an inward current which rapidly depolarizes the membrane towards +30 mV. This initial depolarization or **upstroke** (phase 0; Figure 22.1) is similar to that in nerve and skeletal muscle, and assists transmission to the next myocyte. The Na$^+$ current rapidly inactivates, but, in cardiac myocytes, the initial depolarization activates voltage-gated Ca^{2+} channels (**L-type channels**; threshold approximately −45 mV), through which Ca^{2+} floods into the cell. The resultant inward current prevents the cell from repolarizing, and causes a **plateau phase** (phase 2; Figure 22.1) that is maintained for ~250 ms until the L-type channels inactivate. The cardiac AP is thus much longer than that in nerve or skeletal muscle (~300 ms vs ~2 ms). Repolarization is facilitated by activation of voltage-gated **delayed rectifier** K$^+$ channels (phase 3; Figure 22.1). The plateau and associated Ca^{2+} entry are essential for contraction; blockade of L-type channels (e.g. **dihydropyridines**) reduces force. As the AP lasts almost as long as contraction (Figure 22.2), its *refractory period* (Chapter 5) prevents another AP being initiated until the muscle relaxes; thus cardiac muscle cannot exhibit tetanus (Chapter 17).

The sinoatrial node and origin of the heart beat

The sinoatrial node (SAN) AP differs from that in ventricular muscle (Figure 22.3). The resting potential starts at a more positive value (approximately −60 mV) and decays steadily with time until it reaches a threshold of around −40 mV, when an AP is initiated. The upstroke of the AP is **slow**, as it is not due to activation of fast Na$^+$ channels, but instead slow **L-type Ca^{2+} channels**; the SAN contains no functional fast Na$^+$ channels. The slow upstroke means that conduction between SAN myocytes is slow; this is particularly important in the **atrioventricular node** (**AVN**), which has a similar AP. The rate of decay of the SAN resting potential determines the time it takes to reach threshold and to generate another AP, and hence determines the heart rate; it is therefore called the **pacemaker potential**. The pacemaker potential decays because of a slowly reducing outward K$^+$ current set against inward currents, specifically the "funny" current, I_F. Factors that affect I_F alter the rate of decay and time to reach threshold, and hence the heart rate, and are called **chronotropic agents**. The sympathetic transmitter, noradrenaline (norepinephrine), is *a positive chronotrope* that increases I_F and thus the rate of decay and heart rate, whereas the parasympathetic transmitter, **acetylcholine**, decreases I_F, lengthens the time to reach threshold and decreases heart rate (Figure 22.4).

Action potentials elsewhere in the heart (Figure 22.5). Atria have a similar but more triangular AP compared to the ventricles.

Purkinje fibres in the conduction system are also similar to ventricular myocytes, but have a spike (phase 1) at the peak of the upstroke, reflecting a larger Na$^+$ current that contributes to their fast conduction velocity (Chapter 6). Other atrial cells, AVN, bundle of His and Purkinje system may also exhibit decaying resting potentials that can act as pacemakers. However, the SAN is normally fastest and predominates. This is called **dominance** or **overdrive suppression**.

Excitation–contraction coupling (Figure 22.6)

Contraction. Cardiac muscle contracts when intracellular Ca^{2+} rises above 100 nM. Although Ca^{2+} entry during the AP is essential for contraction, it only accounts for ~25% of the rise in intracellular Ca^{2+}. The rest is released from Ca^{2+} stores in the **sarcoplasmic reticulum** (SR). APs travel down invaginations of the sarcolemma called **T-tubules**, which are close to, but do not touch, the **terminal cisternae** of the SR ❶. During the AP plateau, Ca^{2+} enters the cell and activates Ca^{2+}-sensitive **Ca^{2+} release channels** (ryanodine receptors, RyR) in the SR ❷, allowing stored Ca^{2+} to flood into the cytosol; this is **Ca^{2+}-induced Ca^{2+} release** (CICR). The amount of Ca^{2+} released depends on how much is stored and how much Ca^{2+} enters during the AP. Modulation of the latter is a key way in which cardiac muscle force is regulated (see later). Peak intracellular [Ca^{2+}] normally rises to ~2 μM, although maximum contraction occurs above 10 μM.

Relaxation. Ca^{2+} is rapidly pumped back into the SR (**sequestered**) by the sarco/endoplasmic reticulum Ca^{2+} ATPase (SERCA) ❸. However, Ca^{2+} that entered the myocyte during the AP must also be removed again. This is primarily performed by the **Na$^+$–Ca^{2+} exchanger** (NCX) in the membrane, which pumps one Ca^{2+} ion out in exchange for three Na$^+$ ions, using the Na$^+$ electrochemical gradient as an energy source ❹. This is relatively slow, and continues during diastole. If the latter is shortened, i.e. when the heart rate rises, more Ca^{2+} is left inside the cell and the cardiac force increases. This is the **staircase** or Treppe effect.

Regulation of contractility: inotropic agents (Figure 22.6)

Sympathetic stimulation increases cardiac muscle **contractility** (Chapter 23) because it causes the release of noradrenaline, a **positive inotrope**. Noradrenaline binds to β$_1$-adrenoceptors on the membrane and causes increased Ca^{2+} entry via L-type Ca^{2+} channels during the AP ❺, and thus increases Ca^{2+} release from the SR (❷; see previously). Noradrenaline also accelerates Ca^{2+} sequestration into the SR ❻. The contractility is also increased by slowing the removal of Ca^{2+} from the myocyte. **Cardiac glycosides** (e.g. *digoxin*) inhibit the Na$^+$ pump which removes Na$^+$ from the cell (Chapter 4) ❻. Intracellular [Na$^+$] therefore increases and the Na$^+$ gradient across the membrane is reduced. This depresses Na$^+$–Ca^{2+} exchange ❹, which relies on the Na$^+$ gradient for its motive force, and Ca^{2+} is pumped out of the cell less rapidly. Consequently, more Ca^{2+} is available inside the myocyte for the next beat, and force increases. **Acidosis** (blood pH < 7.3) is **negatively inotropic**, largely because H$^+$ competes for Ca^{2+}-binding sites.

23 Control of cardiac output and Starling's law of the heart

Figure 23.1 Factors affecting cardiac output

Filling pressure of right ventricle (preload)

Resistance to outflow from left ventricle (afterload)

Heart rate contractility

Venous return

Cardiac output

Venous tone

ANS

Arterial tone

Figure 23.2 Ventricular function curves

Sympathetic stimulation ↑contractility

Normal

Heart failure ↓contractility

150

Stroke volume (mL)

0

→ Effect of ↑EDP

0   EDP (mmHg)   10

Figure 23.4 Guyton's analysis

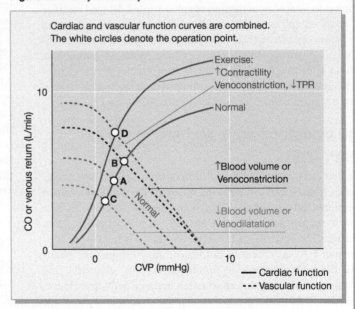

Cardiac and vascular function curves are combined.
The white circles denote the operation point.

Exercise:
↑Contractility
Venoconstriction, ↓TPR

Normal

10

CO or venous return (L/min)

D

B

A

C

Normal

↑Blood volume or Venoconstriction

↓Blood volume or Venodilatation

0

0   CVP (mmHg)   10

— Cardiac function
--- Vascular function

Figure 23.3 Vascular function curves

8

Venous return (L/min)

Normal

↑Blood volume or Venoconstriction

↓Blood volume or Dilation of veins

P$_{MC}$

0

0   CVP (mmHg)   10

8

Venous return (L/min)

Normal

Arterial dilatation ↓TPR

Arterial vasoconstriction ↑TPR

P$_{MC}$

0

0   CVP (mmHg)   10

Physiology at a Glance, Fourth Edition. Edited by Jeremy P.T. Ward and Roger W.A. Linden.
© 2017 John Wiley & Sons, Ltd. Published 2017 by John Wiley & Sons, Ltd. Companion website: www.ataglanceseries.com/physiology

Cardiac output (**CO**) is determined by the heart rate and stroke volume (**SV**): CO = heart rate × SV. SV is influenced by the filling pressure (**preload**), cardiac muscle force, and the pressure against which the heart has to pump (**afterload**). Both the heart rate and force are modulated by the autonomic nervous system (**ANS**) (Figure 23.1). The heart and vasculature form a closed system, so except for transient perturbations **venous return** *must* equal CO.

Filling pressure and Starling's law

The right ventricular end diastolic pressure (**EDP**) is dependent on central venous pressure (**CVP**); left ventricular EDP is dependent on pulmonary venous pressure. EDP and the compliance of the ventricle (how easy it is to inflate) determine the end diastolic volume (**EDV**). As EDP (and so EDV) increases, the force of systolic contraction and thus SV also increases. This is called the **Frank–Starling** relationship, and the graph relating SV to EDP is called a **ventricular function curve** (Figure 23.2). The force of contraction is related to the degree of stretch of cardiac muscle, and **Starling's law of the heart** states: '*The energy released during contraction depends on the initial fibre length*'. As muscle is stretched, more myosin cross-bridges can form, increasing force (**sliding filament theory**; Chapter 15). However, cardiac muscle has a much steeper relationship between stretch and force than skeletal muscle, because stretch also increases the Ca^{2+} sensitivity of troponin (Chapter 15), so more force is generated for the same intracellular Ca^{2+}. The ventricular function curve is therefore steep, and small changes in EDP lead to large increases in SV.

Importance of Starling's law

The most important consequence of Starling's law is that **SV in the left and right ventricles is matched**. If, for example, right ventricular SV increases, the amount of blood in the lungs and thus pulmonary vascular pressure will also increase. As the latter determines left ventricular EDP, left ventricular SV increases due to Starling's law until it again matches that of the right ventricle, when input to and output from the lungs equalize and the pressure stops rising. This represents a rightward shift along the function curve (Figure 23.2). Starling's law thus explains how an increase in CVP, which is only perceived by the right ventricle, can increase CO. It also explains why an increase in afterload (e.g. hypertension) may have little effect on CO. It should be intuitive that an increase in afterload will reduce SV if cardiac force is not increased. However, this means more blood is left in the left ventricle after systole, and also that the outputs of the two ventricles no longer match. As a result, blood accumulates on the venous side and filling pressure rises. Cardiac force therefore increases according to Starling's law until it overcomes the increased afterload and, after a few beats, CO is restored at the expense of an increased EDP.

Autonomic nervous system

The ANS provides an important extrinsic influence on CO. **Sympathetic** stimulation increases heart rate whereas **parasympathetic** decreases it; sympathetic stimulation also increases cardiac muscle force without a change in stretch (or EDV) (i.e. it increases **contractility**; Chapter 22). The ventricular function curve therefore shifts upwards (Figure 23.2). By definition, Starling's law does *not* increase contractility.

Activation of sympathetic nerves also induces arterial and venous vasoconstriction (Chapter 25). An often overlooked point is that these differ in effect. Arterial vasoconstriction increases total peripheral resistance (**TPR**) and impedes blood flow. However, unlike arteries, veins are highly compliant (stretch easily), and contain ~70% of blood volume. Venoconstriction reduces the compliance of veins and hence their capacity (amount of blood they contain), and therefore has the same effect as increasing blood volume, i.e. **CVP increases**. Venoconstriction does not significantly impede flow because venous resistance is very low compared to TPR. Sympathetic stimulation therefore increases CO by increasing heart rate, contractility and CVP.

Postural hypotension. On standing from a prone position, gravity causes blood to pool in the legs and CVP falls. This in turn causes a fall in CO (*due to Starling's law*) and thus a fall in blood pressure. This **postural hypotension** is normally rapidly corrected by the **baroreceptor reflex** (Chapter 25), which causes venoconstriction (partially restoring CVP) and an increase in heart rate and contractility, so restoring CO and blood pressure. Even in healthy people it occasionally causes a temporary blackout (fainting or *syncope*) due to reduced cerebral perfusion. Reduction of ANS function with age accounts for a greater likelihood of postural hypotension as we get older.

Venous return and vascular function curves

Blood flow is driven by the arterial–venous pressure difference, so **venous return** will be *impeded* by a rise in CVP (Figure 23.3). This is at first glance inconsistent with Starling's law if CO *must* equal venous return. However, CVP is only altered by changes in blood volume or its distribution (e.g. venoconstriction), and these also alter the relationship between CVP and venous return (the **vascular function curve**; Figure 23.3). This figure indicates that venous return is maximum when CVP is zero (the flattening of the curve reflects venous collapse at negative pressures). Conversely, venous return will be zero if the heart stops, when pressures equalize throughout the vascular system to a **mean circulatory pressure** (P_{MC}); by definition CVP will equal P_{MC} at this point. P_{MC} is dependent on the vascular volume and compliance, and thus primarily on venous status (see above). Raising blood volume or venoconstriction therefore increases P_{MC} and causes a parallel shift of the vascular function curve; the reverse occurs in blood loss. In contrast, arterial vasoconstriction has insignificant effects on P_{MC} because the volume of resistance arteries is small; it does however reduce venous return due to the increase in TPR (see previously). The net effect is therefore to reduce the slope of the curve, whilst a reduction in TPR increases it.

Guyton's analysis combines vascular and cardiac function curves into one graph (Figure 23.4). The only point where CO and venous return are equal is the intersection of the curves (A); this is thus the **operating point**. If blood volume is now increased, the shift in the vascular function curve leads to a new operating point (B) where both CO and CVP are increased; blood loss does the opposite (C). In exercise, a more complex example, sympathetic stimulation causes both increased cardiac contractility and venoconstriction, but TPR *falls* due to vasodilation in active muscle. Thus both cardiac and vascular function curves shift up, but because of the fall in TPR the latter has a steeper slope (see previously). The new operating point (D) shows that in exercise CO can be greatly increased with only minor changes in CVP.

24 Blood vessels

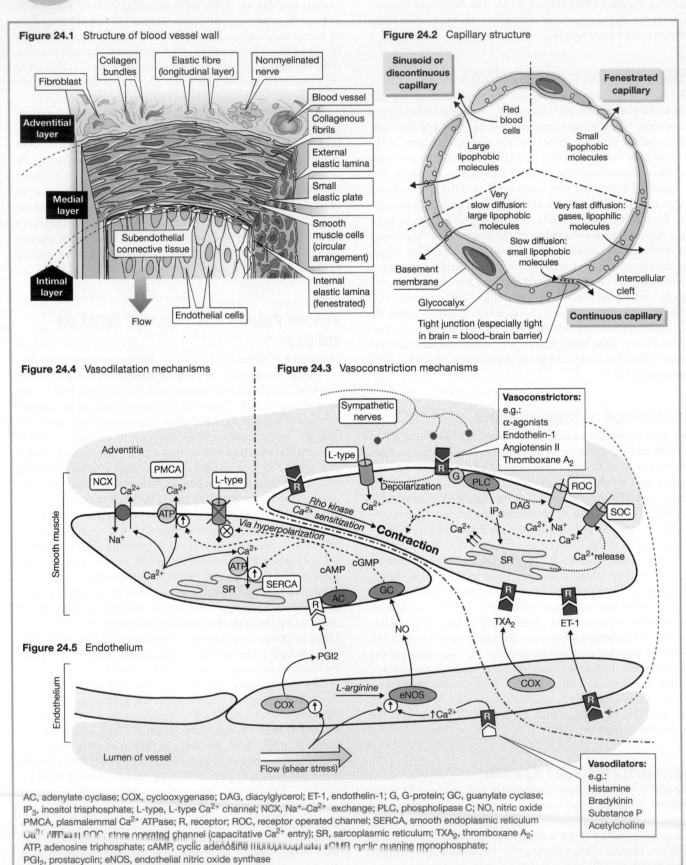

Figure 24.1 Structure of blood vessel wall

Figure 24.2 Capillary structure

Figure 24.4 Vasodilatation mechanisms

Figure 24.3 Vasoconstriction mechanisms

Figure 24.5 Endothelium

AC, adenylate cyclase; COX, cyclooxygenase; DAG, diacylglycerol; ET-1, endothelin-1; G, G-protein; GC, guanylate cyclase; IP$_3$, inositol trisphosphate; L-type, L-type Ca^{2+} channel; NCX, Na$^+$–Ca^{2+} exchange; PLC, phospholipase C; NO, nitric oxide; PMCA, plasmalemmal Ca^{2+} ATPase; R, receptor; ROC, receptor operated channel; SERCA, smooth endoplasmic reticulum Ca^{2+} ATPase; SOC, store operated channel (capacitative Ca^{2+} entry); SR, sarcoplasmic reticulum; TXA$_2$, thromboxane A$_2$; ATP, adenosine triphosphate; cAMP, cyclic adenosine monophosphate; cGMP, cyclic guanine monophosphate; PGI$_2$, prostacyclin; eNOS, endothelial nitric oxide synthase

Structure

The walls of larger blood vessels comprise three layers: an inner **intima** (*tunica intima*) consisting of a thin layer of **endothelial cells**; a thick **media** (*tunica media*) containing **smooth muscle** and **elastin filaments** that provide elastic properties; and an outer **adventitia** (*tunica adventitia*) consisting of fibroblasts and nerves embedded in collagenous tissue (Figure 24.1). The layers are separated by inner and outer **elastic lamina**. In large vessels, the adventitia contains a network of blood vessels called the **vasa vasorum** (*vessel of vessels*) supplying the smooth muscle. Veins have a thinner media than arteries, and contain less smooth muscle. All three layers contain fibrous **collagen**, which acts as a framework to which cells are anchored.

Vascular smooth muscle cells are elongated, 15–100 μm in length, and tend to be orientated in a spiral around the vessel; the lumen therefore narrows as they contract. Cells are connected by **gap junctions**, allowing electrical coupling and depolarization to spread from cell to cell. The structure and functions of smooth muscle are described in Chapter 18.

Capillaries and the smallest venules are formed from a single layer of endothelial cells supported on the outside by a 50–100-nm thick **basal lamina** containing collagen. The luminal surface is covered by a glycoprotein network called the **glycocalyx**. There are three basic types of capillary, varying in permeability (Figure 24.2). **Continuous capillaries** have a low permeability, as junctions between the endothelial cells are very tight and prevent the diffusion of lipophobic molecules of >10 000 Da. They are found in skin, lungs, central nervous system and muscle. **Fenestrated capillaries** have less tight junctions and the endothelial cells are also punctured by 50–100-nm pores (**fenestrae**); they are therefore much more permeable. They are found where large amounts of fluid or material need to diffuse across the capillary wall, including endocrine glands, renal glomeruli and intestinal villa. **Discontinuous capillaries** are found in bone marrow, liver and spleen, and have gaps large enough for red blood cells to pass through. The microcirculation is discussed further in Chapter 26.

Regulation of function and excitation–contraction coupling

Vasoconstriction (Figure 24.3). Most vasoconstrictors bind to receptors and cause a G-protein-mediated elevation in intracellular [Ca^{2+}] (Chapter 7), leading to contraction. Important vasoconstrictors include endothelin-1, angiotensin II (Chapter 38) and the sympathetic transmitter noradrenaline (norepinephrine) (Chapter 8).

Ca^{2+} release. Binding to a receptor activates **phospholipase C**, which generates the second messengers inositol trisphosphate (**IP$_3$**) and diacylglycerol (**DAG**) from membrane phospholipids. IP$_3$ activates receptors that act as Ca^{2+} channels in the **sarcoplasmic reticulum** (SR) causing Ca^{2+} release into the cytoplasm; this may itself activate Ca^{2+} sensitive Ca^{2+} release channels (ryanodine receptors, RyR) and further Ca^{2+} release. Emptying of the SR initiates store operated or *capacitative Ca^{2+} entry* (Chapter 7 and see next paragraph).

Ca^{2+} entry. Vasoconstrictors most commonly cause depolarization, which activates Ca^{2+} entry via **L-type voltage-gated Ca^{2+} channels** as in cardiac muscle (Chapter 22). Unlike cardiac muscle, most types of vascular smooth muscle do not generate action potentials, but instead depolarization is graded, allowing graded entry of Ca^{2+}. **Receptor-operated channels (ROC)** may also be activated, some by DAG, through which both Ca^{2+} and Na$^+$ can enter the cell; the latter contributes to depolarization. Emptying of SR Ca^{2+} stores is detected by STIM (stromal interaction molecule) which activates **store-operated channels (SOC)** such as ORAI in the membrane, causing **capacitative Ca^{2+} entry**.

Many agonists also cause **Ca^{2+} sensitization** of the contractile apparatus, i.e. more force for the same rise in Ca^{2+}. This is mediated by G-protein-mediated activation of **Rho kinase** (Chapter 7), although protein kinase C, which is activated by DAG, may also be involved. The relative importance of the above mechanisms depends on the vascular bed and vasoconstrictor. Most systemic arteries exhibit a degree of **basal** (*myogenic*) **tone** in the absence of vasoconstrictors.

Ca^{2+} removal and vasodilatation (Figure 24.4). Ca^{2+} is pumped back into the SR (*sequestrated*) by the **sarco/endoplasmic reticulum Ca^{2+} ATPase (SERCA)** which can rapidly reduce cytosolic Ca^{2+}. Ca^{2+} is also removed from the cell by a **plasma membrane Ca^{2+} ATPase (PMCA)** and **Na$^+$–Ca^{2+} exchange** (NCX; Chapters 7 and 22). Most endogenous vasodilators cause relaxation by increasing cyclic guanosine monophosphate (cGMP) (e.g. **nitric oxide**, NO) or cyclic adenosine monophosphate (cAMP) (e.g. **prostacyclin** [prostaglandin I$_2$, PGI$_2$]; β-adrenergic receptor agonists). These second messengers act via protein kinase G (PKG) or protein kinase A (PKA), respectively (Chapter 7). Both PKG and PKA lower intracellular Ca^{2+}, partly by stimulating SERCA and PMCA, and partly by hyperpolarizing the membrane (i.e. so voltage-gated Ca^{2+} entry is inhibited). L-type Ca^{2+} channel blocker drugs, such as **verapamil** or **dihydropyridines**, are clinically effective vasodilators.

The endothelium (Figure 24.5)

The endothelium plays a crucial role in the regulation of vascular tone. In response to substances in the blood or changes in blood flow, it can synthesize several important vasodilators, including **NO** and **prostacyclin**, as well as potent vasoconstrictors, such as **endothelin-1** and **thromboxane A$_2$** (TXA$_2$).

NO is synthesized by the endothelial **nitric oxide synthase** (eNOS) from L-arginine. eNOS activity and NO production are increased by factors that elevate intracellular Ca^{2+}, including local mediators such as **bradykinin**, **histamine** and **serotonin**, and some neurotransmitters (e.g. **substance P**). Increased flow (**shear stress**) also stimulates NO production, and additionally activates prostacyclin synthesis. The basal production of NO continuously modulates vascular resistance, as it has been found that inhibition of eNOS causes the blood pressure to rise. NO also inhibits platelet activation and **thrombosis** (inappropriate clotting) (Chapter 10).

Endothelin-1 is an extremely potent vasoconstrictor peptide which is released from the endothelium in the presence of many other vasoconstrictors, including angiotensin II, antidiuretic hormone (ADH; *vasopressin*) and noradrenaline, and may be increased in disease and hypoxia. As endothelin receptor blockade causes a fall in the peripheral resistance of healthy humans, it seems to contribute to the maintenance of blood pressure.

The **eicosanoids** prostacyclin and TXA$_2$ are synthesized by the cyclooxygenase pathway from arachidonic acid, which is made from membrane phospholipids by phospholipase A$_2$ (Chapter 7). In most vessels prostacyclin is most important.

25 Control of blood pressure and blood volume

Figure 25.1 Baroreceptors

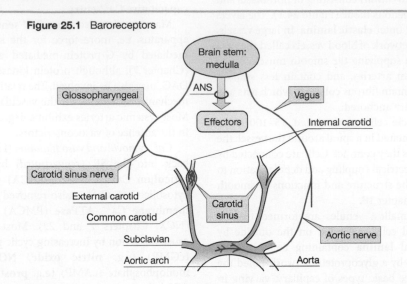

Figure 25.2 Acute control of blood pressure

Figure 25.3 Longer term control of blood pressure and volume

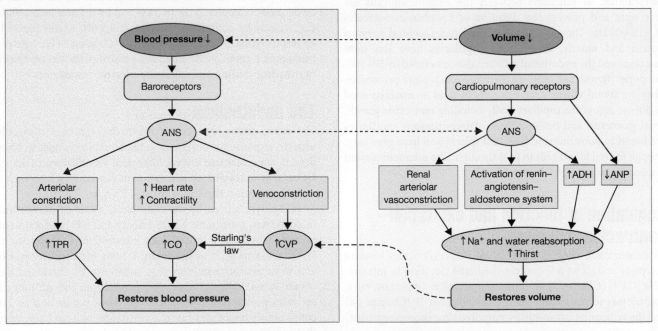

Figure 25.4 Effect of severe (45%) blood loss: Reversible and irreversible cardiovascular shock

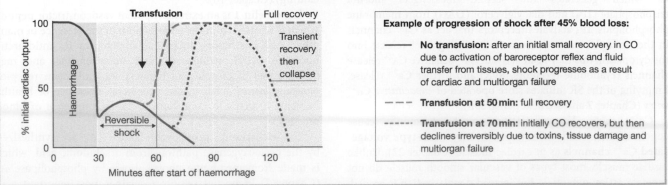

Example of progression of shock after 45% blood loss:

— **No transfusion:** after an initial small recovery in CO due to activation of baroreceptor reflex and fluid transfer from tissues, shock progresses as a result of cardiac and multiorgan failure

--- **Transfusion at 50 min:** full recovery

----- **Transfusion at 70 min:** initially CO recovers, but then declines irreversibly due to toxins, tissue damage and multiorgan failure

Tissues can independently alter their blood flow by changing their vascular resistance. So that this does not have a knock-on effect elsewhere, the pressure head provided by the mean arterial blood pressure (MAP) must be controlled. MAP is determined by the **total peripheral resistance** (TPR) and **cardiac output** (MAP = cardiac output × TPR), which is itself dependent on the **central venous pressure** (CVP) (Chapter 23). CVP is highly dependent on the **blood volume**. Alterations of any of these variables may change MAP.

Effect of gravity. When standing, the blood pressure at the ankle is ~90 mmHg higher than that at the level of the heart, due to the weight of the column of blood between the two. Similarly, the pressure in the head is ~30 mmHg less than that at the level of the heart. Blood pressure is always measured at the level of the heart. Gravity does not affect the driving force between arteries and veins because arterial and venous pressures are affected equally.

Acute regulation of the mean arterial blood pressure: the baroreceptor reflex

Physiological regulation commonly involves **negative feedback**. This requires a **sensor** that detects the controlled variable (e.g. MAP), a **comparator** that compares the sensor output to a **set point**, and a **feedback pathway** driving **effectors** that adjust the variable until the difference between the sensor output and the set point is minimized (Chapter 1). The sensor for MAP is provided by **baroreceptors** (stretch receptors) located in the **carotid sinus** and **aortic arch** (Figure 25.1). A decrease in MAP reduces arterial wall stretch and *decreases* baroreceptor activity, resulting in decreased firing in afferent nerves travelling via the glossopharyngeal and vagus to the medulla of the brain stem, where the activity of the **autonomic nervous system** (ANS) (Chapter 8) is coordinated. Sympathetic nervous activity consequently *increases*, causing an increased heart rate and cardiac contractility (Chapter 23), peripheral vasoconstriction and an increase in TPR, and venoconstriction, which increases CVP (Chapter 24). Parasympathetic activity *decreases*, contributing to the rise in heart rate (Chapter 22). MAP therefore returns to normal (Figure 25.2). An increase in MAP has the opposite effects.

The baroreceptors are most sensitive between 80 and 150 mmHg, and their sensitivity is increased by a large **pulse pressure** (Chapter 19). They also show **adaptation**; if a new pressure is maintained for a few hours, activity slowly returns towards (but not to) normal. The baroreceptor reflex is important for buffering *short-term* changes in MAP, e.g. when muscle blood flow increases rapidly in exercise. Cutting the baroreceptor nerves has a minor effect on average MAP, but fluctuations in pressure are much greater.

Posture. Changes in posture provide a good example of the acute baroreceptor reflex. When standing from a supine position, blood pools in the veins of the legs, causing a fall in CVP; cardiac output and MAP therefore fall (**postural hypotension**; Chapter 23). Baroreceptor firing is reduced and the baroreceptor reflex is activated. *Venoconstriction* reduces blood pooling and helps restore CVP which, coupled with an *increase in heart rate and cardiac contractility*, returns cardiac output towards normal; peripheral *vasoconstriction* assists the restoration of MAP. The transient dizziness or blackout (**syncope**) occasionally experienced when rising rapidly is due to a fall in cerebral perfusion that occurs before cardiac output and MAP can be corrected.

Long-term regulation: control of blood volume (Figure 25.3)

The blood volume is dependent on total body Na^+ and water. These are regulated by the kidneys, and it is therefore strongly recommended that this chapter is read together with Chapter 38, where the renal mechanisms involved are discussed in detail.

The activation of the baroreceptor reflex by a reduction in MAP leads to renal arteriolar constriction mediated by efferent sympathetic nerves. This and the fall in MAP itself cause a reduction in renal perfusion pressure, which reduces glomerular filtration and so inhibits excretion of Na^+ and water in the urine. Sympathetic stimulation and reduced arteriolar pressure also activate the **renin–angiotensin system** (Chapter 38) and thus the production of **angiotensin II**, a potent vasoconstrictor that increases TPR. Angiotensin II also stimulates the production of **aldosterone** from the adrenal cortex, which promotes renal Na^+ reabsorption. The net effect is Na^+ and water retention, and an increase in blood volume (Figure 25.4). Conversely, a rise in MAP increases Na^+ and water excretion.

Changes in blood volume are sensed directly by **cardiopulmonary receptors: veno-atrial receptors** are located around the join between the veins and atria, and **atrial receptors** in the atrial wall. These effectively respond to changes in CVP and *blood volume*. Stimulation (stretch) suppresses the renin–angiotensin system, sympathetic activity and secretion of **antidiuretic hormone** (ADH, vasopressin), but increases release of **atrial natriuretic peptide** (ANP) from the atria. Together, these changes promote renal Na^+ and water excretion and reduce blood volume (Chapters 37 and 38). A fall in blood volume will induce the opposite effects. The cardiopulmonary receptors normally cause **tonic depression** – cutting their efferent nerves increases the heart rate and causes vasoconstriction in the gut, kidney and skeletal muscle, thus raising MAP.

Cardiovascular shock and haemorrhage

Cardiovascular shock. This is an acute condition with inadequate blood flow throughout the body, commonly associated with a fall in MAP. It can result from reduced blood volume (**hypovolumic shock**), profound vasodilatation (**low-resistance shock**) or acute failure of the heart to pump (**cardiogenic shock**). The most common cause of hypovolumic shock is **haemorrhage**; others include severe burns, vomiting and diarrhoea (e.g. cholera). Low-resistance shock is due to the profound vasodilatation caused by bacterial infection (**septic shock**) or powerful allergic reactions (e.g. to bee stings or peanuts; **anaphylactic shock**).

Haemorrhage. Some 20% of the blood volume can be lost without significant problems, as the baroreceptor reflex mobilizes blood from capacitance vessels and maintains MAP. Volume is restored within 24 h because arteriolar constriction reduces the capillary pressure and fluid moves from tissues into the plasma (Chapter 26), urine production is suppressed (see previously) and ADH and angiotensin II stimulate thirst. Greater loss (30–50%) can be survived, but only with transfusion within ~1 h (the '**golden hour**') (Figure 25.4). After this, **irreversible shock** generally develops, which is irretrievable even with transfusion. This is because the reduced MAP and consequent profound peripheral vasoconstriction cause tissue ischaemia and the build-up of toxins and acidity, which damage the microvasculature and heart and lead to *multiorgan failure*.

26 The microcirculation, filtration and lymphatics

Figure 26.1 Structure of the microcirculation

Smooth muscle cells

Small arterioles

Terminal arterioles

Thoroughfare vessels (present in some tissues)

Capillaries

Capillaries

Lymphatic capillaries

Postcapillary venules

Venule

Skin and some other tissues

Most tissues

Figure 26.2 Fluid filtration in capillaries and Starling's equation

P_c, capillary hydrostatic pressure; P_i, interstitial hydrostatic pressure; σ, reflection coefficient; π_p, plasma colloidal osmotic pressure; π_i, interstitial colloidal osmotic pressure

Net flow across capillary wall $\propto (P_c - P_i) - \sigma(\pi_p - \pi_i)$

Reabsorption

Filtration

Fluid enters lymphatics– if excessive due to high P_c causes oedema

Arteriole

Venule

Normal

$P_i = -2\,mmHg$ $\pi_i = 10\,mmHg$

$P_c = 35\,mmHg$ $\pi_p = 27\,mmHg$ $P_c = 15\,mmHg$

Capillary

Low capillary pressure

$P_i = -2\,mmHg$ $\pi_i = 10\,mmHg$

$P_c = 18\,mmHg$ $\pi_p = 27\,mmHg$ $P_c = 8\,mmHg$

Net flow across capillary wall $\propto (P_c - P_i) - \sigma(\pi_p - \pi_i)$

Reabsorption (transient)

Filtration

Note: Reabsorption is transient because it causes π_i to increase (i.e. concentrating interstitial proteins)

Physiology at a Glance, Fourth Edition. Edited by Jeremy P.T. Ward and Roger W.A. Linden.

The **microcirculation** is perhaps the *raison d'être* for the cardiovascular system, as it is here that exchange between blood and tissues occurs. It consists of the smallest (**terminal**) **arterioles** and the **exchange vessels – capillaries** and **small venules** (Chapter 19). Blood flow into the microcirculation is regulated by the vasoconstriction of small arterioles, activated by sympathetic stimulation through numerous nerve endings in their walls (Chapters 8 and 25). Each small arteriole feeds many capillaries via several **terminal arterioles** (Figure 26.1), which are not innervated. Instead, the vasoconstriction of terminal arterioles is mediated by **local metabolic products** (Chapter 27), allowing perfusion to be matched to metabolism. A *few* tissues (e.g. mesenteric, skin) have **thoroughfare vessels** connecting small arterioles and venules directly. Note that the term '*pre-capillary sphincter*' is misleading and should be avoided, as no such anatomical structures exist.

Transcapillary exchange

Water, gases and other substances cross the capillary wall mainly by **diffusion** down their concentration gradients (Chapter 12). O_2 and CO_2 are highly **lipophilic** (soluble in lipids), and can cross the endothelial lipid bilayer membrane easily. This is, however, impermeable to **hydrophilic** ('water-loving', lipid-insoluble) molecules, such as glucose, and **polar** (charged) molecules and ions (electrolytes). Such substances mainly cross the wall of **continuous capillaries** through the gaps between endothelial cells. This is slowed by **tight junctions** between cells and by the **glycocalyx** (Chapter 24), so that diffusion is 1000–10 000 times slower than for lipophilic substances. This **small pore** system also prevents the diffusion of substances greater than 10 000 Da (e.g. plasma proteins). The latter can cross the capillary wall, but extremely slowly; this may involve **large pores** through endothelial cells. **Fenestrated capillaries** (gut, joints, kidneys) are 10-fold more permeable than continuous capillaries because of pores called **fenestrae** (from the Latin for '*windows*'), whereas **discontinuous capillaries** arc highly permeable due to large spaces between endothelial cells, and occur where blood cells need to cross the capillary wall (bone marrow, spleen, liver) (Chapter 24).

Filtration (Figure 26.2)

The capillary walls are much more permeable to water and electrolytes than to proteins (see previously). The concentration of electrolytes (e.g. Na^+, Cl^-), and therefore the osmotic pressure exerted by them (**crystalloid osmotic pressure**), is very similar in plasma and interstitial fluid, and has little effect on fluid movement. The protein concentration in plasma however is greater than that in interstitial fluid, and the component of osmotic pressure exerted by proteins (**colloidal osmotic** or **oncotic pressure**) in the plasma (~27 mmHg) is therefore greater than in the interstitial fluid (~10 mmHg). Water tends to flow from a *low* to a *high* osmotic pressure, but from a *high* to a *low* hydrostatic pressure. The net flow of water across the capillary wall is therefore determined by the balance between the hydrostatic (P) and colloidal osmotic (π) pressures, according to **Starling's equation**, **flow $\propto (P_c - P_i) - \sigma(\pi_p - \pi_i)$**, where $(P_c - P_i)$ is the difference in hydrostatic pressure between capillary and interstitial fluid, and $(\pi_p - \pi_i)$ is the difference in colloidal osmotic pressure between plasma and interstitial fluid; $(\pi_p - \pi_i)$ has an average value of ~17 mmHg. σ is the **reflection coefficient** (~0.9), a measure of how difficult it is for plasma proteins to cross the capillary wall. Note that the interstitial protein concentration, and therefore π_i, differs between tissues; in the lung for example $(\pi_p - \pi_i)$ is ~13 mmHg.

The capillary hydrostatic pressure normally varies from ~35 mmHg at the arteriolar end to ~15 mmHg at the venous end, whereas the interstitial hydrostatic pressure is approximately –2 mmHg. $(P_c - P_i)$ is therefore greater than $\sigma(\pi_p - \pi_i)$ along the length of the capillary, resulting in the **net filtration** of water into the interstitial space (Figure 26.2). Although arteriolar constriction will reduce capillary pressure and therefore lead to the reabsorption of fluid, this will normally be transient due to concentration of interstitial fluid (i.e. increased π_i). A reduction in plasma protein (e.g. *starvation*), or a loss of endothelium integrity and thus diffusion of protein into the interstitial space (e.g. *inflammation*, *ischaemia*), will similarly reduce $(\pi_p - \pi_i)$, leading to enhanced filtration and loss of fluid into the tissues (**oedema**; see below). Oedema is also caused by high venous pressures.

Lymphatics

Fluid filtered by the microcirculation (~8 L per day) is returned to the blood by the **lymphatic system**. Lymphatic capillaries are blind-ended bulbous tubes (diameter, ~15–75 vμm) walled with endothelial cells (Figure 26.1). These allow the entry of fluid, proteins and bacteria, but prevent their exit. Lymphatic capillaries merge into **collecting lymphatics** and then larger lymphatic vessels, both containing smooth muscle and **unidirectional valves**. Lymph is propelled by smooth muscle constriction and compression of the vessels by body movement into **afferent lymphatics** and then the **lymphatic nodes**, where bacteria and other foreign materials are removed by phagocytes. Most fluid is reabsorbed here by capillaries, with the remainder returning via **efferent lymphatics** and the thoracic duct into the subclavian veins. Lymphatics are also important for lipid absorption in the gut.

Oedema

Oedema is swelling of tissues due to excess fluid in the interstitial space. It is caused when filtration is increased to the extent that the lymphatics are unable to remove the fluid fast enough (see above), or by dysfunctional lymphatic drainage (e.g. *elephantiasis*, blockage of lymphatics with filarial nematode worms). **Inflammation** (Chapter 11) causes swelling and oedema because it increases capillary permeability, allowing protein to leak into the interstitium and disrupt the oncotic pressure gradient, so filtration is increased. Reduced venous drainage (increased venous pressure) also increases filtration and can lead to oedema; standing without moving the legs prevents the operation of the **muscle pump** (Chapter 19), local venous pressure rises, and the legs swell. In **congestive heart failure**, reduced cardiac function results in increased pulmonary and central venous pressure (Chapter 23), leading, respectively, to **pulmonary oedema** (alveoli fill with fluid) and **peripheral oedema** (swelling of the legs and liver, and accumulation of fluid in the peritoneum [*ascites*]). Severe protein starvation can cause generalized oedema and a grossly swollen abdomen due to ascites and an enlarged liver (*kwashiorkor*).

27 Local control of blood flow and specific circulations

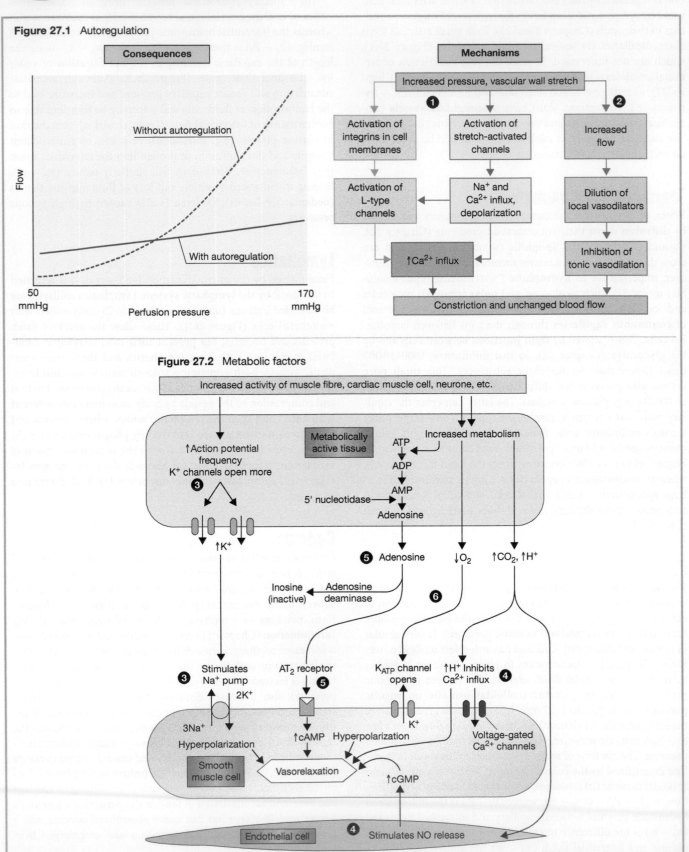

Figure 27.1 Autoregulation

Consequences

Flow vs Perfusion pressure

- Without autoregulation
- With autoregulation

50 mmHg — 170 mmHg

Mechanisms

Increased pressure, vascular wall stretch

1. Activation of integrins in cell membranes → Activation of L-type channels

   Activation of stretch-activated channels → Na$^+$ and Ca^{2+} influx, depolarization → ↑Ca^{2+} influx

2. Increased flow → Dilution of local vasodilators → Inhibition of tonic vasodilation

Constriction and unchanged blood flow

Figure 27.2 Metabolic factors

Increased activity of muscle fibre, cardiac muscle cell, neurone, etc.

Metabolically active tissue

Increased metabolism

ATP → ADP → AMP → Adenosine

5' nucleotidase → AMP

3. ↑Action potential frequency K$^+$ channels open more → ↑K$^+$

5. Adenosine
6. ↓O$_2$
   ↑CO$_2$, ↑H$^+$

Adenosine deaminase → Inosine (inactive)

3. Stimulates Na$^+$ pump — 2K$^+$ — 3Na$^+$ — Hyperpolarization

5. AT$_2$ receptor → ↑cAMP

K$_{ATP}$ channel opens — K$^+$ — Hyperpolarization

4. ↑H$^+$ Inhibits Ca^{2+} influx → Voltage-gated Ca^{2+} channels

Smooth muscle cell → Vasorelaxation ← ↑cGMP

Endothelial cell

4. Stimulates NO release

Physiology at a Glance, Fourth Edition. Edited by Jeremy P.T. Ward and Roger W.A. Linden.

Local control of blood flow

In addition to central control of blood pressure and cardiac output, tissues need to be able to regulate their own blood flow to match their requirements. This is provided by **autoregulation**, **metabolic factors** and **autocoids** (local hormones).

Autoregulation (Figure 27.1). Autoregulation is the ability to maintain a constant flow in the face of variations in arterial pressure between ~50 and 170 mmHg. It is particularly important in the brain, kidney and heart. Two mechanisms contribute to autoregulation. The **myogenic response ❶** involves arteriolar constriction in response to increased pressure and/or distention of the vessel wall. This probably involves activation of transmembrane **integrins** (Chapter 3) in smooth muscle cells, with subsequent opening of voltage-activated L-type Ca^{2+} channels, but **stretch-activated channels** permeable to Ca^{2+} and Na^+ also contribute by causing depolarization, further activation of L-type channels and Ca^{2+} entry. A *reduction* in pressure/stretch has the opposite effects, causing vasorelaxation. The second autoregulation mechanism is due to locally produced **vasodilating factors ❷**. An increase in blood flow dilutes these factors, causing vasoconstriction, whereas decreased blood flow allows accumulation, causing vasodilatation.

Metabolic factors (Figure 27.2). Many factors may contribute to **metabolic hyperaemia** (*increased blood flow*). The most important are K^+, CO_2 and **adenosine**, and in some tissues **hypoxia**. K^+ ❸ is released from active tissues and in ischaemia; local concentrations can increase to >10 mM. It causes relaxation, partly by stimulating the Na^+ pump, thus both increasing Ca^{2+} removal by the Na^+–Ca^{2+} exchanger and hyperpolarizing the cell (Chapter 24). The vasodilatory effects of increased CO_2 (**hypercapnia**) and **acidosis ❹** are mediated largely through increased **nitric oxide** production (Chapter 24) and inhibition of smooth muscle Ca^{2+} entry. **Adenosine ❺** is a potent vasodilator released from heart, skeletal muscle and brain during increased metabolism and hypoxia. It is produced from adenosine monophosphate (AMP), a breakdown product of adenosine triphosphate (ATP), and acts by stimulating the production of cyclic AMP (**cAMP**) in smooth muscle (Chapter 24). **Hypoxia** may reduce ATP sufficiently for K_{ATP} channels (which are inhibited by ATP) to activate ❻, causing hyperpolarization.

Autocoids are mostly important in special circumstances; two examples are given. In **inflammation**, infection and tissue damage initiate release of the vasodilators **histamine**, **bradykinin** and **prostaglandin E₂**, which increase blood flow but also the permeability of exchange vessels, leading to swelling but facilitating access by leucocytes and antibodies to damaged tissues (Chapter 11). The **activation of platelets** during clotting releases the vasoconstrictors **serotonin** and **thromboxane A_2**, so reducing blood loss (Chapter 10).

Specific circulations

Skeletal muscle. This comprises ~50% of the body weight and, at rest, takes 15–20% of cardiac output; during exercise, this can rise to >80%. Skeletal muscle provides a major contribution to the **total peripheral resistance**, and sympathetic regulation of muscle blood flow is important in the **baroreceptor reflex**. At rest, most capillaries are not perfused, as their arterioles are constricted. Capillaries are **recruited** during exercise by dilatation of their arterioles due to local release of K^+, CO_2 and **adenosine** by working muscle (metabolic hyperaemia), which *overrides* sympathetic vasoconstriction. In non-working muscle, the latter reduces blood flow so *conserving* cardiac output. It should be noted that muscular contraction compresses blood vessels and inhibits flow; in rhythmic (**phasic**) activity, metabolic hyperaemia compensates by vastly increasing flow during the relaxation phase. In **isometric** (static) contractions, continuously reduced flow can cause **muscle fatigue**; the consequent large increase in blood flow when contraction ceases is termed **reactive hyperaemia**.

Brain. The occlusion of blood flow to the brain causes unconsciousness within minutes. The brain receives ~15% of cardiac output, and has a high capillary density. The endothelial cells of these capillaries have very tight junctions, and contain membrane transporters that control the movement of substances, such as ions, glucose and amino acids, and tightly regulate the composition of the cerebrospinal fluid. This arrangement is called the **blood–brain barrier**, and is continuous except where substances need to be absorbed or released from the blood (e.g. pituitary gland, choroid plexus). It can cause problems for the delivery of drugs to the brain, particularly antibiotics. The **autoregulation** of cerebral blood flow is highly developed, maintaining a constant flow for blood pressures between 50 and 170 mmHg. CO_2 and K^+ are particularly important metabolic regulators in the brain, and when increased cause a **functional hyperaemia** linking blood flow to activity. Hyperventilation reduces blood P_{CO_2}, and can cause fainting due to cerebral vasoconstriction. Astrocytes surrounding cerebral blood vessels may also link perfusion to neural activity by releasing vasodilators including K^+ and PGE_2.

Coronary circulation. The heart has a high metabolic demand and a dense capillary network. It can extract an unusually high proportion of oxygen from the blood (~70%). In exercise, the reduced diastolic interval (Chapter 21) and increased oxygen consumption demands a greatly increased blood flow, which is achieved under the influence of **adenosine**, K^+ and **hypoxia**. The heart therefore controls its own blood flow by a well-developed **metabolic hyperaemia**. This *overrides* vasoconstriction mediated by sympathetic nerves (Chapters 8 and 24), and is assisted by circulating adrenaline (epinephrine) which causes vasodilatation via β_2-adrenergic receptors.

Pulmonary circulation. This is not controlled by either autonomic nerves or metabolic products, and the most important mechanism regulating flow is **hypoxic pulmonary vasoconstriction**, in which small arteries *constrict* to hypoxia. This is unique to the lung; hypoxia causes vasodilatation elsewhere (see above). Hypoxic pulmonary vasoconstriction diverts blood away from poorly ventilated areas of the lung, thus maintaining optimal **ventilation–perfusion matching** (Chapter 33); conversely, *global hypoxia* due to lung disease or altitude (Chapter 14) detrimentally increases the pulmonary artery pressure (*pulmonary hypertension*).

In health the pulmonary capillary pressure is low (~7 mmHg) compared to systemic capillaries, but fluid filtration still occurs because the interstitial hydrostatic pressure is also low (about −4 mmHg) whereas the interstitial oncotic pressure is high (18 mmHg) (see Chapter 26).

Skin. As the main function of the cutaneous circulation is **thermoregulation**, it is discussed in Chapter 13.

The respiratory system

Chapters

28 Introduction to the respiratory system

Figure 28.1 Respiratory tract

Figure 28.2 Ciliated epithelium in bronchus

Figure 28.3 Alveoli

Figure 28.4 Detailed structure of alveoli

Typical lung volumes for 70 kg male	
Resting tidal volume (TV)	500 mL
Vital capacity (VC)	5500 mL
Inspiratory reserve volume (IRV)	3300 mL
Expiratory reserve volume (ERV)	1700 mL
Total lung capacity (TLC)	7300 mL
Functional residual capacity (FRC)	3500 mL
Residual volume (RV)	1800 mL

Figure 28.5 Lung volumes measured with simple water spirometer

(NB. FRC and RV not directly measurable — you cannot empty your lungs completely!)

Physiology at a Glance, Fourth Edition. Edited by Jeremy P.T. Ward and Roger W.A. Linden.
© 2017 John Wiley & Sons, Ltd. Published 2017 by John Wiley & Sons, Ltd. Companion website: www.ataglanceseries.com/physiology

The **upper respiratory tract** includes the nose, pharynx and larynx; the **lower respiratory tract** starts at the trachea (Figure 28.1). The two **lungs** are enclosed within the **thoracic cage**, formed from the ribs, sternum and vertebral column, with the dome-shaped **diaphragm** separating the thorax from the abdomen. The left lung has two lobes, the right three. The airways, blood vessels and lymphatics enter each lung at the lung root or **hilum**, where the **pulmonary nerve plexus** receives autonomic nerves from the vagus and sympathetic trunk. The vagus contains sensory afferents from **lung receptors** (Chapter 32) and bronchoconstrictor parasympathetic efferents leading to the airways; sympathetic nerves are *bronchodilatory* (Chapter 8). Each lung lobe is made up of several wedge-shaped **bronchopulmonary segments** supplied by their own segmental bronchus, artery and vein. The lungs are covered by a thin membrane (**visceral pleura**), continuous with the **parietal pleura** that lines the inside surface of the thoracic cage. The tiny space between the pleura is filled with lubricating **pleural fluid**.

Airways (Figure 28.1)

The **trachea** divides into two **main bronchi**; their walls contain U-shaped cartilage segments linked by smooth muscle. On entering the lung, the bronchi divide repeatedly into lobar, segmental (generations 3 and 4) and small (generations 5–11) bronchi, the smallest having a diameter of ~1 mm. These all have irregular cartilaginous plates and helical bands of smooth muscle. **Bronchioles** (generations 12–16) lack cartilage and are held open by surrounding lung tissue. The smallest (**terminal**) bronchioles lead to **respiratory bronchioles** (generations 17–19), and thence to **alveolar ducts** and **sacs** (generation 23), the walls of which form **alveoli** and contain only epithelial cells (Figures 28.3 and 28.4). Small pores (**alveolar pores**, *pores of Kohn*) allow pressure equalization between alveoli. Adult human lungs contain ~17 million branches and ~300 million alveoli, providing an exchange surface of ~85 m². The **bronchial circulation** supplies airways down to the terminal bronchioles; respiratory bronchioles and below obtain nutrients from the **pulmonary circulation** (Chapter 19).

Epithelium and airway clearance

The airways from the trachea to the respiratory bronchioles are lined with **ciliated columnar epithelial cells**. **Goblet cells** and **submucosal glands** secrete a 10–15-μm thick, gel-like **mucus** that floats on a more fluid *sol phase* (Figure 28.2). Synchronous beating of the cilia moves the mucus and associated debris to the mouth (**mucociliary clearance**). Factors that increase the thickness or viscosity of the mucus (e.g. *asthma, cystic fibrosis*) or reduce cilia activity (e.g. *smoking*) impair mucociliary clearance and lead to recurrent infections. Mucus contains substances that protect the airways from pathogens (e.g. *antitrypsins, lysozyme, immunoglobulin A*).

Epithelial cells forming the walls of the alveoli and alveolar ducts are unciliated, and largely very thin **type I alveolar pneumocytes** (alveolar cells; *squamous epithelium*) (Figure 28.4). These form the gas exchange surface with the capillary endothelium (**alveolar–capillary membrane**). A few **type II pneumocytes** secrete **surfactant** which reduces the surface tension and prevents alveolar collapse (Chapter 29). **Macrophages** (*mobile phagocytes*) in the airways ingest foreign materials and destroy bacteria; in the alveoli, they take the place of cilia by clearing debris.

Respiratory muscles

The main respiratory muscles are inspiratory, the most important being the **diaphragm**; contraction pulls down the dome, reducing pressure in the thoracic cavity, and thus drawing air into the lungs. The **external intercostal muscles** assist by elevating the ribs and increasing the dimensions of the thoracic cavity. Quiet breathing is normally diaphragmatic; **accessory inspiratory muscles** (e.g. *scalene, sternomastoids*) aid inspiration if airway resistance or ventilation is high. Expiration is achieved by *passive recoil* of the lungs and chest wall, but, at high ventilation rates, this is assisted by the contraction of **abdominal muscles** which speed recoil of the diaphragm by raising abdominal pressure (e.g. exercise).

Lung volumes and pressures (Figure 28.5)

The **tidal volume** (TV) is the volume of air drawn into and out of the lungs during normal breathing; the **resting tidal volume** is normally ~500 mL but, like all lung volumes, is dependent on age, sex and height. The **vital capacity** (VC) is the maximum tidal volume, when an individual breathes in and out as far as possible. The difference in volume between a resting and maximum expiration is the **expiratory reserve volume** (ERV); the equivalent for inspiration is the **inspiratory reserve volume** (IRV). The volume in the lungs after a maximum inspiration is the **total lung capacity** (TLC), and that after a maximum expiration is the **residual volume** (RV).

The **functional residual capacity** (FRC) is the volume of the lungs at the end of a normal breath, when the respiratory muscles are relaxed. It is determined by the balance between *outward elastic recoil* of the chest wall and *inward elastic recoil* of the lungs. These are coupled by the fluid in the small pleural space, which therefore has a negative pressure (**intrapleural pressure**: −0.2 to −0.5 kPa). Perforation of the chest therefore allows air to be sucked into the pleural space, and the chest wall expands while the lung collapses (**pneumothorax**). Diseases that affect lung elastic recoil alter FRC; *fibrosis* increases recoil and therefore reduces FRC, whereas in *emphysema*, where lung structure is lost, recoil is reduced and FRC increases.

During **inspiration**, the expansion of the thoracic cavity makes the intrapleural pressure more negative, causing the lungs and alveoli to expand, and reducing the alveolar pressure. This creates a pressure gradient between the alveoli and the mouth, drawing air into the lungs. During **expiration**, intrapleural and alveolar pressures rise, although, except during forced expiration (e.g. coughing), the intrapleural pressure remains negative throughout the cycle because expiration is normally *passive*.

The **dead space** refers to the volume of the airways that does not take part in gas exchange. The **anatomical dead space** includes the respiratory tract down to the terminal bronchioles; it is normally ~150 mL. The **alveolar dead space** refers to alveoli incapable of gas exchange; in health, it is negligible. The **physiological dead space** is the sum of the anatomical and alveolar dead spaces.

29 Lung mechanics

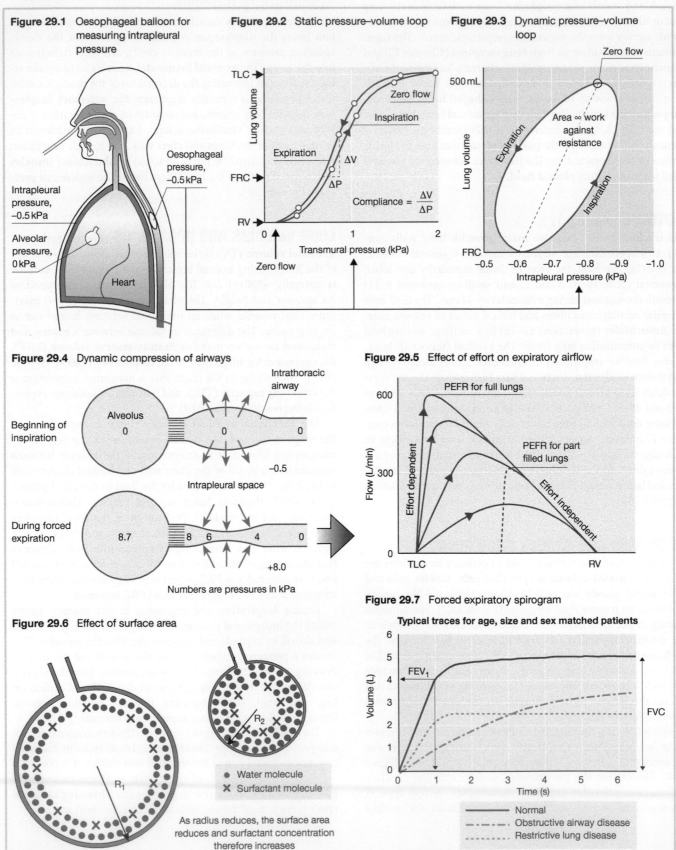

Figure 29.1 Oesophageal balloon for measuring intrapleural pressure

Oesophageal pressure, −0.5 kPa

Intrapleural pressure, −0.5 kPa

Alveolar pressure, 0 kPa

Heart

Figure 29.2 Static pressure–volume loop

TLC

Zero flow

Inspiration

Expiration

ΔV

FRC

ΔP

RV

$$\text{Compliance} = \frac{\Delta V}{\Delta P}$$

0   1   2

Transmural pressure (kPa)

Zero flow

Figure 29.3 Dynamic pressure–volume loop

Zero flow

500 mL

Area ∝ work against resistance

Expiration

Inspiration

FRC

−0.5 −0.6 −0.7 −0.8 −0.9 −1.0

Intrapleural pressure (kPa)

Figure 29.4 Dynamic compression of airways

Intrathoracic airway

Alveolus

Beginning of inspiration

0   0   0

−0.5

Intrapleural space

During forced expiration

8.7   8   6   4   0

+8.0

Numbers are pressures in kPa

Figure 29.5 Effect of effort on expiratory airflow

600

PEFR for full lungs

Flow (L/min)

Effort dependent

300

PEFR for part filled lungs

Effort independent

0

TLC   RV

Figure 29.6 Effect of surface area

R₁

R₂

• Water molecule
✕ Surfactant molecule

As radius reduces, the surface area reduces and surfactant concentration therefore increases

Figure 29.7 Forced expiratory spirogram

Typical traces for age, size and sex matched patients

6

5

4   FEV₁

Volume (L)

3   FVC

2

1

0

0   1   2   3   4   5   6

Time (s)

—— Normal
—·—·— Obstructive airway disease
········ Restrictive lung disease

Physiology at a Glance, Fourth Edition. Edited by Jeremy P.T. Ward and Roger W.A. Linden.
© 2017 John Wiley & Sons, Ltd. Published 2017 by John Wiley & Sons, Ltd. Companion website: www.ataglanceseries.com/physiology

The respiratory muscles have to overcome resisting forces during breathing. These are primarily the **elastic resistance** in the chest wall and lungs, and the resistance to air flow (**airway resistance**).

Lung compliance

Lung compliance (C_L) represents the 'stretchiness' of the lungs, defined as change in volume per unit change in distending pressure ($C_L = \Delta V/\Delta P$). It is the inverse of elastic resistance when there is no air flow (**static compliance**). The pressure distending the lungs (**transmural pressure**) is equal to alveolar–intrapleural pressure (Chapter 28). Intrapleural pressure can be estimated using an oesophageal balloon (Figure 29.1). Alveolar pressure equals mouth pressure (i.e. zero) if no air is flowing. To measure C_L, a subject breathes in steps and intrapleural pressure is measured at each held volume (mouth open). Figure 29.2 shows a typical static **pressure–volume plot**. The inspiratory and expiratory curves are slightly different (*hysteresis*), typical for elastic systems. The **static lung compliance** is the maximum slope, generally just above functional residual capacity (FRC), and is normally ~1.5 L/kPa, although this is dependent on age, size and sex. Compliance is reduced by *fibrosis* (stiffer lungs, greater elastic recoil), and increased in *emphysema* where loss of structure makes them easier to stretch (reduced elastic recoil).

Dynamic compliance is measured during breathing, and therefore includes a component due to **airway resistance**. The dynamic pressure–volume loop (Figure 29.3) is therefore much wider, reflecting the pressure required to suck in or expel air; the *area of the curve* is a measure of work done against airway resistance. The curve has two points where flow is zero (end of inspiration/expiration); the slope of a line between them is the **dynamic compliance**. Though normally similar to static compliance, this can be altered in disease.

Surfactant and the alveolar air–fluid interface

Surface tension of the fluid lining the alveoli contributes to lung stiffness, as attraction of water molecules at the air–fluid interface tends to collapse the alveoli. This is a manifestation of **Laplace's law** (Chapter 12), which shows that the pressure in a bubble (or alveolus) is proportional to the surface tension (T) and radius (P ∝ T/r). A small bubble will therefore have a higher pressure than a larger one and, if connected, will collapse into it. The inward force created by surface tension also tends to suck fluid into the alveoli (**transudation**). These problems are minimized in the lung by **surfactant**, a mixture of **phospholipids** secreted by **type II pneumocytes** (Chapter 28). Surfactant floats on the alveolar fluid surface, and reduces surface tension. As alveoli shrink and the fluid surface area is reduced, surfactant is thus concentrated, further reducing surface tension (Figure 29.6). As the surface area of a sphere ∝ radius^2, the increase in surfactant concentration and reduction in surface tension exceeds the reduction in radius, so alveolar pressure actually falls (P ∝ T/r). Surfactant thus prevents alveolar collapse and helps maintain similar alveolar sizes, and reduces lung stiffness and transudation. Premature babies with insufficient surfactant develop **neonatal respiratory distress syndrome**, with stiff lungs, lung collapse and transudation.

Airway resistance

Flow through the airways is described by **Darcy's law**; flow = ($P_1 - P_2$)/R (Chapter 12), where P_1 is the alveolar pressure, P_2 is the mouth pressure and R is the resistance to air flow. Airway resistance is determined by the airway radius, according to **Poiseuille's law**, and whether the flow is laminar or turbulent (Chapter 12).

Airway resistance is increased by factors that constrict airway smooth muscle (**bronchoconstrictors**). These include reflex release of **muscarinic** neurotransmitters from parasympathetic nerve endings, generally due to the activation of **irritant receptors** (Chapter 32), and mediators released by inflammatory cells (e.g. **histamine**, **prostaglandins**, **leukotrienes**), e.g. in **asthma**. Increased mucus production also narrows the lumen and increases resistance. Sympathetic stimulation, adrenaline (epinephrine) and salbutamol (common asthma therapy) cause **bronchodilatation** via β_2-adrenoceptors on the smooth muscle.

Effect of transmural pressure. Expiration is normally passive (Chapter 32). Forced expiration increases the intrapleural and thus alveolar pressure, increasing the pressure gradient to the mouth and therefore theoretically leading to increased flow. However, although expiration from fully inflated lungs is indeed **effort dependent**, towards the end of the breath, increasing force does not increase flow, i.e. it is **effort independent** (Figure 29.5). This occurs due to the *pressure gradient* between the alveoli and mouth. Midway between them, generally in the bronchi, the pressure in the airway falls below the intrapleural pressure, causing the airway to collapse (**dynamic compression**; Figure 29.4). As there is now no flow, the pressure rises again until it is greater than the intrapleural pressure, and the airway re-opens. This sequence happens repeatedly, producing the brassy sound heard during forced expiration. This does not occur in normal (passive) expiration because intrapleural pressure remains negative throughout. In diseases in which the airways are already narrowed (e.g. *asthma, COPD*), this leads to expiratory wheezing and air trapping.

Lung function tests

Lung volumes can be measured using a simple spirometer (Chapter 28). Airway resistance and lung compliance can be assessed indirectly by measuring the forced expiratory flows and volumes. The easiest and quickest measurement is the **peak expiratory flow rate** (PEFR). PEFR is decreased if the airway resistance is increased (**obstructive disease**), and is commonly used to follow an already diagnosed condition, e.g. asthma. It is, however, dependent on the initial lung volume (Figure 29.5). Plots of **forced expiratory volume against time** provide more information. Subjects breathe out from total lung capacity to residual volume as fast as possible; this is the **forced vital capacity** (FVC), and a typical trace is shown in Figure 29.7. Forced expiratory volume in 1 s (**FEV$_1$**) reflects airway resistance; it is normally expressed as a ratio to FVC (**FEV$_1$/FVC**) to correct for lung volume, and is usually 0.75–0.90. It can be used to distinguish between **obstructive** (increased airway resistance) and **restrictive** (decreased lung compliance) diseases. In asthma, for example, FEV$_1$/FVC is typically <0.7. In restrictive disease (e.g. lung fibrosis), FEV$_1$ and FVC are low, but FEV$_1$/FVC is normal or even increased due to greater elastic recoil (Figure 29.7).

Transport of gases and the gas laws

Figure 30.1 Fractional concentrations and partial pressures

	Dry room air			37°C and 100% humidity (SWVP–saturated water vapour pressure)					
Fractional concentration		Partial pressure (kPa)	Fractional concentration	Inspired air in airways	Partial pressure (kPa)	Fractional concentration	Alveoli air (typical)	Partial pressure (kPa)	
				FH_2O 0.06	H_2O	SWVP 6.3	FH_2O 0.06	H_2O	SWVP 6.3
							FCO_2 0.05	CO_2	PCO_2 5.3
FO_2 0.21	O_2	PO_2 21.2	FO_2 0.20	O_2	PO_2 19.9	FO_2 0.13	O_2	PO_2 13.3
FN_2 0.79	N_2	PN_2 79.8	FN_2 0.74	N_2	PN_2 74.8	FN_2 0.75	N_2	PN_2 76.1
Total 1.0		101	1.0		101	1.0*		101

Barometric pressure (say 101 kPa)

*Error due to rounding

Figure 30.2 Gas partial pressures (kPa) in airways and blood (values x 7.5 for mmHg)

Figure 30.3 Alveolar–capillary membrane

Inhaled air
PO_2 21.2
PCO_2 0.0

Exhaled air
PO_2 15.5
PCO_2 4.3

Inspired air in airways
PO_2 19.9
PCO_2 0.0

Alveolus
PO_2 13.3
PCO_2 5.3

Mixed venous blood (resting)
PO_2 5.3
PCO_2 6.1

Arterial blood
PO_2 13
PCO_2 5.3

Capillary/tissues
PO_2 5.3 or less
PCO_2 6.1 or more

Epithelium

Alveolus

Capillary

Blood flow

Endothelium

Alveolar partial pressure

<0.4 mm

Rate of transfer ∞ (alveolar PO_2 – capillary PO_2)

N_2O

O_2

O_2 (high flow)

(Venous PO_2)

CO

Capillary partial pressure

Time from entering capillary (s)

0   0.25   0.50   0.75

Notes.
Typical values for a resting, young healthy male. Difference between alveolar and arterial PO_2 due to physiological shunts (Chapter 00).
Difference between alveolar and exhaled values due to dead space (Chapter 28). Capillary/tissue values very variable.

Physiology at a Glance, Fourth Edition. Edited by Jeremy P.T. Ward and Roger W.A. Linden.
© 2017 John Wiley & Sons, Ltd. Published 2017 by John Wiley & Sons, Ltd. Companion website: www.ataglanceseries.com/physiology

Dry air contains 78.1% N_2 and 21% O_2; other inert gases account for the balance (0.9%), but are normally pooled with N_2 (i.e. N_2 = 79%). The small amount of CO_2 in air (<0.04%) is usually ignored.

Partial pressures and fractional concentrations (Figure 30.1)

The volume of a fixed amount of gas is inversely proportional to the pressure ($V \propto 1/P$; **Boyle's law**) and proportional to the absolute temperature ($V \propto T$; **Charles' law**). An ideal gas occupies 22.4 L per mole at 1 atm (101 kPa, 760 mmHg) and 0 °C (273 K), and thus the volume of each gas in a mixture is directly proportional to the quantity of that gas in moles. The term **fractional concentration (F)** can therefore be used to denote the relative quantities of gases in any mixture; thus F_{N_2} is 0.79 in *dry* air, and F_{O_2} is 0.21. The **partial pressure** of each gas in a mixture is that part of the total (e.g. barometric) pressure that is exerted by that gas, and is directly proportional to the quantity. Thus, according to **Dalton's law**, the partial pressure of O_2 (P_{O_2}) in dry air is F_{O_2} × barometric pressure (P_B), e.g. 0.21 × 101 kPa × 21.2 kPa. At the summit of Everest, P_B is ~34 kPa, but the relative proportions of gases are the same as at sea level, and so P_{O_2} is 0.21 × 34 kPa = 7.14 kPa.

Water vapour pressure. Water vapour behaves like any other gas, and exerts a partial pressure. The maximum or **saturated water vapour pressure (SWVP)** depends on the temperature: 2.33 kPa at 20 °C and 6.3 kPa at 37 °C. Inspired air quickly reaches body temperature and becomes fully humidified (100% saturated) in the airways. Water vapour dilutes the other gases, so that P_{N_2} and P_{O_2} will be lower than in dry air. Thus, P_{O_2} will be 0.21 × (P_B – saturated water vapour pressure) or, under these conditions, 0.21 × (101 – 6.3) = 19.9 kPa (Figure 30.1). The water vapour content of room air depends on the conditions (e.g. desert vs seaside); 40% humidity denotes 40% of the predicted SWVP for that temperature.

Standardization. From the above and Boyle's and Charles' laws, it should be clear that gas volumes and partial pressures cannot be compared unless corrected to a standardized pressure, temperature and humidity. Two standards are commonly used: standard temperature and pressure, dry gas (STPD), corrected to 1 standard atm (101 kPa), 0 °C and dry gas; and body temperature and pressure (1 atm), saturated with water (BTPS).

Gases dissolved in body fluids

The quantity of gas dissolving in a fluid is described by **Henry's law**: dissolved gas concentration = partial pressure of gas above fluid × **solubility** of that gas in that fluid. The solubility tends to decrease with a rise in temperature, and varies significantly between gases. For example, CO_2 is 20 times more soluble than O_2 in water, so that water exposed to the same partial pressures of CO_2 and O_2 will contain 20 times as much CO_2 as O_2. Henry's law describes an *equilibrium* – increasing the partial pressure of a gas will cause more to dissolve in the fluid until a new equilibrium is reached. The concept of a partial pressure of gas dissolved in a fluid (e.g. P_{O_2} of blood) is sometimes difficult to understand, but merely reflects the partial pressure that would be required to dissolve that amount of gas in the fluid, according to Henry's law. From the above, it can be deduced that the movement of gases between gas and fluid phases (e.g. alveolar air and capillary blood) will be dependent on the **difference in partial pressures** rather than the concentration. Typical values for partial pressures in the airways and blood are shown in Figure 30.2.

Diffusion across the alveolar–capillary membrane (Figure 30.3)

Diffusion is discussed in Chapter 12. The rate of gas flow across the alveolar–capillary membrane = permeability × area × (difference in partial pressures), where the permeability depends on the membrane thickness, gas molecular weight and its solubility in the membrane (Chapter 12). Although CO_2 is larger than O_2, it crosses the membrane faster because it is more soluble in biological membranes. For gas transfer across the lungs, the permeability and area are commonly combined as the **diffusing capacity (D_L)** for that gas, a measure of alveolar–capillary membrane function. Thus, the rate of O_2 transfer = $D_{L}O_2$ × (alveolar P_{O_2} – lung capillary P_{O_2}), or $D_{L}O_2$ = O_2 **uptake from lungs/(alveolar P_{O_2} – lung capillary P_{O_2})**. $D_{L}O_2$ is sometimes called the **transfer factor**. $D_{L}O_2$ cannot be estimated directly, because capillary P_{O_2} cannot be measured. However, the factors affecting O_2 diffusion also affect carbon monoxide (CO) diffusion. CO binds extremely strongly to haemoglobin, and so, if low concentrations of CO are inhaled, CO diffusing into the blood is completely bound to haemoglobin and capillary P_{CO} remains close to zero (Figure 30.3). Thus, $D_{L}CO$ = CO uptake from lungs/alveolar P_{CO}, and can be easily measured as an estimate of alveolar–capillary transfer function. $D_{L}CO$ is reduced by a decrease in lung exchange area (e.g. emphysema) or an increase in alveolar–capillary membrane thickness (e.g. lung fibrosis, oedema).

Diffusion and perfusion limitation (Figure 30.3)

Because CO binds so avidly and rapidly to haemoglobin, at low concentrations its rate of transfer into the blood is not affected by the blood flow, because there is always plenty of haemoglobin. It is thus limited solely by its rate of diffusion across the alveolar–capillary membrane, i.e. transfer is **diffusion limited**. For a poorly soluble gas, however (e.g. the anaesthetic nitrous oxide, N_2O), the partial pressure in the blood rapidly reaches equilibrium with alveolar air, preventing further diffusion. In this case, increased blood flow will increase the rate of transfer, i.e. transfer is **perfusion limited**. O_2 transfer is normally perfusion limited.

Carriage of oxygen and carbon dioxide by the blood

Figure 31.1 O_2 dissociation curve

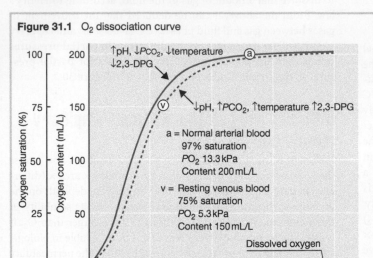

↑pH, ↓PCO$_2$, ↓temperature ↓2,3-DPG

↓pH, ↑PCO$_2$, ↑temperature ↑2,3-DPG

a = Normal arterial blood
97% saturation
PO_2 13.3 kPa
Content 200 mL/L

v = Resting venous blood
75% saturation
PO_2 5.3 kPa
Content 150 mL/L

Dissolved oxygen

Figure 31.2 Anaemia, CO poisoning, fetal haemoglobin (HbF)

HbF

Normal (150 g/L)

[Hb] 150 g/L; COHb 50%

Anaemia (75 g/L)

Figure 31.3 CO_2 dissociation curve

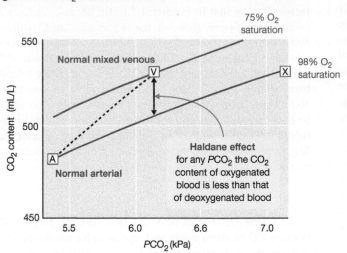

75% O_2 saturation

Normal mixed venous

98% O_2 saturation

Haldane effect
for any PCO$_2$ the CO_2
content of oxygenated
blood is less than that
of deoxygenated blood

Normal arterial

Figure 31.4 How CO_2 is carried in arterial and venous blood

Arterial	Venous
5% Carbamino	30%
87% HCO$_3^-$	60%
8% Dissolved	10%

48 mL CO_2/100 mL

52 mL CO_2/100 mL

Figure 31.5 CO_2 uptake and O_2 delivery in the tissues – role of red cells

Red cell

CO_2 → $CO_2 + H_2O$ →(CA)→ H_2CO_3 → $HCO_3^- + H^+$

Cl$^-$
HCO$_3^-$
Cl$^-$

Chloride shift

Hb

H_2O ← H_2O

Hb.O$_2$

Hb.COOH

Carbamino formation

O_2

CA = carbonic anhydrase
Hb = reduced haemoglobin
HbO$_2$ = oxygenated Hb

Physiology at a Glance, Fourth Edition. Edited by Jeremy P.T. Ward and Roger W.A. Linden.
© 2017 John Wiley & Sons, Ltd. Published 2017 by John Wiley & Sons, Ltd. Companion website: www.ataglanceseries.com/physiology

Oxygen

The resting O_2 consumption in adults is ~250 mL/min, rising to >4000 mL/min during heavy exercise. The O_2 **solubility** in plasma is, however, low and at a Po_2 of 13 kPa blood contains only 3 mL/L of dissolved O_2 in solution. Most O_2 is therefore carried bound to **haemoglobin** in red blood cells. Each gram of haemoglobin can combine with 1.34 mL of O_2 and so, for a haemoglobin concentration [Hb] of 150 g/L, blood can contain a maximum of 200 mL/L of O_2 (**O_2 capacity**). The actual amount of O_2 bound to haemoglobin (**O_2 content**) depends on the Po_2, and the **percentage O_2 saturation** = content/capacity × 100 (Figure 31.1). Each haemoglobin molecule binds up to four O_2 molecules; binding is **cooperative**, so that the binding of each O_2 molecule makes it easier for the next. This steepens the **O_2 haemoglobin dissociation curve**, which describes the relationship between blood O_2 content and Po_2 (Figure 31.1). The curve flattens above ~8 kPa Po_2 as all binding sites become occupied. Thus, for a normal arterial Po_2 (~13 kPa) and [Hb], the blood is ~97% saturated and contains slightly less than 200 mL/L of O_2. Because the dissociation curve is flat in this region, any increase in Po_2 (breathing O_2-enriched air) will have little effect on content. On the steep part of the curve, however (<8 kPa Po_2), small changes in Po_2 will have large effects on content.

Oxygen uptake and delivery. The high Po_2 in the lungs facilitates O_2 binding to haemoglobin, whereas the low Po_2 in the tissues encourages release. The dissociation curve is shifted to the right (reduced affinity, facilitating O_2 release) by a fall in pH, a rise in Pco_2 (**Bohr shift**) and an increase in temperature, which occur in active tissues (Figure 31.1). The metabolic by-product **2,3-diphosphoglycerate** (2,3-DPG) also causes a right shift. In the lungs, Pco_2 falls, the pH consequently rises and the temperature is reduced; these all increase affinity and shift the curve to the left, facilitating O_2 uptake.

Anaemia. This is an abnormally low [Hb]; the O_2 capacity is therefore less and the O_2 content at any Po_2 is reduced (Figure 31.2). Arterial Po_2 and O_2 saturation remain normal. In order to deliver the same amount of O_2 to the tissues, the capillary Po_2 would have to fall further than normal (Figure 31.2), reducing the driving force for O_2 diffusion into the tissues. The latter may become inadequate for metabolism, especially during exercise, although a 50% reduction in [Hb] does not usually cause symptoms at rest.

Carbon monoxide. Carbon monoxide (CO) binds 240 times more strongly than O_2 to haemoglobin and, by occupying O_2-binding sites, reduces the O_2 capacity. However, unlike anaemia, CO also increases the affinity and shifts the dissociation curve to the left, making O_2 release to the tissues more difficult. Thus, if 50% of haemoglobin is bound to CO, Po_2 needs to fall much further than in anaemia to release the same amount of O_2, causing symptoms of severe hypoxia (headache, convulsions, coma, death) (Figure 31.2).

Fetal haemoglobin. Fetal haemoglobin (HbF) binds 2,3-DPG less strongly than does adult haemoglobin (HbA), and so the dissociation curve is shifted to the left. This facilitates the transfer of O_2 from maternal blood to the fetus, where the arterial Po_2 is only ~5 kPa (Figure 31.2).

Carbon dioxide

CO_2 is formed in the tissues and transported to the lungs where it is expired. Blood can carry much more CO_2 than O_2, as can be seen in the **CO_2 dissociation curve** (Figure 31.3). This is also more linear than the O_2 dissociation curve and does not plateau. CO_2 is transported as **bicarbonate, carbamino compounds** and simply **dissolved** in plasma (Figure 31.4).

Bicarbonate. Approximately 60% of CO_2 is carried as bicarbonate. Water and CO_2 combine to form carbonic acid (H_2CO_3) and thence bicarbonate (HCO_3^-): $CO_2 + H_2O \Leftrightarrow H_2CO_3 \Leftrightarrow HCO_3^- + H^+$. The left side of the equation is normally slow, but speeds up dramatically in the presence of **carbonic anhydrase**, found in red cells. Bicarbonate is therefore formed preferentially in red cells, from which it easily diffuses out. Red cells are, however, impermeable to H^+ ions, and Cl^- enters the cell to maintain electrical neutrality (**chloride shift**) (Figure 31.5). H^+ binds avidly to **deoxygenated** (*reduced*) haemoglobin (haemoglobin acts as a buffer), and so there is little increase in $[H^+]$ to impede further bicarbonate formation. Oxygenated haemoglobin does not bind H^+ as well, and so in the lungs H^+ dissociates from haemoglobin and shifts the CO_2–HCO_3^- equation to the left, assisting CO_2 unloading from the blood (Figure 31.5); the reverse occurs in the tissues. This contributes to the **Haldane effect**, which states that, for any Pco_2, the CO_2 content of oxygenated blood is less than that of deoxygenated blood. Thus the red line A–X in Figure 31.3 shows the relationship between CO_2 content and Pco_2 if the blood remained 98% saturated with O_2. Mixed venous O_2 saturation is however ~75%, so as the blood becomes oxygenated in the lungs or deoxygenated in the tissues, the relationship between CO_2 content and Pco_2 actually follows the dashed line A–V.

Carbamino compounds. These compounds are formed by the reaction of CO_2 with protein amino groups: $CO_2 + protein-NH_2 \Leftrightarrow protein-NHCOOH$. The most prevalent protein in blood is haemoglobin, which forms **carbaminohaemoglobin** with CO_2. This occurs more readily for deoxygenated than oxygenated haemoglobin, contributing to the Haldane effect (Figure 31.3). Carbamino compounds account for 30% of CO_2 carriage.

Dissolved carbon dioxide. CO_2 is 20 times more soluble than O_2 in plasma, and ~10% of CO_2 in blood is carried in **solution**.

Hyperventilation and hypoventilation

Doubling the rate of ventilation halves the alveolar and arterial Pco_2. Ventilation is normally closely matched to the metabolic rate as reflected by CO_2 production (Chapter 32). **Hyperventilation** (overventilation) and **hypoventilation** (underventilation) are defined in terms of arterial Pco_2, so that a subject is *hyperventilating* when Pco_2 is <5.3 kPa, and hypoventilating when Pco_2 is >5.9 kPa. Rapid breathing in exercise is *not* hyperventilation, as this is appropriate for increased CO_2 production and Pco_2 does not fall. Hyperventilation cannot normally increase the O_2 content, as arterial haemoglobin is already nearly fully saturated. The fall in Pco_2 (**hypocapnia**) during hyperventilation causes light-headedness, visual disturbances due to cerebral vasoconstriction (Chapter 27) and muscle cramps (tetany). Hyperventilation can be caused by pain, hysteria and strong emotion. Hypoventilation causes a high Pco_2 (**hypercapnia**) and a low Po_2 (**hypoxia**), and may be caused by head injury or respiratory disease.

32 Control of breathing

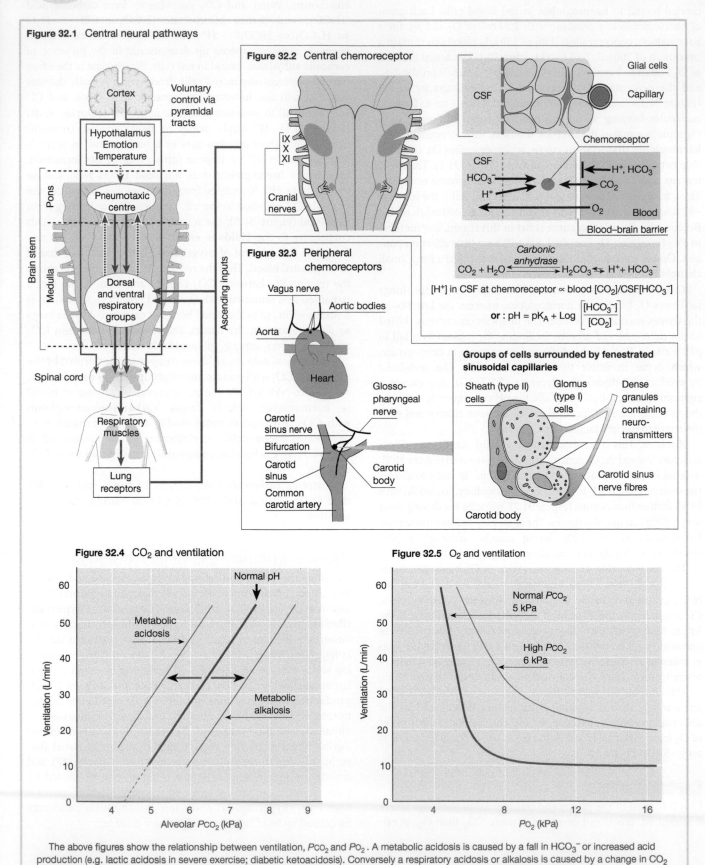

Figure 32.1 Central neural pathways

Cortex — Voluntary control via pyramidal tracts

Hypothalamus Emotion Temperature

Pons — Pneumotaxic centre

Brain stem

Medulla — Dorsal and ventral respiratory groups

Ascending inputs

Spinal cord

Respiratory muscles

Lung receptors

Figure 32.2 Central chemoreceptor

IX X XI

Cranial nerves

Glial cells

Capillary

CSF

Chemoreceptor

CSF
HCO₃⁻
H⁺

H⁺, HCO₃⁻
CO₂
O₂
Blood

Blood–brain barrier

$$CO_2 + H_2O \overset{\textit{Carbonic anhydrase}}{\rightleftharpoons} H_2CO_3 \rightleftharpoons H^+ + HCO_3^-$$

[H⁺] in CSF at chemoreceptor ∝ blood [CO₂]/CSF[HCO₃⁻]

$$or : pH = pK_A + Log \left[\frac{[HCO_3^-]}{[CO_2]}\right]$$

Figure 32.3 Peripheral chemoreceptors

Vagus nerve
Aortic bodies
Aorta
Heart

Glosso-pharyngeal nerve
Carotid sinus nerve
Bifurcation
Carotid sinus
Common carotid artery
Carotid body

Groups of cells surrounded by fenestrated sinusoidal capillaries

Sheath (type II) cells
Glomus (type I) cells
Dense granules containing neuro-transmitters
Carotid sinus nerve fibres
Carotid body

Figure 32.4 CO₂ and ventilation

Normal pH
Metabolic acidosis
Metabolic alkalosis

Ventilation (L/min) vs Alveolar PCO₂ (kPa)

Figure 32.5 O₂ and ventilation

Normal PCO₂ 5 kPa
High PCO₂ 6 kPa

Ventilation (L/min) vs PO₂ (kPa)

The above figures show the relationship between ventilation, P_{CO_2} and P_{O_2}. A metabolic acidosis is caused by a fall in HCO_3^- or increased acid production (e.g. lactic acidosis in severe exercise; diabetic ketoacidosis). Conversely a respiratory acidosis or alkalosis is caused by a change in CO_2

Physiology at a Glance, Fourth Edition. Edited by Jeremy P.T. Ward and Roger W.A. Linden.
© 2017 John Wiley & Sons, Ltd. Published 2017 by John Wiley & Sons, Ltd. Companion website: www.ataglanceseries.com/physiology

Ventilation of the lungs provides O_2 for the tissues and removes CO_2. Breathing must therefore be closely matched to metabolism for adequate O_2 delivery and to prevent a build-up of CO_2. A **central pattern generator** in the brain stem sets the basic rhythm and pattern of ventilation and controls the respiratory muscles. It is modulated by higher centres and feedback from **sensors**, including **chemoreceptors** and **lung mechanoreceptors** (Figure 32.1). The neural networks are complex, as breathing must be coordinated with coughing, swallowing and speech. Control of breathing in exercise is not straightforward.

The brain stem and central pattern generator

The brain stem includes diffuse groups of respiratory neurones in the **pons** and **medulla** that act together as the central pattern generator (Figure 32.1); it is unclear whether there is a single pacemaker region. Some neurones only show activity during inspiration or expiration, and these exhibit **reciprocal inhibition**, i.e. inspiration inhibits expiration and *vice versa*. The medulla contains **dorsal** and **ventral respiratory groups** that receive input from the chemoreceptors and lung receptors and drive the respiratory muscle motor neurones (intercostals, phrenic [diaphragm], abdominal). The medullary respiratory groups also provide ascending input to and receive descending input from the **pneumotaxic centre** in the pons, which is critical for normal breathing. The pneumotaxic centre receives input from the hypothalamus and higher centres, coordinates medullary homeostatic functions with factors such as emotion and temperature, and affects the pattern of breathing. Voluntary control is mediated by cortical motor neurones in the **pyramidal tract**, which bypasses the respiratory neurones in the brainstem.

Chemoreception

Chemoreceptors detect arterial P_{CO_2}, P_{O_2} and pH – P_{CO_2} is the most important. Alveolar P_{CO_2} ($P_A{CO_2}$) is normally ~5.3 kPa (40 mmHg), and $P_A{O_2}$ normally 13 kPa (100 mmHg). An increase in $P_A{CO_2}$ causes ventilation to rise in an almost linear fashion (Figure 32.4). Increased acidity of the blood (e.g. lactic acidosis in severe exercise) causes the relationship between P_{CO_2} and ventilation to shift to the left, and decreased acidity causes a shift to the right. Conversely, P_{O_2} normally stimulates ventilation only when it falls below ~8 kPa (~60 mmHg) (Figure 32.5). However, when a fall in P_{O_2} is accompanied by an increase in P_{CO_2}, the resultant increase in ventilation is greater than would be expected from adding the effects of either alone; there is thus a **synergistic** (more than additive) relationship between P_{O_2} and P_{CO_2} (Figure 32.5).

The **central chemoreceptor** comprises a collection of neurones near the ventrolateral surface of the medulla, close to the exit of the cranial nerves IX and X (Figure 32.2). It responds *indirectly* to blood P_{CO_2}, but does **not** respond to changes in P_{O_2}. Although CO_2 can easily diffuse across the **blood–brain barrier** from the blood into the cerebrospinal fluid (CSF), H^+ and HCO_3^- cannot. As a result, the pH of the CSF around the chemoreceptor is determined by the arterial P_{CO_2} and CSF $[HCO_3^-]$, according to the Henderson–Hasselbalch equation (Figure 32.2). A rise in blood P_{CO_2} therefore makes the CSF more acid; this is detected by the chemoreceptor, which increases ventilation to blow off CO_2. The central chemoreceptor is responsible for ~80% of the response to CO_2 in humans. Its response is delayed because CO_2 has to diffuse across the blood–brain barrier. As the blood–brain barrier is impermeable to H^+, the central chemoreceptor is not affected by blood pH.

The **peripheral chemoreceptors** are located in the carotid and aortic bodies (Figure 32.3). The **carotid bodies** are small distinct structures located at the bifurcation of the common carotid arteries, and are innervated by the carotid sinus nerve and thence the glossopharyngeal nerve. The carotid body is formed from **glomus** (type I) and **sheath** (type II) cells. Glomus cells are chemoreceptive, contain neurotransmitter-rich dense granules and contact carotid sinus nerve axons. The **aortic bodies** are located on the aortic arch and are innervated by the vagus. They are similar to carotid bodies but functionally less important. Peripheral chemoreceptors respond to changes in P_{CO_2}, H^+ and, importantly, P_{O_2}. They are responsible for ~20% of the response to increased P_{CO_2}.

Lung receptors

Various types of lung receptor provide feedback from the lungs to the respiratory centre. In addition, **pain** often causes brief apnoea (cessation of breathing) followed by rapid breathing, and **mechanical** or **noxious** stimulation of receptors in the trigeminal region and larynx causes apnoea or spasm of the larynx.

Stretch receptors. These are located in the bronchial walls. Stimulation (by stretch) causes short, shallow breaths, and delay of the next inspiratory cycle. They provide negative feedback to turn off inspiration. They are mostly **slowly adapting** (continue to fire with sustained stimulation) and are innervated by the vagus. They are largely responsible for the **Hering–Breuer inspiratory reflex**, in which lung inflation inhibits inspiration to prevent overinflation.

Juxtapulmonary (J) receptors. These are located on the alveolar and bronchial walls close to the capillaries. They cause depression of somatic and visceral activity by producing rapid shallow breathing or apnoea, a fall in heart rate and blood pressure, laryngeal constriction and relaxation of the skeletal muscles via spinal neurones. They are stimulated by increased alveolar wall fluid, oedema, microembolisms and inflammation. The afferent nerves are small unmyelinated (C-fibre) or myelinated nerves in the vagus.

Irritant receptors. These are located throughout the airways between epithelial cells. In the trachea they cause cough, and in the lower airways hyperpnoea (rapid breathing); stimulation also causes bronchial and laryngeal constriction. They are also responsible for the deep augmented breaths every 5–20 min at rest, reversing the slow collapse of the lungs that occurs in quiet breathing, and may be involved in the first deep gasps of the newborn. They are stimulated by irritant gases, smoke and dust, rapid large inflations and deflations, airway deformation, pulmonary congestion and inflammation. The afferent nerves are rapidly adapting myelinated fibres in the vagus.

Proprioceptors (position/length sensors). These are located in the Golgi tendon organs, muscle spindles and joints. They are important for matching increased load, and maintaining optimal tidal volume and frequency. They are stimulated by shortening and load in the respiratory muscles (but not diaphragm). Afferents run to the spinal cord via the dorsal roots. It should be noted that input from non-respiratory muscles and joints can also stimulate breathing.

33 Ventilation–perfusion matching and right to left shunts

Figure 33.1 Different types of V_A/Q mismatching

	Normal	Dead space	Dead space effect	Shunt effect	True/anatomical shunt
	V_A = Normal Q = Normal V_A/Q = ~1	V_A = Normal Q = 0 V_A/Q = ∞	V_A = Normal Q = Low V_A/Q = High	V_A = Low Q = Normal V_A/Q = Low	V_A = 0 Q = Normal V_A/Q = 0
		(No perfusion)			(No ventilation)
Blood gases in outflow	PO_2 = normal PCO_2 = normal O_2 content = normal CO_2 content = normal		PO_2 = ↑ PCO_2 = ↓ O_2 content = normal CO_2 content = ↓	PO_2 = ↓ PCO_2 = ↑ O_2 content = ↓ CO_2 content = ↑	PO_2 = ↓ PCO_2 = ↑ O_2 content = ↓ CO_2 content = ↑
Effect of ↑O₂ in inspired air	PO_2 = ↑ O_2 content = nil		PO_2 = ↑ O_2 content = nil	PO_2 = ↑ O_2 content = ↑	PO_2 = nil O_2 content = nil

Figure 33.2 The effect of mixture of high and low V_A/Q regions on arterial blood gases

Small flow with:
High PO_2
Normal O_2 content
Low PCO_2
Low CO_2 content

$\dot{V}_A$ = 4
$\dot{V}_A/\dot{Q}$ = 4
Q = 1

$\dot{V}_A$ = 5
$\dot{V}_A/\dot{Q}$ = 0.3
$\dot{Q}$ = 15

Large flow with:
Low PO_2
Low O_2 content
High PCO_2
High CO_2 content

Combined to give:
Low O_2 content
High CO_2 content
Low PO_2
Slightly high PCO_2

Peripheral and central chemoreceptors

↑Ventilation

Final picture:
Low O_2 content
Normal or low CO_2 content
Low PO_2
Normal or low PCO_2

Figure 33.3 Consequences of right to left shunt on arterial blood gases

O_2 and CO_2 dissociation curves

● Normal
○ With right to left shunt

O_2 and CO_2 content (mL/L)

PO_2/PCO_2 (kPa)

Physiology at a Glance, Fourth Edition. Edited by Jeremy P.T. Ward and Roger W.A. Linden.
© 2017 John Wiley & Sons, Ltd. Published 2017 by John Wiley & Sons, Ltd. Companion website: www.ataglanceseries.com/physiology

Ventilation–perfusion matching (Figure 33.1)

At rest, total alveolar ventilation (V_A) is similar to total pulmonary capillary perfusion (Q), or about 5 L/min. For optimal gas exchange, all regions of the lung should ideally have a **ventilation–perfusion ratio** (V_A/Q) of unity. When there are variations significantly away from unity, either lower or higher, this is referred to as **ventilation–perfusion mismatch**. In a **right to left shunt** (see later), for example, ventilation is zero and V_A/Q = ∞; whereas when an embolism blocks a pulmonary artery, perfusion in the part of the lung fed by that artery is zero, and V_A/Q = 0. Regions of the lung that have a V_A/Q value much greater than unity have excessive ventilation, and blood derived from them will have a high Po_2 and a low Pco_2 (**dead space effect**). Regions with a V_A/Q value much less than unity have a **shunt** or **venous admixture** effect; there is some gas exchange, but the blood has a lower than normal Po_2 and a higher than normal Pco_2.

Effect of ventilation–perfusion mismatch on arterial gases. Regions of high V_A/Q cannot compensate for regions of low V_A/Q. This is because of the way in which O_2 is carried in the blood (Chapter 31). Although regions of high V_A/Q produce blood with a high Po_2, this does not translate to any significant increase in O_2 content, as the haemoglobin in the blood is already close to saturation at the normal Po_2. Conversely, blood derived from regions with a low V_A/Q, especially if Po_2 < 8 kPa, will have a significantly reduced O_2 content (Figure 33.2). Regions of high V_A/Q are also most usually due to insufficient perfusion, so that the amount of blood, and therefore O_2, that such regions contribute to the total will be relatively small. As a result, the combined blood from regions with high and low V_A/Q will have a low O_2 content and a low Po_2, even if total ventilation and perfusion are matched for the whole lung.

The CO_2 content is less severely affected, because overventilated areas can lose extra CO_2 and partly compensate for underventilated areas. Moreover, a rise in Pco_2 will stimulate breathing via the chemoreceptors, allowing CO_2 to be corrected, or even overcorrected if Po_2 is sufficiently low (Chapter 32). Significant V_A/Q mismatching will therefore usually result in arterial blood with a low Po_2 but normal or low Pco_2 (Figure 33.2). Ventilation with O_2-enriched air will improve oxygenation in regions of low V_A/Q, but is not useful for shunts, as the enriched air never reaches the shunted blood. **Hypoxic pulmonary vasoconstriction** (Chapter 27) reduces the severity of V_A/Q mismatch by diverting blood from the affected region to well-ventilated areas.

Effect of gravity

The blood pressure at the base of the lungs is greater than that at the apex (top) because of the weight of the column of blood.

This increased pressure distends the pulmonary blood vessels at the base and the flow is therefore increased. Conversely, blood flow at the apex may be reduced if the pulmonary venous pressure falls below the alveolar pressure, when the vessels will be compressed. The net result is that, on standing, pulmonary blood flow falls progressively on moving from the bottom of the lung to the top.

Gravity also affects the intrapleural pressure, which is thus less negative at the base of the lung than at the apex. Alveoli at the base are therefore less expanded at functional residual capacity, and thus have more potential for expansion during inspiration. As a result, ventilation is greatest at the base of the lung. Although the effects of gravity on perfusion and ventilation partly cancel each other out, ventilation is less affected than perfusion, so that V_A/Q is highest at the apex of the lung and lowest at the base. In the young, this relatively small variation has little effect on blood gases, but in the elderly, it may contribute to a low Po_2.

Right to left shunts

Part of the venous effluent of the bronchial and coronary circulations bypasses the lungs and enters the pulmonary vein and left ventricle, respectively (Chapter 19). Oxygenated blood from the lungs is therefore diluted by venous blood. These are **anatomical right to left shunts** and account for <2% of cardiac output in healthy individuals. Larger shunts can occur in disease when regions of the lung are not ventilated (e.g. lung collapse, pneumonia), or due to **congenital heart malformations**. When calculating the effects of right to left shunts on arterial blood, the blood **content** of O_2 and CO_2 needs to be considered. For a 20% shunt, the 80% of blood passing through the lungs will have normal arterial O_2 and CO_2 contents of 200 and 480 mL/L, respectively, whilst the 20% bypassing the lungs will have normal venous values of 150 and 520 mL/L, respectively. On combination, the blood will contain (200 × 0.8) + (150 × 0.2) = 190 mL/L of O_2, and (480 × 0.8) + (520 × 0.2) = 488 mL/L of CO_2. From the dissociation curves (Figure 33.3), it can be seen that this results in a fall in Po_2 from 13 to 9 kPa, whereas Pco_2 rises only marginally from 5.3 to 5.5 kPa because of the steeper curve. Changes in Pco_2 and Po_2 stimulate the chemoreceptors and increase ventilation (Chapter 32), so that arterial Pco_2 returns to normal. However, increased ventilation cannot increase blood O_2 content, as the haemoglobin of the blood passing through the lungs is already close to saturation. Thus, right to left shunts commonly result in a *low arterial Po_2* but a *normal or low Pco_2*.

The renal system

Part 5

Chapters

34 Introduction to the renal system

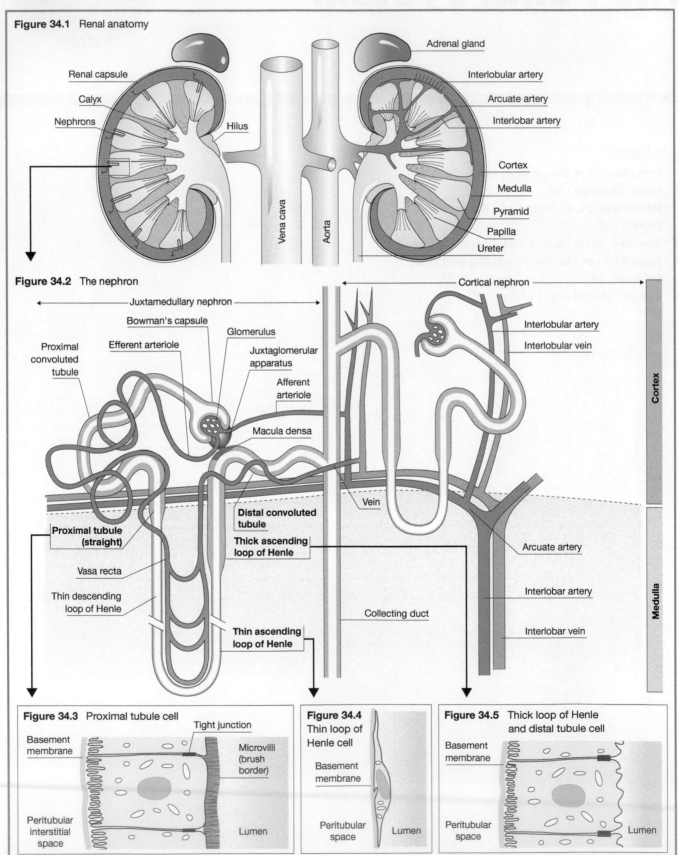

Figure 34.1 Renal anatomy

- Renal capsule
- Calyx
- Nephrons
- Hilus
- Adrenal gland
- Interlobular artery
- Arcuate artery
- Interlobar artery
- Cortex
- Medulla
- Pyramid
- Papilla
- Ureter
- Vena cava
- Aorta

Figure 34.2 The nephron

- Juxtamedullary nephron
- Cortical nephron
- Bowman's capsule
- Glomerulus
- Proximal convoluted tubule
- Efferent arteriole
- Juxtaglomerular apparatus
- Afferent arteriole
- Interlobular artery
- Interlobular vein
- Macula densa
- Cortex
- **Proximal tubule (straight)**
- **Distal convoluted tubule**
- **Thick ascending loop of Henle**
- Vein
- Vasa recta
- Arcuate artery
- Thin descending loop of Henle
- Collecting duct
- Interlobar artery
- **Thin ascending loop of Henle**
- Interlobar vein
- Medulla

Figure 34.3 Proximal tubule cell

- Basement membrane
- Tight junction
- Microvilli (brush border)
- Peritubular interstitial space
- Lumen

Figure 34.4 Thin loop of Henle cell

- Basement membrane
- Peritubular space
- Lumen

Figure 34.5 Thick loop of Henle and distal tubule cell

- Basement membrane
- Peritubular space
- Lumen

Physiology at a Glance, Fourth Edition. Edited by Jeremy P.T. Ward and Roger W.A. Linden.
© 2017 John Wiley & Sons, Ltd. Published 2017 by John Wiley & Sons, Ltd. Companion website: www.ataglanceseries.com/physiology

The kidneys help to maintain the composition of extracellular body fluids, and regulate ions (e.g. Na^+, K^+, Ca^{2+}, Mg^{2+}), acid–base status and body water. They also have an endocrine function. Plasma is **filtered** by capillaries in the **glomerulus** (Chapter 35), and the composition of the filtrate is modified by **reabsorption** and **secretion** in the nephrons. The average urine output is ~1.5 L per day, although this can fall to <1 L per day and increase to nearly 20 L per day.

Gross structure

The kidneys are located on each side of the vertebral column, behind the peritoneum. The renal artery and vein, lymphatics and nerve enter the kidney via the **hilus**, from which the **renal pelvis**, which becomes the **ureter**, emerges (Figure 34.1). The kidney is surrounded by a fibrous **renal capsule**. Internally, the kidney has a dark outer **cortex** surrounding a lighter **medulla**, which contains triangular lobes or **pyramids**. The cortex contains the **glomerulus** and **proximal** and **distal tubules** of the **nephrons**, whilst the **loop of Henle** and **collecting ducts** descend into the medulla (Figure 34.2). Each kidney contains ~800 000 nephrons. The collecting ducts converge in the **papilla** at the apex of each pyramid, and empty into the **calyx** (plural: *calyces*) and thence renal pelvis. Urine is propelled through the ureter into the **bladder** by peristalsis.

The nephron

Each **nephron** begins with a capsule (**Bowman's capsule**) surrounding the glomerular capillaries, which collects filtrate (Figure 34.1), followed by the **proximal tubule**, **loop of Henle**, **distal tubule** and early **collecting duct** (Figure 34.2). There are two types of nephron – those with glomeruli in the outer 70% of the cortex and short loops of Henle (**cortical nephrons**: ~85%), and those with glomeruli close to the cortex–medulla boundary and long loops of Henle (**juxtamedullary nephrons**: ~15%).

The **glomerulus** produces **ultrafiltrate** from plasma (Chapter 35).

The **proximal tubule** is convoluted when it leaves the Bowman's capsule, but straightens before becoming the descending limb of the loop of Henle in the medulla. Its walls are formed from *columnar epithelial* cells with a **brush-border** of *microvilli* on the luminal surface that increases the surface area ~40-fold (Figure 34.3). **Tight junctions** close to the luminal side limit diffusion through gaps between cells. The basal or peritubular side of the cells shows considerable *interdigitation*, which increases the surface area. The term **lateral intercellular space** is often used to describe the space between the interdigitations and basement membrane, and between the bases of adjacent cells. The main function of the proximal tubule is **reabsorption** (Chapter 36).

The thin part of the **loop of Henle** is formed from thin, flat (*squamous*) cells (Figure 34.4), with no microvilli. The **thick ascending loop of Henle** has columnar epithelial cells similar to the proximal tubule, but with few microvilli (Figure 34.5). At the point at which the loop associates with the **juxtaglomerular apparatus** (Chapter 38), after re-entering the cortex, the wall is formed from modified **macula densa** cells (Figure 34.2). The loop of Henle is important for the production of concentrated urine.

The **distal tubule** is functionally similar to the **cortical collecting duct**. Both contain cells similar to those in the thick ascending loop of Henle (Figure 34.5). In the collecting duct, these **principal cells** are interspersed with **intercalated cells** of different morphology and function; these play a role in acid–base balance (Chapter 39). The collecting duct plays an important role in water homeostasis (Chapter 38).

Renal circulation

The kidneys receive ~20% of cardiac output. The renal artery enters via the hilus and divides into **interlobar arteries** running between the pyramids to the cortex–medulla boundary, where they split into **arcuate arteries**. **Interlobular arteries** ascend into the cortex, and feed the **afferent arterioles** of the glomerulus (Figures 34.1 and 34.2). The capillaries of the glomerulus are the site of **filtration**, and drain into the **efferent arteriole** (*not* vein). Afferent and efferent arterioles provide the major resistance to renal blood flow. Efferent arterioles branch into a network of capillaries in the cortex around the proximal and distal tubules (**peritubular capillaries**). Capillaries close to the cortex– medulla boundary loop into the medulla to form the **vasa recta** surrounding the loop of Henle; this provides the only blood supply to the medulla. All capillaries drain into the renal veins. Ninety per cent of the blood entering the kidney supplies the cortex, giving a high blood flow (~500 mL/min/100 g) and a low arteriovenous O_2 difference (~2%). Medullary blood flow is less (20–100 mL/min/100 g).

Regulation of renal blood flow. Differential constriction of afferent and efferent arterioles strongly affects filtration (see previously; Chapter 35). The kidneys exhibit a high degree of **autoregulation** (Figure 34.5), both by the **myogenic** response (Chapter 27) and via the macula densa, which detects high filtration rates and releases adenosine, which constricts afferent arterioles, so reducing filtration. Noradrenaline (norepinephrine) from renal sympathetic nerves constricts both afferent and efferent arterioles, and increases renin and thus the production of angiotensin II (a potent vasoconstrictor) (Chapter 38). Many peripheral vasoconstrictors (e.g. endothelin, angiotensin II) cause the release of vasodilating prostaglandins in the kidney, so protecting renal blood flow.

Hormones and the kidney

Renal function is affected by a variety of hormones that modulate the regulation of ions and water (e.g. **antidiuretic hormone**, **aldosterone**). **Renin** is produced by the juxtaglomerular apparatus and promotes the formation of angiotensin (Chapter 38). **Erythropoietin** is synthesized by interstitial cells in the cortex, and stimulates red cell production (Chapter 9). **Vitamin D** is metabolized in the kidney to its active form (**1,25-dihydroxycholecalciferol**), which is involved in Ca^{2+} and phosphate regulation (Chapters 37 and 51). Various **prostaglandins** are also produced in the kidney, and affect renal blood flow.

Micturition

The constriction of smooth muscle in the bladder wall (**detrusor** muscle) expels urine through the **urethra** (**micturition**, urination). Micturition is initiated by a spinal reflex when urine pressure reaches a critical level, but is strongly controlled by higher (voluntary) centres. The neck of the bladder forms the **internal urethral sphincter**; the **external sphincter** is formed from voluntary skeletal muscle around more distal regions of the urethra.

35 Renal filtration

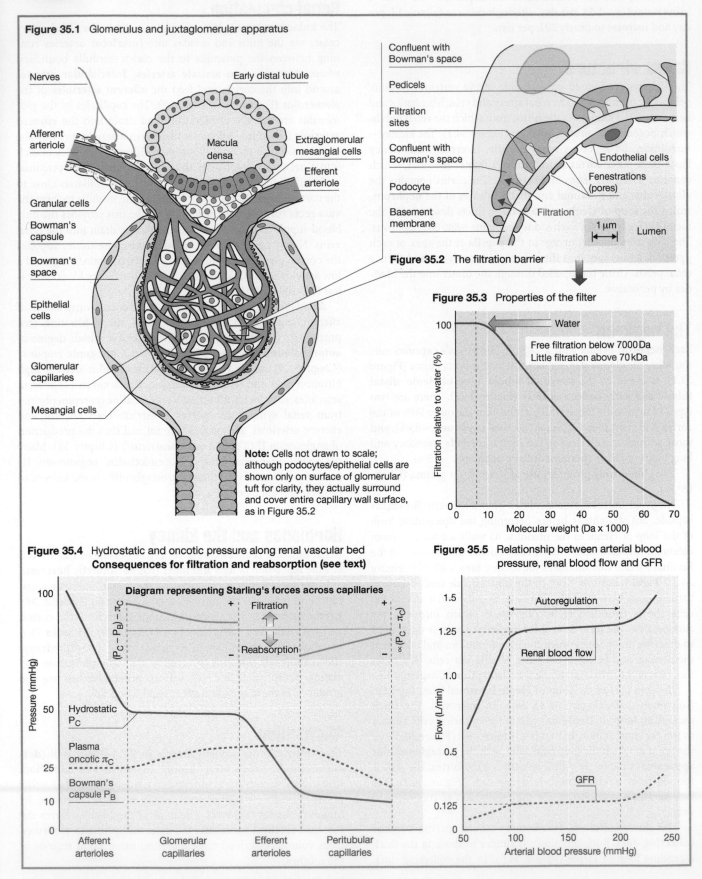

Figure 35.1 Glomerulus and juxtaglomerular apparatus

Nerves
Early distal tubule
Afferent arteriole
Macula densa
Extraglomerular mesangial cells
Efferent arteriole
Granular cells
Bowman's capsule
Bowman's space
Epithelial cells
Glomerular capillaries
Mesangial cells

Note: Cells not drawn to scale; although podocytes/epithelial cells are shown only on surface of glomerular tuft for clarity, they actually surround and cover entire capillary wall surface, as in Figure 35.2

Figure 35.2 The filtration barrier

Confluent with Bowman's space
Pedicels
Filtration sites
Confluent with Bowman's space
Podocyte
Basement membrane
Endothelial cells
Fenestrations (pores)
Filtration
1 µm
Lumen

Figure 35.3 Properties of the filter

Filtration relative to water (%)

Water

Free filtration below 7000 Da
Little filtration above 70 kDa

Molecular weight (Da x 1000)

Figure 35.4 Hydrostatic and oncotic pressure along renal vascular bed
Consequences for filtration and reabsorption (see text)

Diagram representing Starling's forces across capillaries

$(P_C - P_B) - \pi_C$
Filtration
Reabsorption
$\propto (P_C - \pi_C)$

Pressure (mmHg)

Hydrostatic P_C
Plasma oncotic π_C
Bowman's capsule P_B

Afferent arterioles
Glomerular capillaries
Efferent arterioles
Peritubular capillaries

Figure 35.5 Relationship between arterial blood pressure, renal blood flow and GFR

Flow (L/min)

Autoregulation

Renal blood flow

GFR

Arterial blood pressure (mmHg)

Physiology at a Glance, Fourth Edition. Edited by Jeremy P.T. Ward and Roger W.A. Linden.
© 2017 John Wiley & Sons, Ltd. Published 2017 by John Wiley & Sons, Ltd. Companion website: www.ataglanceseries.com/physiology

The structure of the **glomerulus** is shown in Figure 35.1. The walls of the afferent arteriole are associated with *granular cells* that produce **renin** (Chapter 38); there are numerous sympathetic nerve endings. The tuft of glomerular capillaries is surrounded by **Bowman's capsule**, the inner surface of which and the capillaries are covered by specialized epithelial cells (**podocytes**; see below). The glomerulus is interspersed with **mesangial** cells which are **phagocytic** (engulf large molecules) and **contractile**; contraction may limit the filtration area and alter filtration. Mesangial cells are also found between the capsule and **macula densa** (*extraglomerular mesangial cells*; Figure 35.1).

Glomerular filtration

Plasma is filtered in the glomerulus by **ultrafiltration** (i.e. works at the molecular level), and filtrate passes into the proximal tubule. The **glomerular filtration rate** (GFR) is ~125 mL/min in humans. The renal *plasma* flow is ~600 mL/min, so that the proportion of plasma that filters into the nephron (**filtration fraction**) is ~20%. Fluid and solutes have to pass three filtration barriers (Figure 35.2):

1 The **glomerular capillary endothelium**, which is approximately 50 times more permeable than in most tissues because it is **fenestrated** with small (70 nm) pores (Chapter 26).
2 A specialized capillary **basement membrane** containing negatively charged glycoproteins, which is thought to be the main site of ultrafiltration.
3 Modified epithelial cells (**podocytes**) with long extensions (*primary processes*) that engulf the capillaries and have numerous foot-like processes (**pedicels**) directly contacting the basement membrane. The regular gaps between pedicles are called **filtration slits**, and restrict large molecules. Podocytes maintain the basement membrane and, like mesangial cells, may be phagocytic and partially contractile.

The permeability of the filtration barrier is dependent on the molecular size. Substances with molecular weights of <7000 Da pass freely, but larger molecules are increasingly restricted up to 70 000 Da, above which filtration is insignificant (Figure 35.3). Negatively charged molecules are further restricted as they are repelled by negative charges in the basement membrane. Thus, albumin (~69 000 Da), which is also negatively charged, is filtered in minute quantities, whereas small molecules such as ions, glucose, amino acids and urea pass the filter without hindrance. This means that the glomerular filtrate is almost protein free, but otherwise has an identical composition to plasma.

Factors determining the glomerular filtration rate

GFR is dependent on the difference between the **hydrostatic** and **oncotic** (colloidal osmotic, due to proteins) pressures in the glomerular capillaries and Bowman's capsule, as determined by **Starling's equation** (Chapter 26). The glomerular capillary pressure (P_c) is greater than that elsewhere (~45 mmHg) because of the unique arrangement of afferent and efferent arterioles, and low afferent but high efferent resistances. As the pressure in Bowman's capsule (P_B) is ~10 mmHg, the net hydrostatic force driving filtration is (P_c – P_B) or ~35 mmHg. This is opposed by the oncotic pressure of capillary plasma (π_c; ~25 mmHg); the filtrate oncotic pressure is essentially zero (no protein). Thus, GFR $\propto$ (P_c – P_B) – π_c (Figure 35.4). It should be noted that, because the filtration fraction is appreciable (~20%) and proteins are not filtered, the plasma protein concentration and thus π_c will rise as blood traverses the glomerulus, reducing (*but not abolishing*) filtration. In peritubular capillaries, where the hydrostatic pressure is very low, this increase in π_c promotes reabsorption (Figure 35.4).

GFR is therefore strongly dependent on the relative resistance of afferent and efferent arterioles, which is influenced by sympathetic tone and other vasoactive agents. GFR is constant over a wide range of blood pressure (90–200 mmHg) because of the **autoregulation** of renal blood flow (Figure 35.5; Chapter 27). Renal disease, circulating and local vasoconstrictors, and sympathetic activation all reduce GFR, although angiotensin II preferentially constricts *efferent* arterioles, and thus increases GFR (Chapter 38), or rather helps maintain it if blood pressure falls.

Measurement of the glomerular filtration rate and the concept of clearance

If substance X is freely filtered and neither reabsorbed nor secreted in the nephron, the amount appearing in the urine per minute must equal the amount filtered per minute. Thus, if the plasma concentration of X is C_p and the urine concentration is C_u, and the volume of urine passed per minute is V, then $C_p \times$ GFR = $C_u \times$ V, or **GFR = ($C_u \times$ V)/C_p**.

Creatinine, which is steadily released from skeletal muscle, is often used for clinical measurements of GFR because it is freely filtered and not reabsorbed; there is a little secretion, but this introduces only a small error, except when plasma creatinine or GFR is abnormally low. More accurate measurements are made by infusing the polysaccharide **inulin**, which is neither reabsorbed nor secreted.

This is known as a **clearance method**. The term **clearance** can be confusing, as it does not refer to what actually happens but is merely a way of looking at how the kidney deals with a substance. It is defined as the volume of plasma that would need to be completely cleared of a substance per minute in order to produce the amount found in the urine, or: **clearance = ($C_u \times$ V)/C_p** (i.e. the same equation as above). Thus, the **clearance of inulin is equal to GFR**. If a substance is reabsorbed in the nephron, its clearance will be less than the GFR and, if it is secreted, it will be greater than the GFR. Some substances that are normally completely reabsorbed have zero clearance until the reabsorption mechanism becomes saturated (e.g. glucose; Chapter 36).

The **renal plasma flow** (RPF) can be measured in a similar fashion by infusing *para*-**aminohippuric acid** (PAH) which at low concentrations is completely removed from renal blood by both filtration and secretion, so that none remains in the venous outflow. The amount appearing in the urine must therefore equal the amount entering the kidney, and thus the **clearance of PAH is equal to RPF**. The filtration fraction (GFR/RPF; see previously) can therefore be estimated from inulin clearance/PAH clearance. The renal blood flow is equal to RPF/(1 – haematocrit).

36 Reabsorption, secretion and the proximal tubule

Figure 36.1 Transport mechanisms in the proximal tubule

NB. cell morphology simplified (see Figure 34.3)

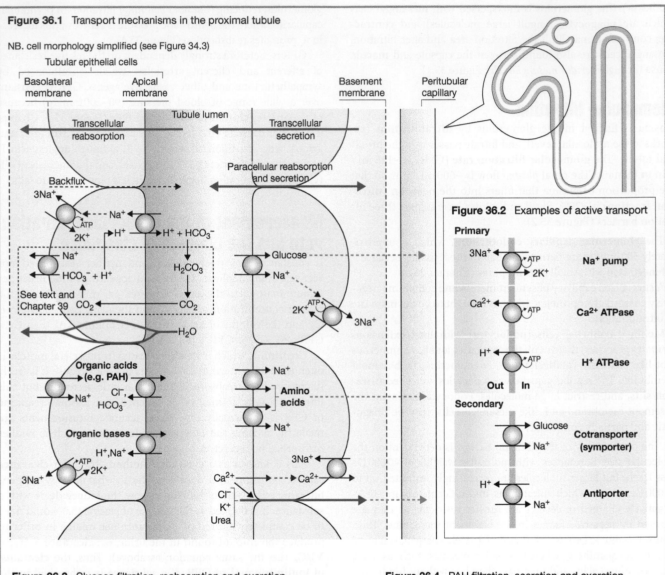

Figure 36.2 Examples of active transport

Figure 36.3 Glucose filtration, reabsorption and excretion

Glucose is normally completely reabsorbed in the proximal tubule but when plasma concentration rises above threshold, glucosetransport saturates as the T_m is reached, and no further reabsorption can occur. Excretion then parallels filtration.

Figure 36.4 PAH filtration, secretion and excretion

Below a plasma concentration of 80 mg/L PAH is almost completely removed from renal blood by filtration and secretion. Above ~100 mg/L the secretory mechanisms saturate as T_m is reached and further excretion is due only to filtration.

Physiology at a Glance, Fourth Edition. Edited by Jeremy P.T. Ward and Roger W.A. Linden.
© 2017 John Wiley & Sons, Ltd. Published 2017 by John Wiley & Sons, Ltd. Companion website: www.ataglanceseries.com/physiology

In a healthy adult, ~180 L of filtrate enters the proximal tubules daily. A significant component must be reabsorbed to prevent the loss of water and solutes. The filtrate is progressively modified as it passes through the nephron by the **reabsorption** of substances into the blood and **secretion** into the tubular fluid. The net reabsorption or secretion of any substance can be determined from its **clearance** (Chapter 35).

Tubular transport processes

Reabsorption and secretion involve the transport of substances across the tubular epithelium; this occurs either by diffusion through tight junctions and lateral intercellular spaces (**paracellular** pathway), driven by concentration, osmotic or electrical gradients, or by **active transport** through the epithelial cells themselves (**transcellular** pathways) (Figure 36.1). The latter usually involves an active process on either the apical or basolateral cell membrane, with passive diffusion across the opposite membrane driven by the concentration gradient so created. The movement of solutes between the peritubular space and capillaries is by **bulk flow and diffusion** (Chapter 12); the movement of water is influenced by **Starling's forces** (Chapter 26).

Active transport involves proteins called **transporters** that translocate substances across the cell membrane (Figure 36.2; Chapter 4). **Primary active transport** uses adenosine triphosphate (ATP) directly, e.g. the **Na$^+$–K$^+$ ATPase** (Na$^+$ pump). **Secondary active transport** uses the concentration gradient created by primary active transport as an energy source. This is most commonly the Na$^+$ gradient created by the *Na$^+$ pump*, and the latter therefore plays a critical role in renal reabsorption and secretion. **Symporters** (or *cotransporters*) transport substances in the same direction as (for example) Na$^+$, whereas **antiporters** transport in the opposite direction (Chapter 4; Figure 36.2).

The rate of *diffusion* across cell membranes is enhanced by **ion channels** and **uniporters** (transporters carrying only one substance), which effectively increase membrane permeability to specific substances; this is termed **facilitated diffusion**, and may be modulated by hormones or drugs.

Tubular transport maximum

There is a limit to the rate at which any transporter can operate, and so, for any substance, there is a maximum rate of reabsorption or secretion, called the **tubular transport maximum (T$_m$)**. For example, glucose is normally completely reabsorbed in the proximal tubule and none is excreted in the urine (see later). However, when the filtrate glucose concentration rises above the **renal threshold**, the transporters start to **saturate**, and glucose appears in the urine (Figure 36.3). Once T$_m$ is reached, excretion increases linearly with filtration. The threshold concentration is somewhat lower than that required to reach T$_m$ because of the variation in transport maxima between nephrons; this is called **splay**. Secretory mechanisms also exhibit T$_m$. For example, at low concentrations, *para*-aminohippuric acid (PAH) is almost completely removed from capillary blood by filtration and secretion (Chapter 35). At higher concentrations secretion becomes saturated, and further excretion is limited to the filtered load (Figure 36.4).

The proximal tubule (Figure 36.1)

Most glucose, amino acids, phosphate and bicarbonate is reabsorbed in the proximal tubule, together with 60–70% of Na$^+$, K$^+$, Ca^{2+}, urea and water. The secretion of H$^+$ and reabsorption of HCO$_3^-$ are discussed in detail in Chapter 39.

Sodium. The concentration of Na$^+$ in the filtrate is ~140 mmol/L (= plasma Na$^+$ concentration), but is much lower in the cytosol of epithelial cells (~10–20 mmol/L), which is also negatively charged. The electrochemical gradient therefore favours the movement of Na$^+$ from the filtrate into the cells, providing the driving force for the secondary transport of other substances. About 80% of Na$^+$ entering proximal tubular cells exchanges for H$^+$ (Na$^+$–H$^+$ antiporter). The secretion of H$^+$ in the proximal tubule plays a critical role in HCO$_3^-$ reabsorption (Figure 36.1; Chapter 39). Na$^+$ is removed from tubular cells by Na$^+$ pumps primarily on the basolateral membrane, thus transporting Na$^+$ into the interstitial fluid. However, only ~20% of transported Na$^+$ diffuses into the capillaries, as there is significant backflux into the tubule via paracellular pathways.

Water. Water is not actively reabsorbed. As Na$^+$ and HCO$_3^-$ are transported from the tubule into the peritubular interstitial fluid, the **osmolality** of the latter increases, whilst that of the tubular fluid decreases. As the proximal convoluted tubule is highly permeable to water, this osmotic pressure difference causes reabsorption of water.

The reabsorption of water increases tubular concentrations of **Cl$^-$**, **K$^+$**, **Ca^{2+}** and **urea**, which therefore diffuse down their concentration gradients into the peritubular space, largely via paracellular pathways. The final two-thirds of the proximal tubule has increased permeability to Cl$^-$, facilitating Cl$^-$ reabsorption. This makes the lumen more positive, enhancing the reabsorption of cations. As the reabsorption of Na$^+$, Cl$^-$, K$^+$, Ca^{2+} and urea in the proximal tubule is closely coupled to the reabsorption of water, their concentrations (and the total osmolality) are similar in the fluid leaving the proximal tubule to those in the filtrate and plasma, although their total quantity and the fluid volume are decreased by ~70%.

Glucose. Glucose is reabsorbed by **cotransport** with Na$^+$ across the apical membrane of epithelial cells, and then diffuses out of the cells into the peritubular interstitium. The T$_m$ for glucose is ~380 mg/min (~21 mmol/min), and the renal threshold is ~11 mmol/L. The appearance of glucose in the urine reflects **hyperglycaemia** (high plasma glucose), a sign of **diabetes mellitus**.

Amino acids. Amino acids are reabsorbed by several Na$^+$-linked symporters, specific for acidic, basic and neutral amino acids.

Phosphate. Phosphate is cotransported with Na$^+$ across the epithelial apical membrane. Its T$_m$ is close to the filtered load, and so an increase in plasma concentration leads to excretion. Phosphate reabsorption is decreased by **parathyroid hormone**.

Organic acids and bases. These include metabolites (e.g. bile salts, urate, oxalate) and drugs (e.g. PAH, penicillins, aspirin) and are secreted. Organic acids are transported from the peritubular fluid into tubular cells by cotransport with Na$^+$, and diffuse into the tubule in exchange for anions (e.g. Cl$^-$, HCO$_3^-$). Organic bases are actively extruded from the apical membrane in exchange for Na$^+$ or H$^+$.

Proteins/peptides. The tiny amount of protein that does escape through the glomerular filter and small peptide hormones (e.g. insulin, growth hormone) are reabsorbed by **endocytosis** and destroyed.

37 The loop of Henle and distal nephron

Figure 37.3
Counter-current multiplier traps Na$^+$ and Cl$^-$ in loop, causing progressive rise in osmolality towards tip. Recycling of urea between collecting ducts, medulla and loop contributes to ↑osmolality. Operation depends on active transport in TAL and differential permeabilities to water and urea

Figure 37.1 Concentration of urine: loop of Henle and distal nephron
TAL: thick ascending limb of loop of Henle; numbers refer to osmolality (mosmol/kg H$_2$O)

	H$_2$O	Urea	
Tubular permeability	+	−	····
	+$_{+ADH}$	+	---
	−	+	▬▬
	+$_{+ADH}$	−	—·—·

Figure 37.4
Vasa recta capillaries

Figure 37.2
Thick ascending loop of Henle

Figure 37.5
Distal tubule/collecting duct: ADH and water reabsorption

Figure 37.6
K$^+$ secretion and Na$^+$ reabsorption in distal tubule

Figure 37.7
Ca^{2+} reabsorption in distal tubule

The loop of Henle and distal nephron allow urine to be **concentrated** through the creation of a **high osmolality** in the medulla, which drives the reabsorption of water from the **collecting ducts**. The distal nephron also regulates K⁺ and Ca²⁺ excretion and acid–base status (Chapter 39).

The loop of Henle

Fluid entering the descending limb of the loop of Henle is isotonic with plasma (~290 mosmol/kg H_2O). The generation of high osmolality in the medulla depends on the **differential permeabilities** to water and solutes in different regions, the **active transport** of ions in the thick ascending limb and the **counter-current multiplier**. The **thin descending limb** is permeable to water but impermeable to urea, whereas the **ascending limb** is impermeable to water but permeable to urea (Figure 37.1); it is also very highly permeable to Na⁺ and Cl⁻. The **thick ascending limb** actively reabsorbs Na⁺ and Cl⁻ from the tubular fluid by means of apical **Na⁺–K⁺–2Cl⁻ cotransporters**; Na⁺ is primarily transported across the basolateral membrane by Na⁺ pumps (some by Na⁺–HCO₃⁻ cotransport), and Cl⁻ by diffusion (Figure 37.2 and **ⓑ**). K⁺ leaks back into the lumen via apical K⁺ channels (**ROMK**, renal outer medullary potassium channel), creating a positive charge that drives the reabsorption of cations (Na⁺, K⁺, Ca²⁺, Mg²⁺) through paracellular pathways. As the thick ascending limb is impermeable to water, the reabsorption of ions reduces the tubular fluid osmolality (to ~90 mosmol/kg H_2O) and increases the interstitial fluid osmolality, creating an osmotic difference of **~200 mosmol/kg H_2O**.

Counter-current multiplier (Figure 37.3). The increased interstitial osmolality causes water to diffuse out of the descending limb, and some Na⁺ and Cl⁻ to diffuse in, concentrating the tubular fluid (Figure 37.3). As this concentrated fluid descends, it travels in the opposite direction to fluid returning from the still higher osmolality regions of the deep medulla. This **counter-current** arrangement creates an osmotic gradient, causing Na⁺ and Cl⁻ to diffuse out of the ascending limb (diluting the ascending fluid), and water to diffuse out of the descending limb (further concentrating the descending fluid). This effect is potentiated by the fact that the ascending limb is impermeable to water, but highly permeable to Na⁺ and Cl⁻, and also by the recycling of **urea** between the collecting ducts and ascending limb, which makes an important contribution to urine concentration (see later). At the tip of the loop of Henle, the interstitial fluid can reach an osmolality of ~**1400 mosmol/kg H_2O**, due in equal parts to NaCl and urea.

The blood supply to the medulla is prevented from dissipating the osmotic gradient between the cortex and medulla by the *counter-current exchanger* arrangement of the **vasa recta** capillaries (Figure 37.4). The vasa recta also removes water reabsorbed from the loop of Henle and medullary collecting ducts. It should be noted that O_2 and CO_2 are also conserved, so that, in the deep medulla, Po_2 is low and Pco_2 is high.

The distal tubule and collecting duct

Fluid entering the distal tubule is *hypotonic* (~90 mosmol/kg H_2O). More Na⁺ is reabsorbed in principal cells via the Na⁺ channel **ENaC**, which is inhibited by atrial natriuretic peptide (**ANP**); expression of ENaC and thus Na⁺ reabsorption is increased by

aldosterone (Chapter 38). The movement of Na⁺ through ENaC is charge compensated by the opposite movement of K⁺ through ROMK (Figure 37.6 and **ⓕ**). The distal tubule and cortical collecting duct are impermeable to urea. They are also impermeable to water, except in the presence of **antidiuretic hormone** (ADH, *vasopressin*) (Chapter 38), which causes water channels (**aquaporins**) to insert into the apical membrane (Figure 37.5 and **ⓔ**). In the presence of ADH, water diffuses into the cortical interstitium, and the tubular fluid becomes concentrated, reaching a maximum osmolality of ~290 mosmol/kg H_2O (i.e. isotonic with plasma). However, the fluid differs from plasma as large quantities of Na⁺, K⁺, Cl⁻ and HCO₃⁻ have been reabsorbed, their place having being taken by **urea**. This is concentrated as water is reabsorbed, because the distal tubule and cortical collecting duct are impermeable to urea.

The **medullary collecting duct** also becomes permeable to water in the presence of ADH. Water is reabsorbed due to the high osmolality of the medullary interstitium (Figure 37.1). The final urine osmolality can therefore reach **1400 mosmol/kg H_2O** under conditions of maximum ADH stimulation; in the absence of ADH, urine is *dilute* (~**60 mosmol/kg H_2O**) (Chapter 38). Although only 15% of nephrons have loops of Henle that pass deep into the medulla, and so contribute to the high medullary osmolality (Chapter 34), the *collecting ducts of all nephrons pass through the medulla and therefore concentrate urine.*

Urea. The **medullary collecting duct** is relatively permeable to urea, which diffuses down its concentration gradient into the medulla and then into the ascending loop of Henle (Figure 37.1). Urea is therefore 'trapped' and partially recycled, so maintaining a high concentration and providing ~50% of the osmolality in the medulla (see previously). ADH increases the permeability of the medullary collecting duct to urea and hence its reabsorption by activating epithelial **uniporters** (*facilitated diffusion*); this further increases the medullary osmolality and allows the production of more concentrated urine.

Potassium. Potassium has largely been reabsorbed by the time the distal tubule is reached, and so excretion is regulated by secretion in the late distal tubule. K⁺ is actively transported into principal cells by basolateral Na⁺ pumps, and passively secreted via **ROMK channels** and **K⁺–Cl⁻ cotransport**; the former is promoted by the negative luminal charge caused by reabsorption of Na⁺ through ENaC (Figure 37.6 and **ⓕ**). Secretion is therefore driven by the concentration gradient between the cytosol and tubular fluid. However, secreted K⁺ will reduce the gradient unless it is washed away, and so **K⁺ excretion is increased as tubular flow increases**. Diuretics therefore often lead to K⁺ loss (Chapter 39). K⁺ secretion is increased by **aldosterone**, which enhances Na⁺ pump activity and apical membrane K⁺ permeability (Chapter 38). Perturbations of K⁺ homeostasis are often associated with acid–base disorders (Chapter 39).

Calcium. Calcium reabsorption in the distal tubule is regulated by **parathyroid hormone** (**PTH**) and **1,25-dihydroxycholecalciferol** (active form of **vitamin D**). PTH activates Ca²⁺ entry channels in the epithelial apical membrane, and a basolateral Ca²⁺ ATPase that is also activated by 1,25-dihydroxycholecalciferol. Ca²⁺ removal is assisted by an Na⁺–Ca²⁺ antiporter. Ca²⁺-binding proteins prevent cytosolic free Ca²⁺ from rising detrimentally (Figure 37.7 and **ⓖ**). PTH also inhibits phosphate reabsorption (Chapter 36). Ca²⁺ regulation is discussed in Chapter 51.

38 Regulation of plasma osmolality and fluid volume

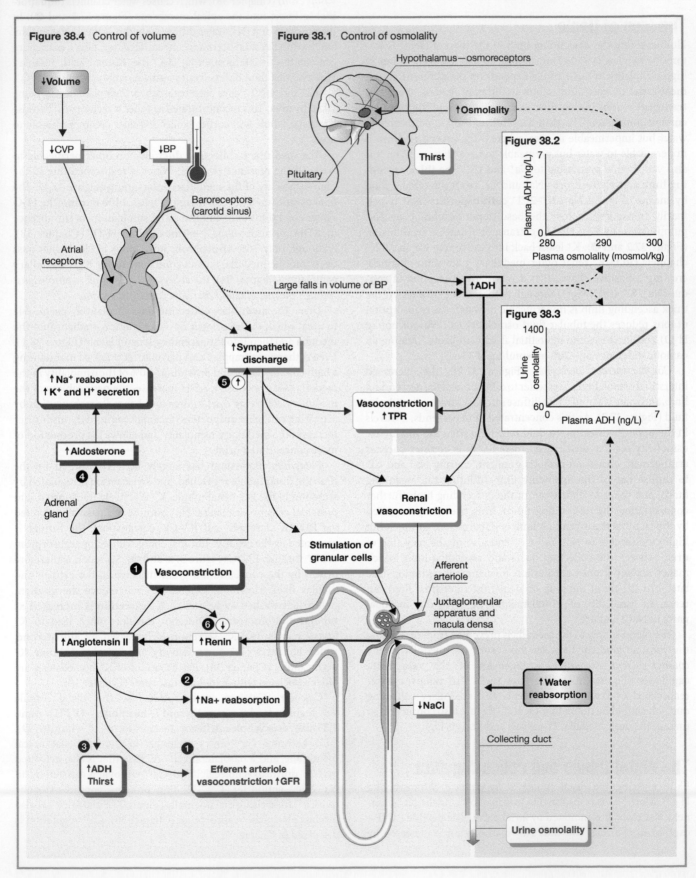

Figure 38.4 Control of volume

Figure 38.1 Control of osmolality

Hypothalamus—osmoreceptors

↑Osmolality

Thirst

Pituitary

Figure 38.2

Plasma ADH (ng/L)

Plasma osmolality (mosmol/kg)

↓Volume

↓CVP → ↓BP

Baroreceptors (carotid sinus)

Atrial receptors

Large falls in volume or BP

↑ADH

Figure 38.3

Urine osmolality

Plasma ADH (ng/L)

↑Na⁺ reabsorption
↑K⁺ and H⁺ secretion

↑Sympathetic discharge

5 ↑

Vasoconstriction
↑TPR

↑Aldosterone

4

Adrenal gland

Renal vasoconstriction

Stimulation of granular cells

1 Vasoconstriction

Afferent arteriole

Juxtaglomerular apparatus and macula densa

6 ↓

↑Angiotensin II ← ↑Renin

2

↑Na+ reabsorption

↑Water reabsorption

↓NaCl

3

↑ADH
Thirst

1

Efferent arteriole vasoconstriction ↑GFR

Collecting duct

Urine osmolality

Physiology at a Glance, Fourth Edition. Edited by Jeremy P.T. Ward and Roger W.A. Linden.

Control of plasma osmolality (Figure 38.1)

Extracellular fluid osmolality must be closely regulated, as alterations cause the swelling or shrinking of all cells, and can lead to cell death. The control of osmolality takes precedence over the control of body fluid volume.

Plasma osmolality is increased in water deficiency and decreased by the ingestion of water. **Osmoreceptors** in the **anterior hypothalamus** are sensitive to changes as small as 1% of plasma osmolality, and regulate **antidiuretic hormone** (**ADH**), also known as **vasopressin**. A rise in osmolality increases ADH release and stimulates **thirst** and water reabsorption; a fall has the opposite effect. ADH is a peptide of nine amino acids formed from a large precursor synthesized in the **hypothalamus** (Chapter 47). ADH is transported from there to the **posterior pituitary** (*neurohypophysis*) within nerve fibres (*hypothalamohypophyseal tract*), where it is stored in **secretory granules**. Action potentials from osmoreceptors cause these to release ADH. ADH binds to V_2 receptors on renal principal cells and increases cyclic adenosine monophosphate (cAMP), causing the incorporation of water channels (*aquaporins*) into the apical membrane (Chapter 37). ADH also causes **vasoconstriction** (including renal) via V_1 receptors.

The relationship between plasma osmolality and ADH release is steep (Figure 38.2), as is the relationship between plasma ADH and urine osmolality (Figure 38.3). Normal urine production is ~60 mL/h (urine osmolality, ~300–800 mosmol/kg H_2O). Maximum ADH reduces the urine volume to a **minimum** of ~400 mL per day (**maximum urine osmolality**, ~1400 mosmol/kg H_2O; this cannot be greater than that in the deep medulla, Chapter 37). In the absence of ADH, urine volume can reach ~25 L per day with a **minimum urine osmolality** of ~60 mosmol/kg H_2O (Chapter 37). ADH is rapidly removed from plasma, falling by ~50% in ~10 min, mainly due to metabolism in the liver and kidneys.

Diabetes insipidus is the production of copious amounts of **hypotonic** (dilute) urine due to defective ADH-dependent water reabsorption. This may be due to a congenital defect in ADH production (*central diabetes insipidus, CDI*), or to a failure to respond to ADH (*nephrogenic diabetes insipidus, NDI*) due to defective ADH receptors or aquaporins.

Control of body fluid volume (Figure 38.4)

As plasma osmolality is strongly regulated by the osmoreceptors and ADH, changes in the major osmotic component of extracellular fluid, i.e. Na^+, will result in changes in extracellular volume. The control of body Na^+ content by the kidney is therefore the main regulator of body fluid volume. Atrial and other low-pressure (cardiopulmonary) stretch receptors (Figure 38.4) detect a fall in central venous pressure (**CVP**), which reflects the blood volume. A fall in volume sufficient to reduce blood pressure activates the **baroreceptor reflex** (Chapter 25). In both cases, increased sympathetic discharge causes peripheral vasoconstriction (increasing total peripheral resistance; TPR), including vasoconstriction of the **renal afferent arterioles**, stimulation of **ADH release** and water reabsorption (see previously), and **release of renin** (see later) from **granular cells** in the juxtaglomerular apparatus (Chapter 34). **Decreased pressure** in the renal afferent arterioles also stimulates renin release, as does reduced NaCl delivery to the **macula densa** in the juxtaglomerular apparatus (Chapter 34) and a reduced glomerular filtration rate (GFR). In extremis, *large* falls in blood volume or pressure will promote ADH release and water retention at the expense of a decreased plasma osmolality.

Renin, angiotensin and aldosterone

Renin cleaves plasma angiotensinogen into angiotensin I, which is converted by **angiotensin-converting enzyme** (ACE) on endothelial cells (primarily in the lung) into **angiotensin II**. Angiotensin II is the primary hormone for Na^+ homeostasis, and has several important functions (Figure 38.4). It is a potent **vasoconstrictor** throughout the vasculature ❶, although in the kidney it preferentially constricts efferent arterioles, thereby increasing GFR (Chapter 35) and protecting GFR from a fall in perfusion pressure. It directly increases Na^+ **reabsorption** in the proximal tubule ❷ by stimulating Na^+–H^+ antiporters (Chapter 36). It stimulates the hypothalamus to increase **ADH secretion** and also causes **thirst** ❸. It stimulates the production of **aldosterone** by the adrenal cortex ❹. Angiotensin II also tends to potentiate sympathetic activity ❺ (*positive feedback*) and inhibit renin production by granular cells ❻ (*negative feedback*). **ACE inhibitors** are important for the treatment of heart failure, when the response to reduced blood pressure leads to detrimental fluid retention and oedema (Chapter 26).

Aldosterone is required for normal Na^+ reabsorption and K^+ secretion. It increases the synthesis of transport mechanisms in the distal nephron, including the Na^+ pump, Na^+–H^+ symporter and K^+ and Na^+ channels in principal cells, and H^+ ATPase in intercalated cells. Na^+ reabsorption and K^+ and H^+ secretion are thereby enhanced (Chapters 37 and 39). As aldosterone acts via **protein synthesis**, it takes hours to have any effect. The production of aldosterone by the adrenal cortex is directly sensitive to small changes in **plasma [K^+]**, suggesting a primary role for K^+ homeostasis.

Atrial natriuretic peptide (**ANP**; *atrial natriuretic factor*) is released from atrial muscle cells in response to stretch caused by increased blood volume (Chapter 25). ANP inhibits ENaC in principal cells of the distal nephron (Chapter 37), suppresses the production of renin, aldosterone and ADH, and causes renal vasodilatation. The net result is increased excretion of water and Na^+.

Diuretics

Osmotic diuretics (e.g. mannitol) cannot be reabsorbed effectively and, consequently, their concentration in tubular fluid increases as water is reabsorbed, limiting further water reabsorption. Thus in uncontrolled **diabetes mellitus**, high plasma glucose saturates glucose reabsorption (Chapter 36) resulting in copious amounts of urine containing glucose. **Diuretic drugs** generally inhibit tubular transport mechanisms. The most potent are **loop diuretics** (e.g. furosemide), which inhibit Na^+–K^+–$2Cl^-$ symporters in the thick ascending loop of Henle, thus preventing the development of high osmolality in the medulla and inhibiting water reabsorption (Chapter 37). The increased flow (and thus increased K^+ secretion), coupled with reduced K^+ reabsorption, enhances K^+ excretion and can cause **hypokalaemia** (low plasma [K^+]). **Aldosterone antagonists** (e.g. spironolactone) and **Na^+ channel blockers** (e.g. amiloride) reduce Na^+ entry in the distal nephron and inhibit K^+ and H^+ secretion; they are weak diuretics, but **K^+ sparing**, and are often given with loop diuretics to reduce K^+ loss. **Alcohol** inhibits ADH release, and so promotes diuresis.

39 Control of acid–base status

Figure 39.1 Relationship between PCO_2, HCO_3^- and pH, and the Henderson–Hasselbalch equation

$$CO_2 + H_2O \overset{CA}{\longleftrightarrow} H_2CO_3 \longleftrightarrow HCO_3^- + H^+$$

$$K = \frac{[HCO_3^-] \times [H^+]}{[H_2CO_3]} \quad \text{(From Law of Mass Action)}$$

CA = carbonic anhydrase
K = dissociation constant
K_A = corrected for $[CO_2]$ instead of $[H_2CO_3]$

$$\log K = \log [H^+] + \log \frac{[HCO_3^-]}{[H_2CO_3]}$$

$$-\log [H^+] = -\log K + \log \frac{[HCO_3^-]}{[H_2CO_3]}$$

Solubility (s) =
0.23 mmol/L/kPa
0.03 mmol/L/mmHg

$$pH = pK + \log \frac{[HCO_3^-]}{[H_2CO_3]}$$

But: $[H_2CO_3] \propto [CO_2]$ $(K_A = 6.1)$
and: $[CO_2] = PCO_2 \times s$ (solubility)

$$pH = 6.1 + \log \frac{[HCO_3^-]}{PCO_2 \times s}$$

Figure 39.2 Davenport diagram: relationship between PCO_2, HCO_3^- and pH

PCO_2 7.8 kPa
PCO_2 5.3 kPa
PCO_2 2.6 kPa

Plasma $[HCO_3^-]$ (mmol/L)

Renal compensation
Metabolic alkalosis
Respiratory acidosis
Respiratory alkalosis
Metabolic acidosis
Respiratory compensation
Blood buffer line

Acidosis ← pH → Alkalosis

Proximal tubule

Figure 39.3 HCO_3^- reabsorption

Lumen | Tubular cells | Interstitial fluid

HCO_3^-

$HCO_3^- + H^+$

H_2CO_3
CA
$H_2O + CO_2$

Na^+
H^+
$3Na^+$
ATP
$2K^+$
HCO_3^-
H_2CO_3
CA
$CO_2 + H_2O$
Na^+
HCO_3^-

$H^+ + NH_3$
Glutamine
NH_3
NH_4^+
Na^+
H^+ + Oxoglutarate
H_2CO_3
CA
$CO_2 + H_2O$
HCO_3^-
NH_4^+
Glucose or CO_2
HCO_3^-

80% → 15% → 5% ⟵ HCO_3^- reabsorption

NH_3

Figure 39.4 Ammonium production

Figure 39.5 Thick ascending loop of Henle

Lumen | Tubular cell | NH_3

Na^+
K^+ or NH_4^+
Cl^-
NH_4^+
Na^+
HCO_3^-
Na^+
ATP
$3Na^+$
$2K^+$
H^+

Collecting duct

Figure 39.6 Acid excretion

Lumen | Intercalated cell

K^+
ATP
H^+
$NH_3 + H^+$
$+$
PO_4
H^+
ATP
H_2CO_3
CA
$CO_2 + H_2O$
Cl^-
HCO_3^-
NH_4^+
Acid excreted

CA, carbonic anhydrase
PO4, phosphate

The pH of arterial blood is 7.35–7.45 ([H$^+$] = 45–35 nmol/L). Metabolism produces ~60 mmol H$^+$ per day, most of which is excreted through the lungs as CO_2, formed by the reaction of H$^+$ with HCO$_3^-$ (bicarbonate) (Figure 39.1). The kidneys conserve and replace HCO$_3^-$ lost in this way, and fine tune H$^+$ excretion. Physiological **buffers** maintain a low *free* [H$^+$] and prevent large swings in pH.

Buffers

Buffers are **weak acids** (HA) or **bases** (A$^-$) that can donate or accept H$^+$ ions. The ratio between buffer pairs (e.g. carbonic acid, H_2CO_3, and bicarbonate, HCO$_3^-$) is determined by [H$^+$] and the **dissociation constant** (K) for that buffer pair: K = ([H$^+$][A$^-$])/[HA], or pH = pK + log([A$^-$]/[HA]) (the **Henderson–Hasselbalch equation**). Thus, an increase in [A$^-$] or a decrease in [HA] will increase pH (more alkaline), and a decrease in pH will decrease the ratio [A$^-$]/[HA]. Buffers work best when the pH is close to their **pK value**, the pH at which the ratio [A$^-$]/[HA] is unity. Bicarbonate and carbonic acid (formed by the combination of CO_2 with water, greatly potentiated by **carbonic anhydrase**, CA; Figure 39.1) are the most important buffer pair in the body, although haemoglobin provides ~20% of buffering in the blood; phosphate and proteins provide intracellular buffering. Buffers in urine (ammonia and phosphate) allow the excretion of large quantities of H$^+$.

Although the HCO$_3^-$ system has a pK value of 6.1, and is theoretically a poor buffer at pH 7.4, it is physiologically effective because CO_2 (and therefore H_2CO_3) and HCO$_3^-$ are precisely controlled by the lungs (Chapter 32) and kidney, respectively. These fix the HCO$_3^-$/ H_2CO_3 ratio and therefore the pH, and the latter determines the ratio of all other buffer pairs. The relationship between pH, Pco$_2$ and [HCO$_3^-$] is described in Figures 39.1 and 39.2. The line BAC is the **buffer line** for whole blood; changes in Pco$_2$ alter HCO$_3^-$ and pH along this line. Point A denotes normal conditions (pH 7.4, [HCO$_3^-$] = 24 mM, Pco$_2$ = 5.3 kPa).

Proximal renal tubule

Bicarbonate is freely filtered, and so filtrate [HCO$_3^-$] is ~24 mmol/L (as in plasma). Less than 0.1% of filtered HCO$_3^-$ is normally excreted in the urine, ~80% being reabsorbed in the proximal tubule. HCO$_3^-$ is not transported directly. Filtered HCO$_3^-$ associates with H$^+$ secreted by epithelial **Na$^+$–H$^+$ antiporters** to form H_2CO_3, which rapidly dissociates to CO_2 and H_2O in the presence of **carbonic anhydrase**. CO_2 and H_2O diffuse into the tubular cells, where they recombine into H_2CO_3, which dissociates to H$^+$ and HCO$_3^-$. HCO$_3^-$ is transported into the interstitium largely by **Na$^+$–HCO$_3^-$ symporters** (Figure 39.3). For each H$^+$ secreted into the lumen, one HCO$_3^-$ and one Na$^+$ enter the plasma. H$^+$ is recycled, so that there is little net H$^+$ secretion at this stage. A further 10–15% of HCO$_3^-$ is similarly reabsorbed in the thick ascending loop of Henle. In total, about 4000–5000 mmol of HCO$_3^-$ is reabsorbed per day.

Ammonia is produced in tubular cells by the metabolism of glutamine, which leads to the generation of HCO$_3^-$ and glucose or CO_2. NH_3 diffuses into the tubular fluid, or as NH_4^+ is transported by the Na$^+$–H$^+$ antiporter. In the tubular fluid, NH_3 gains H$^+$ to form NH_4^+, which cannot diffuse through membranes (Figure 39.4). About 50% of NH_4^+ secreted by the proximal tubule is reabsorbed in the thick ascending loop of Henle, where it substitutes for K$^+$ in the Na$^+$–K$^+$–2Cl$^-$ symporter (Chapter 37), and passes into the medullary interstitium (Figure 39.5). Here, NH_4^+ dissociates into NH_3 and H$^+$, and NH_3 re-enters the collecting duct by diffusion. The secretion of H$^+$ in the collecting duct (see later) leads to conversion back to NH_4^+, which is trapped in the lumen and excreted.

Distal renal tubule

The secretion of H$^+$ in the distal tubule promotes the reabsorption of any remaining HCO$_3^-$. The combination of H$^+$ with NH_3 (see previously) and phosphate prevents H$^+$ recycling and allows acid excretion. In the early distal nephron, H$^+$ secretion is predominantly by Na$^+$–H$^+$ exchange, but more distally secretion is via **H$^+$ ATPase** and **H$^+$–K$^+$ ATPase** in **intercalated cells**, which contain plentiful carbonic anhydrase. As secreted H$^+$ is derived from CO_2, HCO$_3^-$ is formed and returns to the blood (Figure 39.6).

In summary, in the proximal nephron, H$^+$ secretion promotes HCO$_3^-$ reabsorption. In the distal nephron, secretion leads to the combination of H$^+$ with urinary buffers (phosphate, NH_3), and thus the generation of HCO$_3^-$ and acid excretion. As a result of this, tubular fluid becomes more acid as it moves through the nephron. H$^+$ secretion is proportional to intracellular [H$^+$], which is itself related to extracellular pH. A fall in blood pH will therefore stimulate renal H$^+$ secretion.

Acid–base regulation and compensation

Respiratory acidosis and **alkalosis** refer to alterations in pH caused by changes in Pco$_2$ (i.e. ventilation). **Metabolic acidosis** and **alkalosis** refer to changes not related to Pco$_2$ (i.e. increased acid production, diet, renal disease, diabetic ketoacidosis). Thus, hypoventilation increases Pco$_2$ and causes respiratory acidosis, denoted by the move from A to B in Figure 39.2. A *sustained* respiratory acidosis (e.g. *respiratory failure*) can be **compensated** by increased renal excretion of H$^+$ and reabsorption of HCO$_3^-$. The [HCO$_3^-$]/Pco$_2$ ratio is thus restored, and the pH returns towards normal. This **renal compensation** is denoted by the arrow B–D in Figure 39.2). Similarly, **metabolic acidosis** (G) may be compensated by increased ventilation and reduced Pco$_2$ (G–E) (**respiratory compensation**), initiated by the detection of acid pH by the chemoreceptors (Chapter 32). Renal mechanisms are slow because their capacity for handling H$^+$ and HCO$_3^-$ is smaller than that of the lungs for handling CO_2.

K$^+$ homeostasis and acid–base status

Hypokalaemia (low plasma [K$^+$]) is associated with metabolic alkalosis, due to stimulation of ammonia production, Na$^+$–H$^+$ exchange and H$^+$–K$^+$ ATPase, all of which enhance H$^+$ secretion. This is potentiated by aldosterone (Chapter 38). Hyperkalaemia has the opposite effect, and inhibits NH_4^+ reabsorption by competition at the Na$^+$–K$^+$–2Cl$^-$ symporter. Changes in acid–base status can affect K$^+$ homeostasis for similar reasons.

The gut and metabolism

Part 6

Chapters

40 Gastrointestinal tract: overview and the mouth

Figure 40.1 The gastrointestinal tract

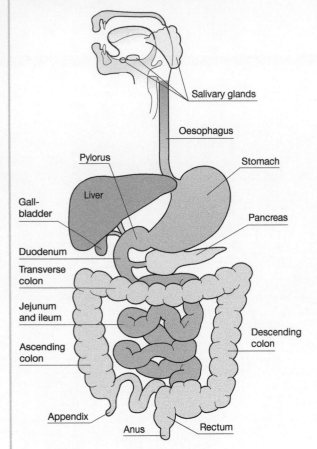

Salivary glands
Oesophagus
Pylorus
Stomach
Liver
Gall-bladder
Pancreas
Duodenum
Transverse colon
Jejunum and ileum
Descending colon
Ascending colon
Appendix
Anus
Rectum

Figure 40.2 Cross-section of gastrointestinal tract

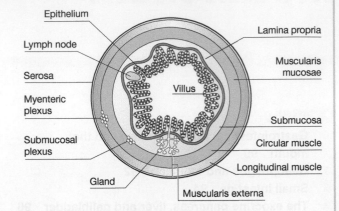

Epithelium
Lymph node
Serosa
Myenteric plexus
Submucosal plexus
Gland
Villus
Lamina propria
Muscularis mucosae
Submucosa
Circular muscle
Longitudinal muscle
Muscularis externa

Figure 40.4 Swallowing. Movement of food from the mouth through to pharynx and upper oesophagus

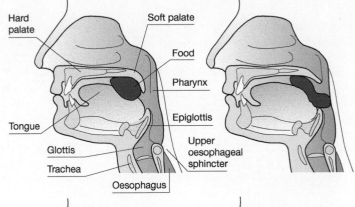

Hard palate
Soft palate
Food
Pharynx
Epiglottis
Tongue
Upper oesophageal sphincter
Glottis
Trachea
Oesophagus

Figure 40.3 Saliva

Salivary flow rates (whole mouth)

- Resting flow rates
  Mean SD: 0.3 0.22 mL/min
- Stimulated flow rates
  Mean SD: 1.7 2.1 mL/min
- Total daily flow rates
  Between 500–1000 mL/day

Saliva in the mouth is hypotonic (more water when compared with extracellular fluid) and contains over 99% water

Composition of saliva

- **Parotid glands** (serous acini) watery proteinaceous saliva, rich in electrolytes and enzymes (amylase) but little mucus
- **Sublingual glands** (mucous acini) viscous mucus saliva rich in mucins, antibodies and antigens, proteins and carbohydrates
- **Submandibular glands** (mixed serous and mucous acini) containing electrolytes, enzymes and mucus-secreting cells
- **Minor salivary glands** (mainly mucous acini)

Constituents of whole mouth saliva at rest and stimulated

Constituent	Rest	Stimulated
Sodium	8 mmol/L	32 mmol/L
Potassium	21 mmol/L	22 mmol/L
Chloride	8 mmol/L	18 mmol/L
Bicarbonate	3 mmol/L	20 mmol/L
Amylase	0.6 mmol/L	1.2 mmol/L
Total protein	2.6 g/L	3.2 g/L
Osmolality	85 mosmol/kg	127 mosmol/kg

Contributions of different glands

Unstimulated		Stimulated	
Parotid	20%	Parotid	50%
Submandibular	65%	Submandibular	30%
Sublingual	7–8%	Sublingual	10%
Minor glands	7–8%	Minor glands	10%

The **gastrointestinal (GI) tract** is responsible for the breakdown of food into its component parts so that they can be absorbed into the body. It is made up of the **mouth, oesophagus, stomach** and **small and large intestines**. The **salivary glands, liver, gallbladder** and **pancreas** are organs distinct from the GI tract, but all secrete juices into the tract and aid the digestion and absorption of the food (Figure 40.1).

Structure

Different regions of the tract are concerned with **motility** (transport), **storage, digestion, absorption** and **elimination of waste**, and these functions of the GI tract are controlled by **neuronal, hormonal** and **local regulatory mechanisms**.

The walls of the GI tract have a general structure that is similar along most of its length, although this is modified as function varies. This basic structure is shown in Figure 40.2. It comprises the **mucosal layer**, made up of epithelial cells (which can be involved in either the process of secretion or absorption depending on their location in the GI tract), and the **lamina propria**, consisting of loose connective tissue, collagen and elastin, blood vessels and lymph tissue, and a thin layer of smooth muscle called the **muscularis mucosa** which, when contracting, produces folds and ridges in the mucosa. The **submucosal layer** comprises a second layer of connective tissue, but also contains larger blood and lymphatic vessels and a network of nerve cells called the **submucosal plexus (Meissner's plexus)**. This is a dense plexus of nerves innervated by the autonomic part of the nervous system which can function as an independent nervous system – the **enteric nervous system**. Below the submucosa is the **muscularis externa**. This comprises a thick **circular layer** of smooth muscle around the GI tract which, when it contracts, produces a constriction of the lumen. Below this layer of muscle is another thinner layer of muscle arranged in a **longitudinal** manner which, when it contracts, results in shortening of the tract. Between these two layers of muscle is a second nerve plexus, called the **myenteric plexus (Auerbach's plexus)**, which is also part of the enteric nervous system. The outermost layer of the GI tract is the **serosa**, another connective tissue layer covered with squamous mesothelial cells.

Saliva and mastication

The GI tract starts in the mouth, where food is initially **chewed (masticated)** and mixed with salivary secretions. **Mastication** is the process of systematic mechanical breakdown of food in the mouth. The amount of mastication necessary in order to swallow the food depends on the nature of the ingested food: solid foods are subjected to vigorous chewing, whereas softer foods and liquids require little or no chewing and are transported almost directly into the oesophagus by swallowing. Mastication is necessary for some foods, such as red meats, chicken and vegetables, to be fully absorbed by the rest of the GI tract. However, fish, eggs, rice, bread and cheese do not require chewing for complete absorption in the tract.

Mastication involves the coordinated activity of the **teeth, jaw muscles, temporomandibular joint, tongue** and other structures, such as the **lips, palate** and **salivary glands**. The forces developed between the teeth during mastication have been measured to be about 150–200 N; however, the maximum biting force developed between the molar teeth is almost 10 times this value.

During mastication three pairs of glands, the **parotid, submandibular** and **sublingual**, secrete saliva. Saliva is **hypotonic**, and its composition differs between glands and whether they are resting or stimulated (Figure 40.3). The major functions of saliva are: to **moisten** and **lubricate** the mouth, particularly during eating and speech; to **dissolve** food molecules so that they can react with taste receptors; to **ease swallowing**; to begin **digestion** of polysaccharides (complex sugars) with **amylase**; and to **protect** the oral cavity by coating the teeth with a proline-rich protein or pellicle that can serve as a protective barrier on the tooth surface. Saliva also contains immunoglobulins and antimicrobials that have a protective role in avoiding bacterial infections.

Formation of saliva is in two stages. Stimulation of **acinar** epithelial cells causes Ca^{2+}-dependent activation of basolateral K^+ channels and apical Cl^- channels. The consequent efflux of Cl^- (negative charge) causes Na^+ to follow through paracellular routes (between cells), and drawing water into the luminal space by osmotic force, creating an isotonic fluid. In the second stage, as this fluid moves through the glandular ducts Na^+ and Cl^- are reabsorbed (by ENaC and Cl^--HCO_3^- exchange) and HCO_3^- and K^+ secreted, ending up with a **hypotonic** saliva. As flow rates increase these latter processes become less effective, so saliva osmolality increases. Acinar cells also secrete the other components of saliva (e.g. enzymes, mucins). Acinar cell ionic content is restored by basolateral Na^+-K^+-$2Cl^-$ cotransporters and Na^+-pumps.

Control of salivary secretion is mediated via sympathetic and parasympathetic nerves to the glands, and depends on reflex responses which, in humans, have been shown to be elicited by the stimulation of gustatory (taste) receptors and periodontal and mucosal mechanoreceptors during mastication. Although it was thought that olfactory afferent stimulation (smell) also had a general reflex effect on salivary secretion, it has now been shown that this reflex operates via the submandibular/sublingual glands and not the parotid in humans. The sight and thought of food in humans have very little effect on salivary production. The perception of an increased salivary production is thought to be related to the sudden awareness of saliva already present in the mouth.

Swallowing

Swallowing occurs in a number of phases. The first phase is **voluntary** and involves the formation of a bolus of food by chewing and tongue movements (backwards and upwards), which push the food into the pharynx. The remaining phases are not voluntary, but **reflex responses** initiated by the stimulation of mechanoreceptors with afferents in the **glossopharyngeal (IX) and vagus (X) nerves** to the medulla and pons (brain stem); here, there is a group of neurones (the 'swallowing centre') which coordinates the complex sequence of events that eventually delivers the bolus into the oesophagus. The **soft palate** elevates to prevent food from entering the **nasal cavity**, respiration is inhibited, the **larynx** is raised, the **glottis** is closed and the food pushes the tip of the **epiglottis** over the tracheal opening, preventing food from entering the trachea. As the bolus enters the **oesophagus**, these changes reverse, the larynx opens and breathing continues (Figure 40.4).

41 Oesophagus and stomach

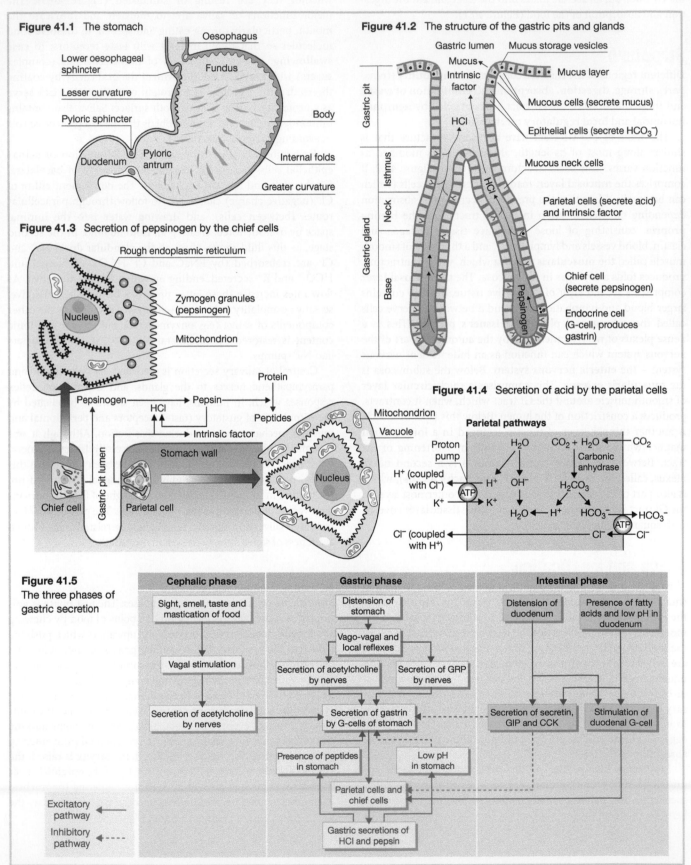

Figure 41.1 The stomach

- Oesophagus
- Lower oesophageal sphincter
- Fundus
- Lesser curvature
- Pyloric sphincter
- Body
- Duodenum
- Pyloric antrum
- Internal folds
- Greater curvature

Figure 41.2 The structure of the gastric pits and glands

- Gastric lumen
- Mucus storage vesicles
- Mucus
- Intrinsic factor
- Mucus layer
- HCl
- Mucous cells (secrete mucus)
- Epithelial cells (secrete HCO_3^-)
- Mucous neck cells
- Parietal cells (secrete acid) and intrinsic factor
- Chief cell (secrete pepsinogen)
- Endocrine cell (G-cell, produces gastrin)
- Pepsinogen
- Gastric pit
- Isthmus
- Neck
- Base
- Gastric gland

Figure 41.3 Secretion of pepsinogen by the chief cells

- Rough endoplasmic reticulum
- Nucleus
- Zymogen granules (pepsinogen)
- Mitochondrion
- Pepsinogen → HCl → Pepsin
- Intrinsic factor
- Stomach wall
- Protein
- Peptides
- Chief cell
- Gastric pit lumen
- Parietal cell
- Mitochondrion
- Vacuole
- Nucleus

Figure 41.4 Secretion of acid by the parietal cells

Parietal pathways

- Proton pump
- H_2O
- $CO_2 + H_2O$ → CO_2
- Carbonic anhydrase
- H^+ (coupled with Cl^-)
- H^+
- OH^-
- H_2CO_3
- K^+ — ATP — K^+
- H_2O ← H^+
- HCO_3^- — ATP — HCO_3^-
- Cl^- (coupled with H^+)
- Cl^- — Cl^-

Figure 41.5 The three phases of gastric secretion

Cephalic phase	Gastric phase	Intestinal phase
Sight, smell, taste and mastication of food	Distension of stomach	Distension of duodenum / Presence of fatty acids and low pH in duodenum
Vagal stimulation	Vago-vagal and local reflexes	
	Secretion of acetylcholine by nerves / Secretion of GRP by nerves	
Secretion of acetylcholine by nerves	Secretion of gastrin by G-cells of stomach	Secretion of secretin, GIP and CCK / Stimulation of duodenal G-cell
	Presence of peptides in stomach / Low pH in stomach	
	Parietal cells and chief cells	
	Gastric secretions of HCl and pepsin	

Excitatory pathway →
Inhibitory pathway ---→

It is possible to swallow food and drink and for it to enter the stomach while standing on one's head or experiencing zero gravity. A ring of skeletal muscle called the **upper oesophageal sphincter** usually closes the **pharyngeal end** of the **oesophagus**. During the **oesophageal phase of swallowing**, this sphincter is relaxed, allowing the bolus of food to pass through it. Immediately afterwards, the sphincter closes. Once in the oesophagus, the bolus is propelled the 25 cm (approximately) to the **stomach** by a process called **peristalsis**, a coordinated wave of relaxation in front of the bolus and contraction behind the bolus of the circular and longitudinal muscle layers of the oesophagus, forcing the food into the stomach in about 5 s. Before the bolus enters the stomach, it passes through another sphincter, the **lower oesophageal sphincter**, formed from a ring of smooth muscle which relaxes as the peristaltic wave reaches it. The **swallowing centres in the medulla** produce a sequence of events that lead to both efferent activity to **somatic nerves** (innervating skeletal muscle) and **autonomic nerves** (innervating smooth muscle). This sequence of events is influenced by afferent receptors in the oesophagus wall sending impulses back to the medulla. The sphincters and the peristaltic waves are principally controlled by activity in the **vagus nerve** and aided by a high degree of coordination of the activity within the **enteric nerve plexuses** within the tract itself.

Once the bolus of food passes through the lower oesophageal sphincter, it enters the **stomach** (Figure 41.1). The **main functions of the stomach** are to **store** food temporarily (as it can be ingested more rapidly than it can be digested) to chemically and mechanically **digest** food using acids, enzymes and movements, to **regulate the release** of the resulting **chyme** into the small intestine, and to secrete a substance called **intrinsic factor** which is essential for the absorption of vitamin B_{12}. The stomach lies immediately below the diaphragm and, like the rest of the gastrointestinal tract, it has longitudinal and circular muscle layers and nerve plexuses in its walls; however, within the mucosa are specialized secretory cells that line the gastric glands or pits (Figure 41.2). When empty, the stomach has a volume of approximately 50 mL; however, when fully distended, its volume can be as much as 4 L. **Proteins** in the food are broken down into **polypeptides** in the stomach by enzymes called **pepsins**. These enzymes are produced in an inactive form called **pepsinogens** by the **chief cells** in the gastric mucosa, and are converted into active pepsins by the acid environment in the stomach (Figure 41.3). The acid in the stomach is **hydrochloric acid** and is produced by a specialized group of cells called **parietal cells**. The stomach can secrete as much as 2 L of acid per day, and the concentration of H^+ ions in the stomach is estimated to be about 1 million times higher than that in the blood. This concentration of H^+ ions requires a very efficient exchange of intracellular H^+ for extracellular K^+ using energy provided by the breakdown of adenosine triphosphate (ATP). This is achieved using a protein known as the **proton pump** or the H^+–K^+ ATPase protein (Figure 41.4).

The gastric mucosa does not digest itself because it is protected by an **alkaline, mucin-rich fluid** secreted by the gastric glands, which acts as a mucosal barrier by bathing the gastric epithelial cells. In addition, local mediators, such as **prostaglandins**, are released when the mucosa is irritated, and these increase the thickness of the **mucous layer** and stimulate the production of **bicarbonate** which neutralizes the acid.

Control of gastric secretions

Gastric secretions occur in basically three phases: **cephalic, gastric** and **intestinal** (Figure 41.5). The **cephalic phase** is brought about by the **sight, smell, taste** and **mastication** of food. At this stage, there is no food in the stomach and acid secretion is stimulated by the activation of the vagus and its actions on the **enteric plexus. Postganglionic parasympathetic fibres** in the **myenteric plexus** cause the release of **acetylcholine (ACh)** and stimulate the release of gastric juices from the gastric glands. Vagal stimulation also causes the release of a hormone called gastrin from cells in the antrum of the stomach called **G-cells**. **Gastrin** is secreted into the bloodstream and, when it reaches the gastric glands, it stimulates the release of **acid** and **pepsinogens**. Both vagal activity and gastrin also stimulate the release of **histamine** from mast cells, which, in turn, acts on **parietal cells** to produce more acid.

When food arrives in the stomach, it stimulates the **gastric phase** of secretion of **acid, pepsinogen** and **mucus**. The main stimuli for this phase are the **distension** of the stomach and the **chemical** composition of the food. Mechanoreceptors in the stomach wall are stretched and set up local myenteric reflexes and also longer vagovagal reflexes. Both cause the release of **ACh** which stimulates the release of **gastrin, histamine** and, in turn, **acid, enzymes** and **mucus**. Stimulation of the **vagus** also releases a specific peptide, **gastrin-releasing peptide (GRP)**, which mainly acts directly on the **G-cells** to release **gastrin**. Whole proteins do not affect gastric secretions directly, but their breakdown products, such as **peptides** and **free amino acids**, do so by **directly stimulating gastrin secretion**. A **low pH** (more acid) in the stomach **inhibits** gastrin secretion; therefore, when the stomach is empty or after food has entered it and acid has been secreted for some time, there is an inhibition of acid production. However, when food first enters the stomach, the **pH rises** (less acid) and this leads to a **release of the inhibition** and causes a **maximum secretion of gastrin**. Thus, gastric acid secretion is **self-regulating**.

The **gastric phase** normally lasts for about 3 h and the food in the stomach is converted into a sludge-like material called **chyme**. The **chyme** enters the first part of the small intestine, the **duodenum**, through the **pyloric sphincter**. The presence of chyme in the **pyloric antrum** distends it and causes antral contractions and opening of the sphincter. The rate at which the stomach empties depends on the volume in the antrum and the fall in the pH of the chyme, both leading to an increase in emptying. However, **distension** of the duodenum, the **presence of fats** and a **decrease in pH** in the duodenal lumen all cause **an inhibition of gastric emptying**. This mechanism leads to a precise supply of chyme to the intestines at a rate appropriate for it to be digested properly.

(For a description of the intestinal phase of gastric secretion, see Chapter 42.)

42 Small intestine

Figure 42.1 Intestinal villi

Microvilli

Epithelial cells

Capillaries

Nerve fibre

Arteriole

Villus

Lumen

Lacteal

Venule

Crypt

Muscularis mucosae

Artery

Nerve

Vein

Lymph duct

The small intestine is the main site for the digestion of food and the absorption of the products of this digestion. It is a tube, 2.5 cm in diameter and approximately 4 m in length, and comprises the **duodenum**, **jejunum** and **ileum**.

When **chyme** first enters the duodenum, there is a continuation of gastric secretion thought to be due to the activation of **G cells** in the **intestinal mucosa** (see **intestinal phase**; Figure 41.5). This is short lived as the duodenum becomes more distended with further gastric emptying. A series of reflexes is initiated which inhibits the further release of **gastric juices**. A number of **hormones** are involved in these reflex responses. **Secretin** is released in response to acid stimulation; it reaches the stomach via the bloodstream and inhibits the release of

gastrin. The presence of **fatty acids**, due to the breakdown of fats in the duodenum itself, releases two polypeptide hormones, called **gastric inhibitory peptide (GIP)** and **cholecystokinin (CCK)**, which inhibit the release of both **gastrin** and **acid**. Both secretin and CCK, however, stimulate the release of **pepsinogen** from the **chief cells**, thereby aiding protein digestion. Together with **mechanoreceptors** in the duodenum via vagal and local reflex pathways, the release of **secretin** and CCK has also been implicated in the control of **gastric emptying**. The chyme that first enters the duodenum is **acidic, hypertonic** and **only partly digested**; at this early stage, the nutrients formed cannot be absorbed. There is an **osmotic** movement of water across the freely permeable wall which leads to the contents becoming isotonic. The acidity is neutralized by the addition of both **bicarbonate** secreted by the **pancreas** and **bile** from the **liver**, and further digestion of the chyme is performed by the addition of enzymes from the pancreas, liver and intestine itself.

The lining of the small intestine is folded into many small, finger-like projections called **villi** (Figure 42.1). Between the villi lie some small glands, called **crypts**, which can secrete up to 3 L of **hypotonic** fluid per day. The surface of the villi is covered with a layer of **epithelial cells** which, in turn, have many small projections called **microvilli** (collectively called the **brush border**) that project towards the lumen of the intestine. The small intestine is particularly adapted for the absorption of nutrients. It has a huge surface area (about the size of a tennis court), and the chyme is forced into a circular motion as it passes through the tract, facilitating mixing and therefore digestion and absorption. There is a constant turnover of epithelial cells within the gastrointestinal (GI) tract, with the small intestine epithelium totally replacing itself approximately every 6 days.

Each **villus** contains a single, blind-ended lymphatic vessel, called a **lacteal**, and also a **capillary network**. Most nutrients are absorbed into the bloodstream via these vessels. The venous drainage from the small intestine, large intestine, pancreas and also from some parts of the stomach passes via the **hepatic portal vein** into the liver; here, it passes through a second capillary bed to be further processed before returning to the circulation.

Absorption of nutrients

The small intestine absorbs **water**, **electrolytes**, **carbohydrates**, **amino acids**, **minerals**, **fats** and **vitamins**. The mechanisms by which movement from the lumen to the circulation occurs are variable. Nutrients move between the GI tract and the blood by passing through and around the epithelial cells. As the contents of the intestine are isotonic with body fluids and mostly have the same concentration of the major electrolytes, their absorption is active. **Water** cannot be moved directly, but follows osmotic gradients set up by the transport of ions. The major contributor to this osmotic gradient is the **sodium pump**. **Na^+–K^+ ATPase** is located on the blood side of the epithelial cell (**basolateral membrane**), and hydrolysis of adenosine triphosphate (ATP) to adenosine diphosphate (ADP) leads to the expulsion of three Na^+ ions from the cell in exchange for two K^+ ions. Both of these are against the concentration gradients, leading to a **low concentration of Na^+** and a **high concentration of K^+** within the cells. The low intracellular concentration of Na^+ ensures a movement of Na^+ from the intestinal contents into the cell by both **membrane channels** and **transported protein mechanisms**. Na^+ is then rapidly transported out of the cell again by the **basolateral Na^+–K^+ pump**. K^+ leaves the cell, again via the basolateral membrane, down its concentration gradient. This outward movement of K^+ is linked to an outward movement of Cl^-, against its concentration gradient, Cl^- having entered down its concentration gradient like Na^+ via the luminal membrane. These movements set up an osmotic gradient between the lumen and the blood, leading to water absorption following the movement of Na^+ and Cl^- from the lumen into the cell across the luminal membrane.

Carbohydrates are absorbed mostly in the form of **monosaccharides** (glucose, fructose and galactose). They are broken down into monosaccharides by enzymes released from the brush border (**maltases, isomaltases, sucrase** and **lactase**). The monosaccharides are transported across the epithelium into the bloodstream by means of cotransporter molecules that link their inward movement with that of Na^+ down its concentration gradient. At the basolateral membrane, monosaccharides leave the cell either by **simple diffusion** or by **facilitated diffusion** down the concentration gradient.

The **polypeptides** produced in the stomach are broken down into **oligopeptides** in the small intestine by enzymes (**proteases**) secreted by the pancreas: **trypsin** and **chymotrypsin**. These are further broken down into **amino acids** by another pancreatic enzyme, **carboxypeptidase**, and an enzyme located on the luminal membrane epithelial cells, **aminopeptidase**. The **free amino acids** enter the epithelial cells by secondary active transport coupled to the movement of Na^+ and a number of different cotransporter mechanisms.

Two very important minerals that are absorbed from the diet are **calcium** and **iron**. **Intracellular calcium** concentrations are low and any **free calcium** in the diet can cross the luminal membrane down a steep concentration gradient through channels or by a carrier mechanism. In the cell, it binds to a protein which carries it to the basolateral membrane, where it is actively transported against the concentration gradient by a **Ca^{2+} ATPase** with the hydrolysis of ATP, or by an **Na^+–Ca^{2+} antiporter** linked with the movement of Na^+ down its concentration gradient into the cell and the removal of Ca^{2+} from it.

Most **dietary iron** is in the **ferric** (Fe^{3+}) form which **cannot** be absorbed; however, in the **ferrous** (Fe^{2+}) form, it forms soluble complexes with **ascorbate** and other substances and **can be readily absorbed**. These complexes are transported across the membrane by a carrier protein and, once in the cell, bind with a variety of substances including **ferritin**. A second carrier protein transports the iron across the basolateral membrane into the bloodstream.

Fats and lipids

Fat digestion occurs almost entirely in the small intestine. The major enzyme is a **pancreatic enzyme** called **lipase** which breaks fat down into **monoglycerides** and **free fatty acids**. However, before the fat can be broken down, it has to be **emulsified**, which is a process by which the larger lipid droplets are broken down into much smaller droplets (about 1 μm in diameter). The main emulsifying agents are the **bile acids, cholic acid** and **chenodeoxycholic acid**. The free fatty acids and monoglycerides form tiny particles (4–5 nm in diameter) with the bile acids, called **micelles**. The outer region of the micelle is **hydrophilic** (water-attracting), whereas the inner core contains the **hydrophobic** (water-repelling) part of the molecule. This arrangement allows the micelles to enter the aqueous layers surrounding the **microvilli**, and the **monoglycerides, free fatty acids, cholesterol** and **fat-soluble vitamins** can then diffuse passively into the duodenal cells, leaving the bile salts within the lumen of the gut until they reach the ileum, where they are reabsorbed. Once within the epithelial cells, the fatty acids and monoglycerides are reassembled into fats by a number of different metabolic pathways. They then enter the lymphatic system via the **lacteals** and eventually reach the bloodstream through the **thoracic duct**.

The **fat-soluble vitamins**, A, D, E and K, essentially follow the pathways for fat absorption. The remaining **water-soluble vitamins** are mainly absorbed by diffusion or mediated transport. The exception is **vitamin B_{12}**, which must first bind with **intrinsic factor** (secreted from the parietal cells in the stomach wall). When bound, vitamin B_{12} attaches to specific sites on the epithelial cells in the **ileum** where a process of endocytosis leads to absorption.

43 The exocrine pancreas, liver and gallbladder

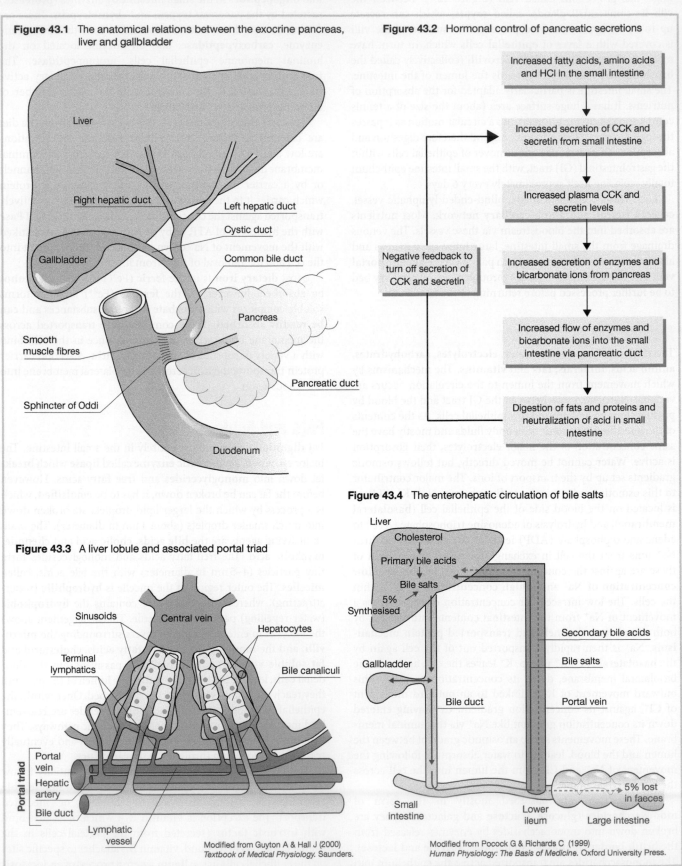

Figure 43.1 The anatomical relations between the exocrine pancreas, liver and gallbladder

Liver

Right hepatic duct

Left hepatic duct

Cystic duct

Gallbladder

Common bile duct

Pancreas

Smooth muscle fibres

Pancreatic duct

Sphincter of Oddi

Duodenum

Figure 43.2 Hormonal control of pancreatic secretions

Increased fatty acids, amino acids and HCl in the small intestine

Increased secretion of CCK and secretin from small intestine

Increased plasma CCK and secretin levels

Negative feedback to turn off secretion of CCK and secretin

Increased secretion of enzymes and bicarbonate ions from pancreas

Increased flow of enzymes and bicarbonate ions into the small intestine via pancreatic duct

Digestion of fats and proteins and neutralization of acid in small intestine

Figure 43.3 A liver lobule and associated portal triad

Sinusoids

Central vein

Hepatocytes

Terminal lymphatics

Bile canaliculi

Portal triad

Portal vein

Hepatic artery

Bile duct

Lymphatic vessel

Modified from Guyton A & Hall J (2000)
Textbook of Medical Physiology. Saunders.

Figure 43.4 The enterohepatic circulation of bile salts

Liver

Cholesterol

Primary bile acids

Bile salts

5%
Synthesised

Secondary bile acids

Bile salts

Gallbladder

Bile duct

Portal vein

Small intestine

Lower ileum

Large intestine

5% lost in faeces

Modified from Pocock G & Richards C (1999)
Human Physiology: The Basis of Medicine. Oxford University Press.

Physiology at a Glance, Fourth Edition. Edited by Jeremy P.T. Ward and Roger W.A. Linden.
© 2017 John Wiley & Sons, Ltd. Published 2017 by John Wiley & Sons, Ltd. Companion website: www.ataglanceseries.com/physiology

The pancreas

The **exocrine pancreas** secretes a major digestive fluid called **pancreatic juice**. This juice is secreted into the duodenum via the pancreatic duct that opens into the gastrointestinal (GI) tract at the same site as the **common bile duct** (see later). When food is present in the duodenum, a small sphincter (**sphincter of Oddi**) relaxes, allowing both bile and pancreatic secretions to enter the tract (Figure 43.1).

Pancreatic juice is made up of a number of **enzymes**, secreted by the **acinar** cells of the pancreas, which break down the major constituents in the diet. The enzymes include **pancreatic amylase**, which breaks down carbohydrates to monosaccharides; **pancreatic lipase**, which breaks down fats to glycerol and fatty acids; **ribonuclease** and **deoxyribonuclease**, which are involved in the breakdown of nucleic acids and free mononucleotides; and a variety of **proteolytic enzymes** (**trypsin**, **chymotrypsin**, **elastase** and **carboxypeptidase**), which break down proteins into small peptides and amino acids. The hormone **cholecystokinin (CCK)**, released into the bloodstream by the duodenal cells in response to the presence of amino acids and fatty acids in the chyme, is responsible for the secretion of the pancreatic enzymes from the acinar cells of the pancreas. The other major secretions, besides the enzymes, are **water** and **bicarbonate ions**. The volume of pancreatic juice secreted precisely neutralizes the acid content of the chyme delivered by the stomach to the intestines. This is caused by the acid in the duodenum releasing **secretin** from its walls into the bloodstream. **Secretin** stimulates the production of water and bicarbonate ions from the duct system and, in particular, from the **epithelial cells** lining the duct. Approximately 1 L of pancreatic juice is secreted per day from a normal individual (Figure 43.2).

The liver

The **liver** is the largest organ of the body, weighing over 1 kg in the normal adult. The **functions of the liver** can be divided into two broad categories. First, it is involved with the processing of absorbed substances, both nutrient and toxic. In other words, it is responsible for the **metabolism** of a vast range of substances produced by the digestion and absorption of food from the intestine. Second, it has an important **exocrine function** in that it is involved in: (i) the production of bile acids and alkaline fluids used in the digestion and absorption of fats and for the neutralization of gastric acid in the intestines; (ii) the breakdown and production of waste products following digestion; (iii) the detoxification of noxious substances; and (iv) the excretion of waste products and the detoxification of substances in bile.

The majority of waste metabolites and detoxified substances are excreted from the body in the bile, from the GI tract, or via secretions from the liver into the bloodstream for subsequent excretion by the kidney. The relationship between the liver, gallbladder and duodenum is shown in Figure 43.1. The **liver** consists of four lobes, with each lobe made up of tens of thousands of hexagonal **lobules**, 1–2 mm in diameter, which are the functional unit of the liver. Each lobule (Figure 43.3) consists of a **central vein** that eventually becomes part of the **hepatic vein**. Surrounding the central vein are single columns of liver cells (**hepatocytes**) radiating outwards; between the hepatocytes are small **canaliculi** which begin as blind-ended structures at the end nearer the central vein, but drain into the **bile duct** on the periphery of the lobule. At each of the six corners of the lobules lies a 'portal triad' comprising branches of the **hepatic artery**, the **portal vein** and the **bile duct**. The bile ducts eventually drain into the **terminal bile duct**.

Bile and the gallbladder

The **hepatocytes** secrete a fluid called **hepatic bile**. It is isotonic and resembles plasma ionically. It also contains **bile salts**, **bile pigments**, **cholesterol**, **lecithin** and **mucus**. This fraction of bile is called the **bile acid-dependent fraction**. As it passes along the bile duct, the bile is modified by the epithelial cells lining the duct by the addition of **water** and **bicarbonate ions**; this fraction is called the **bile acid-independent fraction**. Overall, the liver can produce 500–1000 mL of bile per day. The bile is either discharged directly into the duodenum or stored in the **gallbladder**. The bile acid-independent fraction is made at the time it is required, i.e. during digestion of the chyme. The bile acid-dependent fraction is made when the bile salts are returned from the GI tract to the liver, and is then stored in the gallbladder when the sphincter of Oddi is closed. About 95% of the bile salts that enter the small intestine in bile are recycled and reabsorbed into the portal circulation by active transport mechanisms in the distal ileum (the so-called **enterohepatic circulation**; Figure 43.4). Many of the bile salts are returned unaltered, some are broken down by intestinal bacteria into **secondary bile acids** and then reabsorbed, and a small proportion escapes reabsorption and is excreted in the faeces.

The **gallbladder** not only stores the bile, but also concentrates it by removing non-essential solutes and water, leaving the bile acids and pigments. The process of concentration is mainly by active transport of Na^+ ions into the intercellular spaces of the lining cells and this, in turn, draws water, HCO_3^- and Cl^- ions from the bile and into the extracellular fluid, thereby concentrating the bile held in the gallbladder.

The formation of bile is stimulated by **bile salts**, **secretin**, **glucagons** and **gastrin**. The release of bile stored in the gallbladder, however, is stimulated by the secretion of **CCK** into the bloodstream when chyme enters the duodenum and, to a lesser extent, by the actions of the **vagus nerve**. Within a few minutes of a meal, particularly when fats are consumed, the muscles of the gallbladder contract; this forces the contents into the duodenum through the now relaxed sphincter of Oddi. CCK relaxes the sphincter and stimulates the pancreatic secretions at the same time. The gallbladder empties completely 1 h after a fat-rich meal and maintains the level of bile acids in the duodenum above that necessary for the function of the micelles.

44 Large intestine

Figure 44.1 The structure of the large intestine

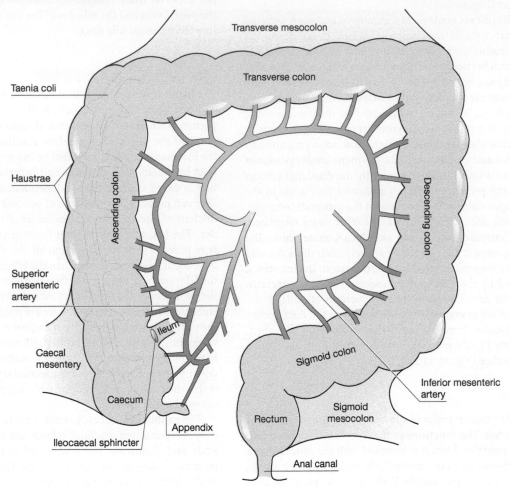

Figure 44.2 Absorption and secretion in the epithelial cells of the colon

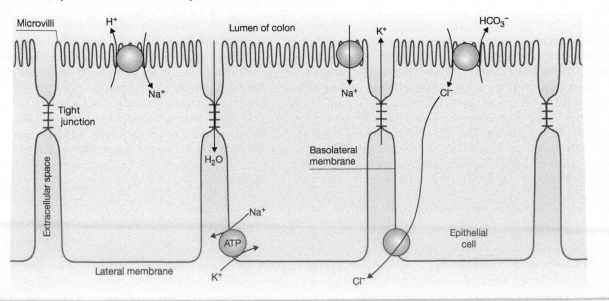

Physiology at a Glance, Fourth Edition. Edited by Jeremy P.T. Ward and Roger W.A. Linden.
© 2017 John Wiley & Sons, Ltd. Published 2017 by John Wiley & Sons, Ltd. Companion website: www.ataglanceseries.com/physiology

The **large intestine** comprises the **caecum, ascending, transverse, descending** and **sigmoid colon, rectum** and **anal canal** (Figure 44.1). It is approximately 1.2 m in length and between 6 and 9 cm in diameter. Approximately 1.5 L of chyme enters the large intestine per day through a sphincter called the **ileocaecal sphincter**. Distension of the terminal ileum results in the opening of the sphincter and distension of the caecum causes it to close, thereby maintaining the optimum rate of entry to maximize the main function of the large intestine, which is to absorb most of the water and electrolytes. The initial 1.5 L is reduced to about 150 g of **faeces** consisting of 100 mL of water and 50 g of solids.

The muscle layers of the large intestine are slightly different from those found in the rest of the gastrointestinal (GI) tract. It still has a powerful circular muscle layer, but its **longitudinal muscle layer** is concentrated into **three bands** called the **taeniae coli**. The caecum and the ascending and transverse colon are innervated by **parasympathetic** branches of the **vagus**; the descending and sigmoid colon, rectum and anal canal are innervated by **parasympathetic** branches of the **pelvic nerves** from the sacral spinal cord. These parasympathetic fibres innervate the intramural plexuses. The **sympathetic** nerves via the superior mesenteric plexus, and via the inferior mesenteric and the superior hypogastric plexuses, innervate the proximal and distal parts of the large intestine, respectively. The rectum and anal canal are innervated via the inferior hypogastric plexus. Stimulation of the parasympathetic fibres causes segmental contraction, whereas stimulation of the sympathetic fibres stops colonic activity. The **internal** and **external anal sphincters** usually keep the anal canal closed and are controlled both **reflexly** and **voluntarily**. The **internal sphincter** is made up of **circular smooth muscle**, and the more distal **external sphincter** is composed of **striated muscle** which is innervated by motor fibres from the **pudendal nerve**.

Movement of the chyme through the large intestine involves both **mixing** and **propulsion**. However, as the main function is to store the residues of food and to absorb water and electrolytes from it, the movements are slow and sluggish (approximately 5–10 cm/h). Chyme usually remains in the colon for up to 20 h. The mixing movement is called **haustration** and the sac-like compartments in the colon caused by this process are called **haustra**. The contents of the haustra are often shunted back and forth from one to another in a process called **haustral shuttling**. This aids the exposure of chyme to the mucosal surface and helps the reabsorption of water and electrolytes. In the distal parts of the colon, the contractions are slower and less propulsive, and eventually the faeces collect in the descending colon.

Several times a day there is an increase in activity within the colon, in which there is a vigorous propulsive movement, the **mass movement**. This results in the emptying of a large proportion of the content of the proximal colon into the more distal parts. This **mass movement** is initiated by a complex series of intrinsic reflex pathways started by the distension of the stomach and duodenum soon after the consumption of a meal.

Defecation

When a critical mass of faeces is forced into the rectum, the desire for **defecation** is experienced. This sudden distension of the rectum walls produced by the final mass movement leads to a **defecation reflex**. This reflex comprises a contraction of the rectum, relaxation of the internal anal sphincter and, initially, contraction of the external anal sphincter. This initial contraction is soon followed by a reflex relaxation of the sphincter initiated by an increase in the peristaltic activity in the sigmoid colon and pressure in the rectum. The faeces are then expelled. This reflex relaxation can be overridden by higher centre activity, leading to a voluntary control over the sphincter which can delay the expulsion of faeces. The prolonged distension of the rectum then leads to a **reverse peristalsis**, which empties the rectum into the colon and removes the urge to defecate until the next mass movement and/or a more convenient time.

The chyme that enters the large intestine is **isotonic**; however, in the colon more water than electrolytes is absorbed, leading to water being absorbed against a concentration gradient. The process is controlled by Na^+–K^+ **ATPases** located in the basolateral and lateral membranes of the epithelial cells that line the walls (Figure 44.2). The mucosal surface of the large intestine is relatively smooth with no villi (only microvilli); however, crypts are present and the majority of cells are **columnar** absorptive cells with a large number of mucous-secreting goblet cells. Na^+ is extruded by the membrane pumps into the extracellular spaces. **Tight junctions** at the luminal side of the cells prevent the diffusion of Na^+ and Cl^- from the extracellular spaces into the lumen; this leaves a hypertonic solution close to the lumen, causing water to diffuse from the contents of the lumen. The electrolytes are absorbed by a variety of mechanisms similar to those described for the small intestine. Essentially, there is a net movement of K^+ and HCO_3^- ions from the blood into the large intestine because of the potential difference set up by the asymmetrical absorption of Na^+ and Cl^- across the cell wall.

Gut microflora

Most of the **bacteria** that are present in the GI tract are found in the large intestine, because the acid environment in the rest of the tract destroys most of the so-called microflora. Ninety-nine per cent of the bacteria are anaerobic and most are lost in the faeces (which is said to contain 10^{11} bacteria per gram). The **bacteria** are involved in the **synthesis** of **vitamins K, B$_{12}$, thiamine** and **riboflavin**, the **breakdown** of **primary** to **secondary bile acids** and the **conversion** of **bilirubin** to **non-pigmented metabolites**, all of which are readily absorbed by the GI tract. The bacteria also break down cholesterol, some food additives and drugs.

Endocrinology and reproduction

Part 7

Chapters

45 Endocrine control

Table 45.1 Tissues involved in endocrine control systems. The top half of the table shows the products of classical glandular tissue; the bottom half lists some of the other organs that release hormones

Secreting tissue	Main hormone(s)	Main target tissue(s)	Discussed in chapter
Glands			
Anterior pituitary (P)	Adrenocorticotrophic hormone (ACTH)	Adrenal cortex (M)	52
	Growth hormone (GH)	Liver, bones, muscle (G)	50
	Follicle-stimulating hormone (FSH)	Gonads (R)	
	Luteinizing hormone (LH)	Gonads (R)	53
	Prolactin	Mammary glands (R)	56
	Thyroid-stimulating hormone (TSH)	Thyroid gland (G, M)	48
Intermediate pituitary (P)	Melanotrophin-stimulating hormone (MSH)	Melanocytes (H)	47
Posterior pituitary (P)	Antidiuretic hormone (ADH)	Kidney (H)	38
	Oxytocin	Mammary glands	56
		Uterus (R)	55
Pineal (A)	Melatonin	Hypothalamus (H)	
Thyroid (A)	Thyroxine (T4)	Most tissues (G, M)	49
	Tri-iodothyronine (T3)	Most tissues (G, M)	
	Calcitonin	Bones, gut (H)	51
Parathyroid (P)	Parathyroid hormone (PTH)	Bones, gut (H)	51
Pancreas (P)	Insulin	Liver, muscle, adipose	46
	Glucagon	tissue (G, M, H)	
Adrenal cortex (S)	Corticosteroids (including cortisol)	Multiple (G, M)	52
	Aldosterone	Kidney (H)	38 and 52
Adrenal medulla (A)	Adrenaline (epinephrine)	Multiple (H, M)	52
	Noradrenaline (norepinephrine)	Multiple (H, M)	
Gonads: male (S)	Testosterone	Testes (R)	53
Gonads: female (S)	Oestradiol	Ovaries, uterus (R)	53 and 55
	Progesterone	Ovaries, uterus (R)	
	Human chorionic gonadotrophin (hCG)	Uterus (R)	55
Placenta (P, S)	Oestradiol	Ovaries, uterus (R)	
	Progesterone	Ovaries, uterus (R)	
Non-glands			
Brain (P, A)	Hypothalamic-releasing hormones	Anterior pituitary gland (H, R, M)	47
	Growth factors	Various (M)	
Heart (P)	Atrial natriuretic peptide (ANP)	Kidney	38
Kidney (P, S)	Erythropoietin (EPO)	Bone marrow (M)	9
	1,25-Dihydroxycholecalciferol	Gut, kidney (H)	51
	Renin	Plasma proteins (H)	38
Liver (P)	Insulin-like growth factor-1 (IGF-1)	Various (M)	50
Adipose tissue (P)	Leptin	Hypothalamus (M)	47
Gastrointestinal tract (P, A)	Gastrin	Gut (H, M)	40–44
	Secretin		
	Cholecystokinin (CCK)		
	Vasoactive intestinal polypeptide (VIP)		
	Gastrin-releasing peptide (GRP)		
Immune cells (P)	Cytokines	Hypothalamus (H, M)	11
Platelets (P)	Growth factors	Various (G)	49
Various sites (P)	Growth factors	Various (G)	49
	Neurotrophins	Neurones (G)	

Molecules: A, modified amino acid; P, peptide/protein; S, steroids/sterols.
Functions: H, homeostasis; R, reproduction; G, growth and development; M, metabolism.

Physiology at a Glance, Fourth Edition. Edited by Jeremy P.T. Ward and Roger W.A. Linden.

© 2017 John Wiley & Sons, Ltd. Published 2017 by John Wiley & Sons, Ltd. Companion website: www.ataglanceseries.com/physiology

Multicellular organisms must coordinate the diverse activities of their cells, often over large distances. In animals, such coordination is achieved by the nervous and **endocrine** systems, the former providing rapid, precise but short-term control and the latter providing generally slower and more sustained signals. The two systems are intimately integrated and in some places difficult to differentiate. Endocrine control is mediated by **hormones**, signal molecules usually secreted in low concentrations (10^{-12}–10^{-7} M) into the bloodstream, so that they can reach all parts of the body. Other types of chemical communication are mediated over smaller distances. Chemical signals can act locally on neighbouring cells (paracrine signals) or can act on the same cell that produced the signal (autocrine signals); **juxtacrine** communication requires direct physical contact between signal chemicals on the surface of one cell and receptor molecules on the surface of a neighbour. Many hormones are secreted by discrete glands (Table 45.1), while others are released from tissues with other primary functions. For instance, several of the cytokines released by immune cells (Chapter 11) act at some distance from their site of release and can fairly be considered as hormones.

Features of hormonal signalling

Hormonal molecules can be: (i) **modified amino acids** (e.g. adrenaline [norepinephrine]; Chapter 52); (ii) **peptides** (e.g. somatostatin; Chapter 47); (iii) **proteins** (e.g. insulin; Chapter 46); or (iv) derivatives of the fatty acid cholesterol, such as **steroids** (e.g. cortisol; Chapter 52; Table 45.1). Protein and peptide hormones are cleaved from larger gene products, whereas smaller molecules require the precursor to be transported into endocrine cells so that it can be modified by sequences of enzymes to generate the final product (e.g. Chapter 42). Most hormones are stored in intracellular membrane-bound **secretory granules**, to be released by a **calcium-dependent mechanism** similar to the release of neurotransmitters from nerve cells (Chapter 8; Figure 48.2) when the cell is activated. However, thyroid hormones and steroids, which are highly lipid soluble, cannot be stored in this way. Most steroids are made immediately before release, whereas the thyroid hormones are bound within a glycoprotein matrix (Chapter 48). After secretion, some hormones bind to **plasma proteins**. In most cases this involves non-specific binding to albumin, but there are **specific binding proteins** for some hormones, such as cortisol or testosterone. A hormone bound to a plasma protein cannot reach its site of action and is protected from metabolic degradation, but is freed when the plasma level of the hormone falls. The bound fraction thus acts as a reservoir that helps to maintain steady plasma levels of the free hormone.

Hormones exert their effects by interactions with **specific receptor proteins** and will act only on cells carrying those receptors. Most protein and peptide hormones activate cell surface receptors that are coupled to guanosine triphosphate-binding proteins (**G-proteins**) (Chapter 7) or that have **intrinsic tyrosine kinase** activity (e.g. Chapter 46). Receptors for lipid-soluble hormones (steroids, thyroid hormones) are usually *inside* the target cell, and modify gene transcription directly (e.g. Chapter 48). Because they are in the bloodstream, free hormones can reach all of the tissues that bear the appropriate receptors. Endocrine signals therefore provide a good way of inducing simultaneous changes in multiple organs, and most hormones have effects in more than one tissue. A corollary of this position is that many physiological processes are influenced by more than one hormone, as will become clear in subsequent chapters. Hormones are **inactivated** by metabolic transformation by enzymes, usually in the liver or at the site of action. It is a general rule that the smaller the hormone, the more rapid its inactivation.

Control of hormones

Endocrine secretion can be controlled by the nervous system, other endocrine glands, or respond directly to levels of metabolites in the environment of the gland, and most are subject to all of these types of control. A common feature of hormonal control systems is a heavy reliance on **negative feedback loops**. Almost all hormones feed back to inhibit their own release, providing a direct method of moderating the output of hormone into the blood (Chapters 47–56). A less common feature of endocrine systems, associated only with reproductive functions, is *positive feedback*, whereby the release of a hormone leads to events that further promote release (Chapters 53, 54 and 56). The carriage of hormones in the blood provides a limit on how quickly hormones produce their effects. The relatively slow nature of hormonal signalling puts limits on the types of physiological processes that can be controlled by hormones. They fall into four broad categories: (i) **homeostasis**; (ii) **reproduction**; (iii) **growth and development**; and (iv) **metabolism**. These systems work over time-scales that range from a few minutes (e.g. milk ejection; Chapter 56) to years (growth; Chapter 50).

46 Control of metabolic fuels

Figure 46.1 Feedback control of plasma glucose by insulin and glucagon

Failure of insulin release
Hyperglycaemia
Ketoacidosis, coma, death

Anabolic state

↑ Insulin
↓ Glucagon

High glucose, fatty acids
and amino acids

Eating

Uptake of glucose and fatty acids
by liver, muscle and adipose cells,
activation of anabolic systems

Activation of catabolic systems,
release of glucose and fatty acids
by liver cells

'Normal' levels of glucose, fatty
acids and amino acids

Stress
exercise
growth

↓ Insulin
↑ Glucagon

Fasting

Low glucose, fatty acids
and amino acids

Catabolic state

Excess insulin, hypoglycaemia,
coma, death

Figure 46.2 Glucose-evoked release of insulin
from pancreatic β cell

Glucose
transporters

Glucose

GLUT-2

Glucose

Metabolic
conversion

ATP

Closes

↓ K⁺ efflux

↑ Ca²⁺ entry

Insulin -
containing
granules

Insulin

Exocytosis
of insulin

E_m increases
(depolarization)

Opens

Voltage-gated
Ca²⁺ channel

ATP-gated
K⁺channel

Figure 46.3 Insulin stimulates translocation of glucose
transporters to membranes of target cells

Insulin receptor

Tyrosine kinase element

IRS-1

Grb2

PI-3 kinase

Glucose
transporters

Ras

GLUT-4

GLUT-4

GLUT-1

GLUT-1

Golgi apparatus

Glucose
transporters

MAPKK

MAPK

IRS-1 = Insulin receptor substrate 1

Grb2 = A coupling protein

Ras = An intracellular GTPase

PI-3 = Phosphatidylinositol-3

MAPK(K) = Mitogen activated protein kinase (kinase)

Animal cells utilize glucose and fatty acids as fuels to generate the energy-rich molecule adenosine triphosphate (ATP) (Chapter 3). The blood levels of these molecules must be carefully controlled to ensure a steady supply of fuel to active tissues, a task that is complicated by the tendency of many animals (not ruminants) to eat discrete meals rather than continuously. Immediately after a meal, circulating levels of fuel molecules rise and any excess to immediate requirements is stored. This requires the transport of the molecules into cells (primarily **liver**, **skeletal muscle** and the fat-storing cells of **adipose tissues**) and the synthesis of storage molecules, such as **glycogen**, a polymer of glucose, **triglycerides** (fats) and, to a lesser extent, proteins. As time after a meal increases, the consumption of blood glucose and fatty acids necessitates the activation of tissue energy stores. Glycogen is broken down into glucose, triglycerides are converted into free fatty acids and ketone bodies and, if the fast is prolonged, proteins are catabolized to provide a supply of amino acids that can be converted to glucose (**gluconeogenesis**). The body thus alternates between two states, which can be described as **anabolic**, in which storage molecules are manufactured, and **catabolic** in which the same molecules are broken down (Figure 46.1). Switching between these states is controlled mainly by hormones, with the pancreatic proteins **insulin** and **glucagon** being the prime movers of the anabolic and catabolic processes, respectively. In addition, growth hormone (Chapter 50), cortisol, adrenaline (epinephrine) and noradrenaline (norepinephrine) (Chapter 52) can stimulate catabolic processes (Figure 46.1).

Control of appetite and body weight

This is a complex process which is centrally mediated by the brain (hypothalamus). Food in the intestine stimulates release of **cholescystokinin** (CCK), **glucagon-like peptide-1** (GLP-1) and **peptide YY** which suppress appetite (**satiety signals**). Over a longer period, **leptin** secretion by adipose tissue (fat deposits) also reduces appetite. A fall in food intake and fasting inhibits these signals, but stimulates secretion of **ghrelin** from the stomach, leading to increased appetite and the sensation of hunger. Unfortunately for some, long-term fasting (i.e. dieting) upregulates **orexigenic** (appetite stimulating) and downregulates **anorexigenic** (appetite suppressing) pathways in the hypothalamus, which is why it is so difficult for those on diets to maintain their initial weight loss.

Insulin and glucagon

These hormones are made in the endocrine tissues of the pancreas, known as the **islets of Langerhans**. Three main types of cell have been identified within the islets: peripherally located α (also known as A) cells, which manufacture and secrete **glucagon**; centrally located β (or B) cells for the production and release of **insulin**; and δ (or D) cells that synthesize and liberate **somatostatin**. The exact role of somatostatin has not been established, but it may be involved in controlling the release of the other two hormones. Insulin release is stimulated initially during eating by the parasympathetic nervous system and gut hormones, such as secretin (Chapter 42), but most output is driven by the rise in plasma glucose concentration that occurs after a meal

(Figures 46.1 and 46.2). Circulating fatty acids, ketone bodies and amino acids augment the effect of glucose. The major action of insulin is to stimulate glucose uptake, with the subsequent manufacture of glycogen and triglycerides by adipose, muscle and liver cells. Its effects are mediated by a **receptor tyrosine kinase** (RTK; Figure 46.3; Chapters 7 and 50). The enzyme activates an intracellular pathway that results in the translocation of the glucose transporter GLUT-4 and to a lesser extent GLUT-1 to the plasma membrane of the affected cell, to facilitate the entry of glucose (Figure 46.3). Insulin thus decreases plasma glucose. Insulin release is reduced as the blood glucose concentration falls, and is further inhibited by catecholamines (Chapter 52) acting at β-cell α$_2$-adrenoceptors (Chapters 8 and 52). Glucagon release patterns tend to be the mirror image of those of insulin. Low blood glucose initiates glucagon release directly and also drives nervous and hormonal release of catecholamines, which activate β-adrenoceptors (Chapters 8 and 52) on α cells to augment glucagon release. Glucagon acts on guanosine triphosphate-binding protein (G-protein)-coupled receptors that stimulate the production of intracellular cyclic adenosine monophosphate (cAMP) (Chapter 7). In liver cells, this results in the inhibition of glycogen synthesis and the activation of glycogen breakdown systems. Similar effects are obtained in muscle cells to increase circulating levels of glucose. There are interactions between glucagon and insulin within the islets: insulin inhibits α-cell release of glucagon, but glucagon *stimulates* the release of insulin, an effect that ensures a basal level of insulin release irrespective of glucose levels. The two hormones operate as part of a classical negative feedback system (Figure 46.1; Chapter 1), in which the α and β cells act as combined sensors–comparators, and their hormones activate the effector tissues.

Diabetes mellitus

This disease is caused by failure of β-cell function, either by **autoimmune attack**, in which the immune system (Chapter 11) misidentifies the cells as non-self and destroys them, or by pathologies, such as **obesity**, that impair insulin release. The former type of disease is usually early onset and is treated with insulin (**insulin-dependent diabetes**), whereas the latter develops later and is treated by diets that lower blood glucose levels or drugs that stimulate insulin release (**non–insulin-dependent diabetes**). Untreated, the condition leads to chronically high levels of plasma glucose (**hyperglycaemia**), overloading the kidney glucose transporters so that glucose begins to appear in the urine (Chapter 36). The osmotic effect of glucose leads to excess production of urine (**polyuria**) that tastes sweet (this used to be the diagnostic test for diabetes, and gives the disease its name; Latin *mellitus* = sweet). Long-term hyperglycaemia drives excessive lipolysis by liver cells, leading to a build-up of ketone bodies and the condition known as **ketoacidosis** (Chapter 39). This disrupts brain function, causing coma and eventually death. A sharp fall in blood glucose (**hypoglycaemia**) caused by excessive insulin administration starves the brain of its main metabolic fuel and, by a sad irony, can also lead to coma and death (Figure 46.1). Long-term complications of diabetes include damage to small blood vessels, especially in the retina and renal nephron (diabetic retinopathy and nephropathy). This is at least partly due oxidative stress as a result of the hyperglycaemia.

The hypothalamus and pituitary gland

Figure 47.1 The pituitary gland: relationships with some hypothalamic neurones

Gonadotrophin-releasing hormone (ventromedial hypothalamus/medial preoptic area)

Antidiuretic hormone/oxytocin (supraoptic)

Superior hypophyseal artery

Antidiuretic hormone/oxytocin (paraventricular)

Corticotrophin-releasing hormone (paraventricular)

Somatostatin (periventricular)

Median eminence

Portal vessels

Inferior hypophyseal artery

⭐ Magnocellular neurone

⬟ Parvocellular neurone

→ Direction of blood flow

Anterior pituitary (adenohypophysis)

Posterior pituitary (neurohypophysis)

Figure 47.3 General model for a hypothalamic-anterior pituitary control axis

Other brain areas → Hypothalamus ←

Hypophysiotropic hormones (+ve or −ve)

Portal vessels

Anterior pituitary cells

General circulation

Pituitary hormone

Target glands → Target gland hormone → Target tissues

Sensory feedback

Physiological effects

Hormonal feedback (negative)

Figure 47.2 Hypophysiotropic control of the anterior pituitary

Hypothalamic hypophysiotropic hormones and their origins

?		Ventromedial hypothalamus	Arcuate nucleus		Paraventricular nucleus				Periventricular nucleus
Melanotrophin-releasing factor	Melanotrophin-inhibitory factor	Gonadotrophin-releasing hormone	Growth hormone-releasing hormone	Dopamine (prolactin inhibitory factor)	Oxytocin	Antidiuretic hormone	Corticotrophin-releasing hormone	Thyrotrophin-releasing hormone	Somatostatin

Anterior pituitary hormones

Melanocyte-stimulating hormone	Luteinizing hormone	Follicle-stimulating hormone	Growth hormone	Prolactin	Adreno-corticotrophic hormone	Thyroid-stimulating hormone

Pigmentation | Reproduction | Growth | Lactation | Stress | Metabolism

→ Stimulatory   ------→ Inhibitory

Physiology at a Glance, Fourth Edition. Edited by Jeremy P.T. Ward and Roger W.A. Linden.

© 2017 John Wiley & Sons, Ltd. Published 2017 by John Wiley & Sons, Ltd. Companion website: www.ataglanceseries.com/physiology

The **pituitary gland**, which is under the direct control of the brain from the **hypothalamus**, provides endocrine control of many major physiological functions. The hypothalamus is composed of a number of nuclei (collections of cell bodies) and vaguely defined 'areas', and surrounds the **third ventricle** at the base of the medial forebrain. The most important hypothalamic areas for endocrine function are the **paraventricular, periventricular, supraoptic** and **arcuate nuclei**, and the **ventromedial hypothalamus**. Some of the hypothalamic neurones can secrete hormones (a process called *neurosecretion*), releasing chemicals in exactly the same way as other nerve cells (Chapter 8), albeit that their signals are liberated into the bloodstream rather than into synapses (Figure 47.1) The pituitary is located immediately beneath the hypothalamus and comprises three divisions: the **anterior pituitary**, the **intermediate lobe** (almost vestigial in humans) and the **posterior pituitary** (Figures 47.1 and 47.2). The anterior pituitary develops from tissues originating in the roof of the mouth, is non-neural and is sometimes known as the **adenohypophysis**. The posterior gland is really an extension from the hypothalamus itself, consists of neural tissue and is referred to as the **neurohypophysis**. All pituitary hormones are either peptides or proteins. As befits their developmental origins, the adeno- and neurohypophyses are controlled in different ways.

The anterior pituitary and intermediate lobe

The adenohypophyseal hormones and their actions are listed in Figure 47.1. They are released under the control of chemical signals (**hypothalamic releasing or inhibiting hormones**) originating from small (**parvocellular**) neurones with their cell bodies in the hypothalamus (Figures 47.1, 47.2 and 47.3). These hormones are peptides or proteins released into the blood at the **median eminence** (Figure 47.1) when the appropriate parvocellular neurones are electrically active. The hypothalamic hormones are transported directly to the anterior pituitary via the **hypophyseal portal vessels** (Figure 47.1). The portal vessels carry hypophysiotropic signals directly to the anterior pituitary to stimulate *or* inhibit the release of pituitary hormones by the activation of receptors on specific groups of pituitary cells (Figure 47.2). It should be noted that some hypothalamic hormones control more than one pituitary hormone. Figure 47.3 illustrates the basic principles that underlie the control of anterior pituitary hormones; this is a form of chemical cascade

that allows for the precise control of pituitary output with two stages of signal amplification: first, at the pituitary itself, where tiny amounts of hypothalamic hormones control the release of larger quantities of pituitary hormone; and then at the final target gland, where the pituitary signals stimulate the release of still larger quantities of hormones such as steroids. The cascade allows for feedback control of hormone release at several points. The final hormone (and often some of the intermediate signals) inhibits further activity in the axis to provide the fine regulation of hormone release (Figure 47.3). This is a characteristic feature of anterior pituitary control systems.

The posterior pituitary

The posterior gland secretes two peptide hormones: **oxytocin** and **antidiuretic hormone** (ADH; also known as **vasopressin**). The hormones are manufactured in the cell bodies of large (**magnocellular**) neurones in the supraoptic and paraventricular nuclei of the hypothalamus, and are transported down the axons of these cells to their terminals on capillaries originating from the **inferior hypophyseal artery** within the posterior pituitary gland (Figure 47.1). When magnocellular neurones are activated (see Chapters 38, 55 and 56), they release oxytocin or ADH into the general circulation, from whence they can reach the relevant target tissues to produce the required effect. The signals that drive the release of posterior gland hormones are entirely neural, so that the hormones are said to be involved in **neuroendocrine reflexes**. These hormones operate over shorter time courses (minutes) than most endocrine events (hours to days). The release of ADH is controlled by conventional negative feedback mechanisms based on plasma osmolality and blood volume (Chapter 38). Oxytocin, however, is involved in *positive* feedback mechanisms (Chapters 55 and 56).

Pulsatile release of pituitary hormones

Hormones released from the hypothalamus tend to appear in the blood in discrete pulses, rather than as continuous secretions. This is achieved by the synchronous activation of hormone-releasing neurones of the hypothalamus. As will be seen in later chapters, episodic release has profound implications for the operation of the endocrine system. It also raises a number of interesting and as yet unanswered questions as to how many separate and more or less widely scattered neurones can be activated simultaneously to give rise to pulsatile release.

48 Thyroid hormones and metabolic rate

Figure 48.1 Structures of tri-iodothyronine (T₃) and thyroxine (T₄)

Figure 48.3 The hypothalamic–thyroid axis

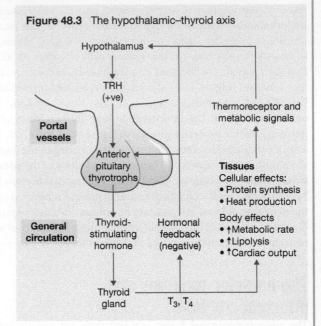

Figure 48.2 Manufacture and release of thyroid hormones

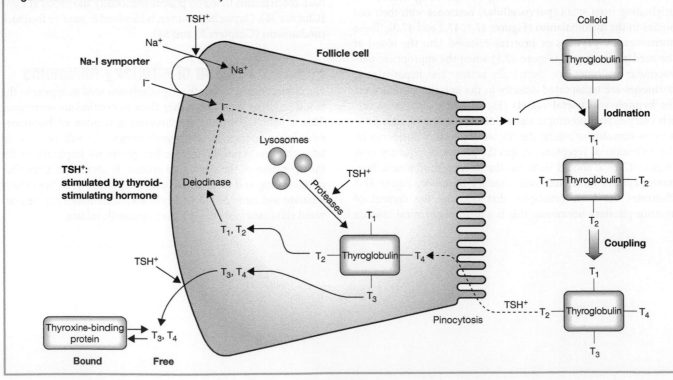

The thyroid gland is attached to the anterior surface of the trachea just below the larynx. It releases two iodine-containing hormones, **thyroxine** (also known as T_4) and **tri-iodothyronine** (T_3; Figure 48.1), the main effect of which is to increase heat production (**thermogenesis**) throughout the body and thereby induce an increase in metabolic rate. The hormones also have a crucial role in growth and development.

Synthesis and release

The thyroid gland is formed from clusters of cells (**follicles**) that surround a gel-like matrix or colloid, the primary constituent of which is the glycoprotein **thyroglobulin**. The follicle cells actively accumulate iodide (I^-) ions by means of an Na^+–I^- symporter (Chapter 4) driven by the inward sodium gradient (Figure 48.2). The formation of T_3 and T_4 occurs in two steps: (i) the amino acid tyrosine is iodinated to form mono- (T_1) or di-iodotyrosine (T_2) (Figure 48.1); (ii) T_2 is then coupled to T_1 or T_2 by thyroperoxidase to form the thyroid hormones. This process occurs with the tyrosine residues attached to thyroglobulin, so that, at any one time, this protein is festooned with molecules of T_1, T_2, T_3 and T_4 (Figure 48.2). The thyroid hormones and their intermediates are highly lipophilic and would escape from the gland were they not incorporated into thyroglobulin, which thus acts as a nucleus for the manufacture of the hormones and as a storage site. The hormones are released under the control of **thyroid-stimulating hormone** (TSH) from the anterior pituitary, which is obligatory for normal thyroid function. TSH release is itself regulated by **thyrotropin-releasing hormone** (TRH) from the hypothalamus in response to thermoreceptor (Chapter 13) and metabolic signals, and circulating levels of T_3 and T_4 detected by both the hypothalamus and pituitary (negative feedback) (Chapter 47; Figure 48.3). Under the action of TSH, thyroid follicle cells pinch off small quantities of colloid by **pinocytosis**. Lysozymal protease enzymes then act on the thyroglobulin to liberate the iodinated compounds into the cell and thence into the bloodstream (Figure 48.2). Free T_1 and T_2 are deiodinated by enzymatic action before they can leave the cell. The average plasma concentration of T_3 is roughly one-sixth of that of T_4, and much of that derives from deiodinated T_4. Most of the thyroid hormones in the blood are bound to thyroxine-binding protein and are thus unavailable to their receptors, which are located *inside* target cells, attached directly to deoxyribonucleic acid (DNA). The small amounts of free T_3 and T_4 in plasma readily cross the cell membranes to bind to thyroid hormone receptors (the most important of which is **TR-α_1**). Thyroid receptors are linked to a DNA sequence known as the **thyroid-response element** (TRE) which initiates the transcription of thyroid-responsive genes. T_3 is some 10 times more potent than T_4 in activating TR-α_1 and consequently mediates most thyroid hormone actions, notwithstanding its lower levels in plasma. Thyroid receptors are present in almost all tissues, with particularly high levels in the liver and low levels in the spleen and testes.

Physiological roles of thyroid hormones

Basal levels of thyroid hormone release are essential to maintain a normal metabolic rate. Situations requiring increased heat production, for instance when the core temperature falls, lead to enhanced activation of the thyroid axis. The effects take up to 4 days to reach a maximum, a slow time course that is characteristic of hormones acting through nuclear receptors. The primary action of thyroid hormones is an increase in the synthesis of Na^+–K^+ ATPase (Chapter 4), an enzyme that consumes large amounts of metabolic energy, to increase heat production. The hormones may also enhance the production of **uncoupling proteins** (UCPs). These molecules act in mitochondria to divert the H^+ ion gradient generated by the electron transport chain (**non-shivering thermogenesis**; Chapter 13), so that it produces heat rather than driving adenosine triphosphate (ATP) synthase. Although UCP-1 is found only in brown fat, a tissue that is uncommon in adult humans, two other members of the family (UCP-2 and UCP-3) are present in muscle and other tissues, and may thus contribute to thyroid-stimulated thermogenesis (Chapter 13). Other important actions of thyroid hormones include a generalized increase in protein turnover (i.e. breakdown *and* synthesis), an increase in cardiac output caused by the enhancement of the effects of adrenaline (epinephrine) at β-adrenoceptors (Chapters 8 and 52), and a strong lipolytic effect that arises from the potentiation of responses to cortisol, glucagon, growth hormone and adrenaline. These actions can be described as generally catabolic (Chapter 46), but it should be noted that low doses of thyroid hormones have an overall anabolic action and that the hormones are essential to normal postnatal growth.

Disorders of the thyroid gland

Lack of dietary iodide or a failure of iodide uptake mechanisms in the thyroid gland produces the conditions of **hypothyroidism**. In fetal and neonatal life, underproduction of thyroid hormones causes inadequate somatic and neural development and gives rise to **cretinism**, a condition characterized by subnormal stature and mental ability. In adults, the main symptoms of thyroid insufficiency are lethargy, sluggishness and an intolerance to cold. In severe cases, there is excess production of water-retaining mucoproteins in subcutaneous tissues, giving rise to tissue bloating, known as **myxoedema**. Such conditions are treated with injections of T_4. When the cause of hypothyroidism is an insufficiency of iodide intake, cells of the thyroid gland undergo hypertrophy and the gland becomes enlarged to form a **goitre**. This (now very uncommon) condition is treated by ensuring an adequate supply of dietary iodide. The overproduction of T_3 and T_4 leads to **hyperthyroidism** (Graves' disease), characterized by **exophthalmia** (bulging eyes), increased behavioural excitability, tremor, weight loss and chronic tachycardia (high heart rate). The last of these symptoms can eventually lead to ventricular arrhythmias and/or heart failure, and so treatment, usually surgical removal of part of the gland or antithyroid drugs, is highly recommended.

49 Growth factors

Figure 49.1 The cell cycle and growth factors

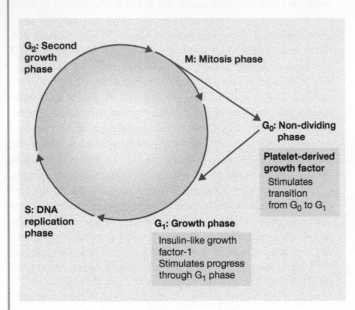

Figure 49.3 The serine–threonine kinase transduction pathway

(i) TGFβ binds to Type II TGFβ receptor

(ii) Dimerization with a Type I TGFβ receptor which is phosphorylated (P)

(iii) Serine–threonine kinase (S-TK) binds SMAD2 (or 3), which is phosphorylated

(iv) Phosphorylated SMAD2 (or 3) dissociates from receptor and dimerizes with SMAD4

(v) Dimerized SMADs bind to DNA and activate other gene regulatory proteins to alter gene expression

Figure 49.2 Intracellular systems activated by receptor tyrosine kinases

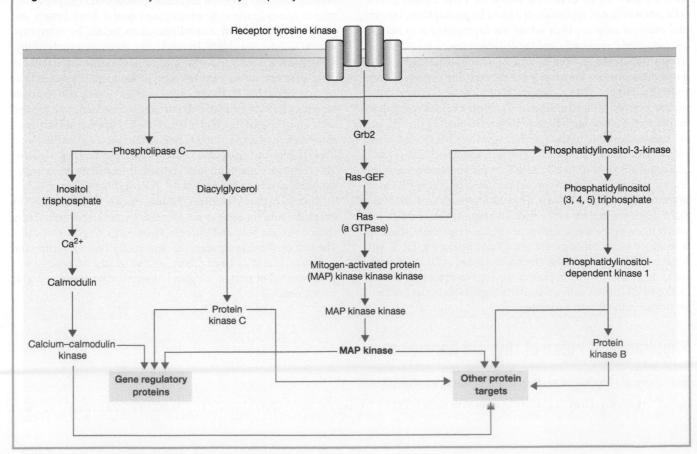

Physiology at a Glance, Fourth Edition. Edited by Jeremy P.T. Ward and Roger W.A. Linden.

For an embryo to develop into an adult, its cells must increase in number by the process of division (**mitosis**) and grow in size (**hypertrophy**). As they mature, cells develop specializations according to the tissue of which they are a part (**differentiation**). In tissue development, excess production of cells is the norm, so that the final shaping of organs depends on programmed death (**apoptosis**) of supernumerary cells. Some tissues, such as nerve and skeletal muscle, reach a stage of terminal differentiation in adulthood and undergo no further cell division. However, most cells in the adult retain the ability to divide, allowing tissues (e.g. blood vessels, bones) to remodel or repair themselves as required. Some cells face particularly high rates of attrition (e.g. enterocytes in the gut lining, skin cells, hair follicles) and are produced continuously throughout life. The processes of mitosis, cell growth and apoptosis are controlled by a large number of systemic and local peptide hormones, known as **growth factors** (Chapter 45). To varying extents, these factors stimulate mitosis (they are **mitogens**), promote growth (a **trophic** effect) and inhibit apoptosis (promote cell **survival**).

Growth factor families and their receptors

Growth factors are classified into a number of families based on common amino acid sequences and the types of receptor that they activate. **Neurotrophins**, which include **nerve growth factor** (**NGF**), are important chemical signals in the development of the nervous system and are potent survival factors for neurones in adults. The **epidermal growth factor** (**EGF**) family includes EGF itself and transforming growth factor-α (TGFα), both of which are mitogens in a wide range of tissues, including the gut and skin. **Fibroblast growth factors** (**FGF-1–24**) are strongly mitogenic and induce the production of new blood vessels (**angiogenesis**). The **transforming growth factor-β** (**TGFβ**) superfamily includes a number of bone-transforming proteins (Chapter 46) and is crucial in embryogenesis and the development and remodelling of structural tissues. The origins of **platelet-derived growth factor** (**PDGF**) are self-explanatory. It stimulates division, growth and survival in a number of cell types, and is important in tissue repair after injury. **Insulin** and **insulin-like growth factors** (**IGF-1** and **IGF-2**) have similar structures but rather different actions: insulin promotes anabolic activity generally (Chapter 43), whereas the IGFs are mitogenic, trophic and act as survival factors for several cell types. Numerous other hormones have mitogenic properties, e.g. the stimulation of red blood cell production by **erythropoietin** (Chapter 9) and white cell production by **cytokines** (Chapter 11) means that these hormones are also described as growth factors.

Mitosis occurs during the **cell cycle** (Figure 49.1). Some mitogens, including PDGF, stimulate transition from the non-dividing state (G_0) into the growth phase of the cycle (G_1), whereas others, such as EGF and IGF-1, stimulate progress through G_1. With the exception of TGFα, erythropoietin and the cytokines, growth factors work by activating receptor tyrosine kinases (Chapters 7 and 46; Figure 49.2). Binding of the hormone leads to phosphorylation of the tyrosine residues of a number of important intracellular proteins, including phospholipase C, Grb2 and phosphatidylinositol-3 kinase, eventually leading to the production of more kinases: **protein kinases C and B**, **calcium-calmodulin kinase** (**CAM kinase**) and **mitogen-activated protein kinase** (**MAP kinase**) (Figure 49.2). These enzymes have many targets within the cell, but MAP kinase, in particular, enters the nucleus and activates immediate to early genes, such as *c-fos* and *c-jun*. The products of these genes are transcription factors, driving the expression of further genes, such as those that produce G_1 **cyclins**, proteins that are required for cell division. The MAP kinase pathway appears to be the main intracellular signalling system for the stimulation of mitosis. The TGFβ family exerts its effects through **receptor serine–threonine kinases** that phosphorylate their target proteins at serine and threonine residues (Chapter 7). The pathway activated by these receptors involves proteins called **SMADs** (the name is derived from genes that code for similar proteins in *Drosophila melanogaster* [fruit fly] and *Caenorhabditis elegans*, a nematode worm). SMAD2 and/or SMAD3 is phosphorylated while it is attached to the receptor; it then dissociates to dimerize with SMAD4, forming a complex that directly activates gene regulatory proteins (Figure 49.3). Growth hormone, erythropoietin and the cytokines activate receptors that signal through **Janus kinases** (**JAKs**; Chapter 50).

Growth factors and cancer

Cell division and growth are strictly controlled so that organs do not invade the space needed for other tissues. When this process is deranged, cancers are formed. Cancer cells do not recognize the normal constraints of organ growth or the limits to the number of divisions to which cells are normally subjected, and are unusually mobile. These features make cancer cells extremely dangerous, as they supplant healthy tissues and cause fatal damage to physiological systems. Cancerous growths start with mutations in particular genes (**oncogenes**) that impact on cell division and/or apoptosis. *Ras* genes, which produce the Ras GTPases that are key mediators in the MAP kinase pathway (Figure 49.2), are commonly found to be defective in human tumours. In view of the importance of this pathway in mitogenesis, it is not difficult to see how the abnormal activation of these genes could lead to excessive cellular proliferation. In this situation, the signals involved in normal tissue growth provide the driving force for tumour growth and survival. EGF, in particular, has been associated with the maintenance of colorectal and breast cancers, and anti-EGF drugs are showing some promise as tumour-controlling agents.

50 Somatic and skeletal growth

Figure 50.1 Control of growth hormone release

Sleep/wake cycle, stress → Hypothalamus ←

Somatostatin (–ve)   GHRH (+ve)

Portal vessels

Anterior pituitary somatotrophs

Growth hormone

Hormonal (negative) feedback

General circulation

Liver → IGF-1 → Bones, muscle, cartilage

Skeletal and muscular growth, protein synthesis

Metabolic signals

Muscle, adipocytes → ?Protein synthesis
?Blood glucose
?Lipolysis

Figure 50.2 Cellular mechanism of action of growth hormone

(i) Growth hormone receptor

(ii) GH binding causes receptor dimerization

(iii) STATs bind to receptor to be phosphorylated (P) by JAKs (Janus kinases)

(iv) Phosphorylated STATs dissociate from receptor and dimerize

(v) Dimerized STATs regulate gene expression by binding to DNA

Figure 50.3 The main features of bone

Epiphysis

Diaphysis

Marrow
• Source of all bone and blood cells

Cartilage/forming bone
• Osteoblasts lay down collagen/proteoglycan matrix
• Calcified in adults (trabecular)

Growth plate
• Maturing chondrocytes (least mature nearest the marrow)
• Calcified in adults

Trabecular bone
• Calcified, open texture
• Osteocytes in spaces within bone matrix
• Osteoblasts
• Osteoclasts

Cortical bone
• Calcified, dense texture
• Osteocytes in spaces within bone matrix
• Osteoblasts
• Osteoclasts

Figure 50.4 The normal pattern of somatic growth

Growth (% maximum) vs Age (years)

Growth and development are entirely under endocrine control. The key signals involved in these processes are **growth hormone**, thyroid hormones (Chapter 48), sex steroids (Chapters 53 and 54) and growth factors (Chapter 49). Normal growth depends on the interplay between all of these factors. In development, there are two periods of particularly rapid growth: during pregnancy and up to the 2 years immediately after birth, and around the time of puberty (Figure 50.4).

Growth hormone

Growth hormone (GH; also known as **somatotrophin**) provides the main drive for growth. It is a protein released from pituitary somatotrophs under hypothalamic control (Figure 50.1) that stimulates growth in muscles, bones and connective tissue. It is essential for normal growth both before and after birth. The release of the hormone increases immediately after birth before subsiding to a low level for most of prepubertal life. There is another surge in release around the time of puberty, after which plasma concentrations again fall and then continue to decline steadily into old age. The release of the hormone varies throughout the day, with the highest levels achieved during deep sleep. The episodic appearance of growth hormone in the blood is driven by hypothalamic **growth hormone-releasing hormone (GHRH)**, and **somatostatin (SST)**, which inhibits growth hormone release (Chapter 47; Figure 53.1). The growth hormone receptor is linked to an intracellular enzyme, **Janus kinase-2 (JAK-2)** (Figure 50.2). Once activated, this enzyme binds and phosphorylates **signal transduction and activation of transcription (STAT)** proteins, which consequently modify gene transcription (Chapter 7). To provide energy for growing tissues, growth hormone has an anti-insulin action in increasing plasma glucose and stimulating lipolysis (Chapter 46). However, its overall effect is anabolic, increasing protein synthesis in many tissues. Most of its effects on growth arise from the stimulation of the release of insulin-like growth factor-1 (IGF-1) (Chapter 49) into the circulation, mainly from the liver. The lifetime release of growth hormone is regulated by the genetic factors that determine body size, but full expression of its effects requires adequate supplies of metabolic fuels and the presence of the other hormones mentioned above. In the short term, it is also liberated in response to stress and exercise.

The overproduction of growth hormone in children is associated with **gigantism**, and underproduction with **dwarfism**, which is much more common. Dwarfism is currently treated with human growth hormone manufactured by genetically engineered bacteria. Growth retardation can also result from defects in the GH receptor, or problems with IGF-1 production or action. Excess growth hormone release in adults leads to disproportionate growth of the bones of the face and limb extremities, a condition known as **acromegaly**.

Bone growth and remodelling

The bones are a major target for growth hormone. They are composed of an organic matrix made up of the structural protein **collagen**, combined with glycoproteins, that forms a framework within which the mineral **hydroxyapatite** $[Ca_{10}(PO_4)_6(OH)_2]$ is deposited. There are two main varieties of bone structure. **Cortical** or compact bone has a dense structure and provides most of the strength of the skeleton. It forms the outer layer of all bones and is particularly prevalent in the **diaphyses** (shafts) of limb bones. **Trabecular** or spongy bone has a more open structure than cortical bone and surrounds the marrow. Axial bones, such as the vertebrae, and the ends (**epiphyses**) of long bones are largely composed of trabecular matrix (Figure 50.3). In development, bones grow from the interface between the epiphysis and the diaphysis (the **growth plate**). The elongation of bones involves the laying down of new collagen matrix at the growth plate by rapidly dividing **chondrocytes**, followed by **calcification** (hydroxyapatite deposition) through the action of **osteoblasts**. When growth is complete at about 20 years of age (Figure 50.4), the growth plate itself becomes calcified and bone elongation ceases. This stage is known as **epiphyseal closure**, a process driven by the high levels of sex steroids present at puberty. Even in adults, bones remain dynamic structures, with substantial proportions of the skeleton (25% of trabecular bone and 3% of cortical bone) being replaced by new growth every year. Osteoblasts develop into **osteocytes**, cells with numerous processes that settle into spaces in the bone matrix. Osteocytes maintain the integrity of the matrix, but can also secrete acids that dissolve hydroxyapatite and thus provide free Ca^{2+} to the circulation when required (Chapter 51). **Osteoclasts** are large cells similar to macrophages (Chapter 11) that remove old bone matrix so that it can be replaced by new material. Osteoblasts, osteocytes and osteoclasts are all present in mature bone. The collective activity of these cells allows bone to be remodelled throughout life to cope with changes in skeletal stresses, and plays an essential role in the repair of broken bones. All bone cells differentiate from bone marrow stem cells. Systemic IGF-1 and locally produced IGF-1 and IGF-2 (Chapter 49) stimulate the division, differentiation and matrix-secreting activity of osteoblasts and chondrocytes (which are also involved in cartilage formation), whereas members of the transforming growth factor-β (TGFβ) family of growth factors are thought to provide the same stimuli for osteoclasts.

Osteoporosis

After the menopause women lose bone mass, leading to a weakening of the skeleton with a consequent increase in the likelihood of fractures in older women. This is due to the reduced secretion of sex steroids from the ovaries (Chapter 53), which normally suppress the production of the cytokine **interleukin-6 (IL-6)** in bones. High levels of IL-6 stimulate the differentiation of osteoclasts, so that bone resorption outstrips the laying down of new matrix and more bone is removed than is replaced. The condition can be successfully treated by the administration of oestrogen (**hormone replacement therapy**). Recent evidence suggests that bone destruction in **rheumatoid arthritis** may also be driven by cytokines.

51 Control of plasma calcium

Figure 51.1 Control of plasma calcium

Figure 51.2 Biosynthesis of 1,25-dihydroxycholecalciferol

Physiology at a Glance, Fourth Edition. Edited by Jeremy P.T. Ward and Roger W.A. Linden.

© 2017 John Wiley & Sons, Ltd. Published 2017 by John Wiley & Sons, Ltd. Companion website: www.ataglanceseries.com/physiology

In cells, Ca^{2+} ions are used to trigger many key physiological events, including muscle contraction (Chapter 15), the release of neurotransmitters (Chapter 8), the release of hormones (Chapters 46 and 47), secretion from exocrine glands and the activation of many important intracellular enzymes, such as the calcium-calmodulin kinases (CAM kinases) (Chapter 49) and nitric oxide synthase (Chapters 24 and 54). Ca^{2+} ions are triggers in so many crucial events that free intracellular Ca^{2+} must be maintained at a very low level (Chapter 2). Most is stored in the endoplasmic reticulum or mitochondria. External to cells, Ca^{2+} ions contribute to the blood clotting cascade (Chapter 10) and the normal functioning of Na^+ ion channels (Chapter 4). When extracellular Ca^{2+} is too low, Na^+ channels open spontaneously, leading to involuntary contractions of skeletal muscles, described as **hypocalcaemic tetany**. This is the clinical sign of low plasma Ca^{2+}. It is evident that Ca^{2+} levels in plasma must be very carefully controlled, a function performed by the coordinated activity of three hormones: **parathyroid hormone** (**PTH**), **1,25-dihydroxycholecalciferol** (**1,25-(OH)$_2$D**) and **calcitonin** (Figure 51.1).

Parathyroid hormone and calcitonin

PTH, a peptide of 84 amino acids, is the major controller of free calcium in the body. It is released from **chief cells** of the four (or more) **parathyroid glands** located immediately behind the thyroid gland, when the plasma concentration of Ca^{2+} decreases. This is detected by a calcium-sensing receptor protein (CaSR) expressed by chief cells. When Ca^{2+} ions bind to the receptor, intracellular levels of cyclic adenosine monophosphate (cAMP) (Chapter 3) decrease and the release of PTH is *inhibited*. PTH increases the plasma levels of Ca^{2+} by activating specific membrane receptors in bone, gut and kidney. In bone, the immediate effect of PTH is to stimulate **osteocytic osteolysis** of bone crystals to release Ca^{2+} ions (Chapter 50). After a longer time, PTH also increases osteoclast activity (Chapter 50) to gain access to more of the bone mineral. In the gut, PTH, acting in concert with 1,25-(OH)$_2$D, enhances the absorption of Ca^{2+} ions. In the kidney, the same combination of hormones enhances the reabsorption of Ca^{2+} from the renal tubules and simultaneously decreases the reabsorption of PO_4^{3-} ions (Chapter 37). PTH also stimulates the kidney to produce more 1,25-(OH)$_2$D. Thus, PTH leads the response to a fall in plasma Ca^{2+} by releasing ions stored in bone, conserving ions filtered by the kidney and enhancing the intake of new ions from the gut (Figure 51.1). The effects of PTH are in each case mediated by stimulating an increase in cAMP in the target cells. **Calcitonin** is a 32-amino acid peptide released from C cells of the thyroid gland in response to high levels of plasma Ca^{2+} ions. C cells carry the same Ca^{2+} receptor as parathyroid chief cells. Calcitonin inhibits bone resorption by osteocytes and may inhibit reabsorption in the kidney, so reducing plasma levels of the ion. The fact that complete removal of the thyroid gland causes no obvious problems with calcium homeostasis has led some physiologists to doubt the significance of this hormone in the normal control of Ca^{2+} ions.

Vitamin D and 1,25-dihydroxycholecalciferol

Vitamin D is an umbrella term for two molecules: **ergocalciferol** (vitamin D$_2$) and **cholecalciferol** (vitamin D$_3$), a derivative of provitamin D (dehydrocholesterol; Figure 51.2). The primary source of supply is the diet, with ergocalciferol derived from plants and yeasts and cholecalciferol from animal (particularly dairy) products. Unusually for a vitamin, cholecalciferol can be manufactured within the body via a reaction that is enabled by ultraviolet irradiation of the skin. The D vitamins are then converted to the active form 1,25-(OH)$_2$D in the kidney (Figure 51.2). The final reaction is the slowest step in the process and therefore regulates the speed of the entire chain of reactions (i.e. it is rate limiting); it is under the influence of PTH. 1,25-(OH)$_2$D has a steroid-like structure and is sometimes referred to as a **sterol**. Its receptors are members of the superfamily of steroid receptors and are located *inside* target cells. The hormone–receptor complex binds to response elements on deoxyribonucleic acid (DNA) to drive the transcription of genes. **Calcium-binding protein**, which promotes calcium transport across epithelia (Chapter 37), is the product of one of the genes activated by 1,25-(OH)$_2$D. The major action of 1,25-(OH)2D is to enable Ca^{2+} absorption from the gut. Without the hormone, Ca^{2+} uptake is severely impaired to the point at which intake of the hormone is insufficient to maintain body stores. This leads to the increased release of PTH and resorption of bone. A lack of D vitamins in children leads to inadequate calcification of bones, which become malformed. This leads to the characteristically bowed limbs seen in **rickets**. This condition was common in the early part of the 20th century, but was virtually eliminated in the UK by the introduction of free school milk. However, recent evidence suggests vitamin D deficiency is more common in the UK than previously thought, and impairs the function of the immune system. Severe vitamin D deficiency in adults leads to bone wasting, a condition known as **osteomalacia**, with symptoms similar to those of osteoporosis (Chapter 50). 1,25-(OH)$_2$D also promotes the reabsorption of Ca^{2+} from the kidney tubules (Chapter 37). The effects of this hormone are generally augmented in the presence of PTH.

Other hormones affecting calcium

Growth-promoting hormones (growth hormone, thyroid hormones and sex steroids) tend to promote the incorporation of calcium into bones (Chapter 50). Excess corticosteroids (Chapter 52) inhibit calcium uptake from the gut and reabsorption from the kidney.

52 The adrenal glands and stress

Figure 52.1 The adrenal glands

- Zona glomerulosa (aldosterone)
- Zona fasciculata (cortisol)   } Cortex
- Zona reticularis (DHEA)
- Medulla (catecholamines)

Renal artery

Kidney

Figure 52.3 Adrenal steroids derived from cholesterol

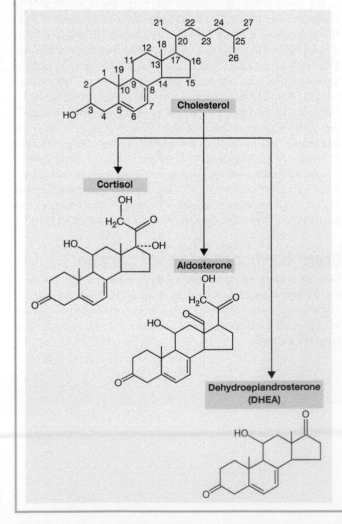

Cholesterol

Cortisol

Aldosterone

Dehydroepiandrosterone (DHEA)

Figure 52.2 Synthesis of catecholamine hormones

Tyrosine   Dihydroxyphenylalanine (DOPA)   Dopamine

Catechol nucleus

Tyrosine hydroxylase   DOPA decarboxylase

Dopamine-β-hydroxylase

Phenylethanolamine-N-methyl transferase

Production stimulated by cortisol

Adrenaline   **Noradrenaline**

Figure 52.4 Responses to stress

Potential pathological outcomes of chronic stress

Stress

Depression
Hippocampus → (−) → Amygdala

(−) → Hypothalamus → Medulla (brain stem)

CRH

Portal vessels

(−) → Anterior pituitary

ACTH

Adrenal cortex   Adrenal medulla

Sympathetic nerves   Parasympathetic nerves

Cortisol

Catecholamines

Anti-inflammatory immunosuppression   Glycolysis Lipolysis Gluconeogenesis   ↑Cardiac output and blood pressure   ↑Gastric acid secretion

Susceptibility to infection   **Chronic hypertension**   **Peptic ulcers**

The adrenal glands are located just above each kidney (hence the name; Figure 52.1) and consist of two endocrine tissues of distinct developmental origins. The inner core (the **adrenal medulla**) releases the catecholamine hormones **adrenaline** (epinephrine) and **noradrenaline** (norepinephrine). It develops from neuronal tissue and is functionally part of the **sympathetic nervous system** (Chapter 8). The outer layers of the gland (the **adrenal cortex**) originate from mesodermal tissue and secrete steroid hormones, primarily under the control of the anterior pituitary gland (Chapter 47). Removal of the adrenal glands in animals results in death within a few days, which is thought to result from the loss of the ability to cope with **stress**.

The adrenal medulla

The **chromaffin cells** of the adrenal medulla manufacture and secrete **noradrenaline** (20%) and **adrenaline** (80%). These catecholamine hormones are derived from tyrosine by a series of steps catalysed by specific enzymes (Figure 52.2). The production of the rate-limiting enzyme, **phenylethanolamine-N-methyl transferase**, is stimulated by **cortisol**, providing a direct link between the functioning of the medulla and cortex. The secretion of catecholamines is stimulated by sympathetic preganglionic neurones located in the spinal cord (Chapter 8), so that the adrenal medulla functions in concert with the sympathetic nervous system, of which noradrenaline is the main neurotransmitter. Catecholamine release contributes to normal physiological functions, but is enhanced by stress (see later). Adrenaline and noradrenaline act through guanosine triphosphate-binding protein (G-protein)-coupled **adrenoceptors**. These are classified as α_1, α_2 and β_1–β_3. The hormones have the same effects in tissues as the stimulation of sympathetic nerves, with important stress-related responses being vasoconstriction (α_1), increased cardiac output (β_1) and increased glycolysis and lipolysis (β_2, β_3). These actions support increased physical activity. Noradrenaline has equal potency at all adrenoceptors, but adrenaline, at normal plasma concentrations, will only activate β-receptors (NB: higher levels do stimulate α-receptors). **Phaeochromocytoma** is a tumour of the adrenal medulla that leads to the excess production of catecholamines, with high blood pressure as the most immediately threatening symptom. It is treated by α-adrenoceptor antagonists and/or surgery.

The adrenal cortex

The cortex is made up of three zones of tissue: the outer **zona glomerulosa**, which releases **aldosterone**; the **zona fasciculata**, which produces **cortisol** and several related but less important hormones; and the inner **zona reticularis**, which secretes the androgen **dehydroepiandrosterone (DHEA)**. All of these secretions are steroids (Figure 52.3). Aldosterone is referred to as a **mineralocorticoid** as it controls the reabsorption of Na^+ and K^+ ions in the kidney (Chapter 38), whereas DHEA and its metabolite, **androstenedione**, provide an important source of androgens for females, contributing to hair growth and libido (Chapter 53). Cortisol and its analogues (such as cortisone) have powerful effects on glucose metabolism and are collectively classified as **glucocorticoids**,

although they do have some mineralocorticoid actions. The release of cortisol and DHEA is stimulated by **adrenocorticotrophic hormone (ACTH)** liberated from the pituitary gland (Chapter 47; Figure 52.4), whereas the secretion of aldosterone is stimulated by angiotensin II and raised plasma $[K^+]$ (Chapter 38). The effects of cortisol are mediated by intracellular receptors that translocate to the cell nucleus after binding the hormone. The cortisol–receptor complex binds to **glucocorticoid response elements** on deoxyribonucleic acid (DNA) to initiate gene transcription.

Cortisol is released during the course of normal physiological activity. The pattern of secretion is pulsatile, driven by activity in corticotrophin-releasing hormone (CRH) neurones of the hypothalamus (Chapter 47). There is usually a surge in cortisol release in the hour after waking. The primary stimulus for the increased release of glucocorticoids is **stress**, which is the result of exposure to adverse situations. The **stress response** is driven by the **amygdala**, part of the forebrain that stimulates: (i) activity in hypothalamic CRH neurones; (ii) activity in the sympathetic nervous system; (iii) activity in the parasympathetic nerves that cause acid secretion in the stomach (Chapter 41); and (iv) the feeling of fear (Figure 52.4). The stress response evolved to cope with immediate threats, such as predators, to which the appropriate physiological reaction is to prepare for physical activity. The actions of the two parts of the adrenal gland are complementary in this respect. Catecholamines are released from the medulla to produce a rapid increase in cardiac output and the mobilization of metabolic fuels. Corticosteroids produce a slower, more sustained response, increasing the amount of glucose in the plasma (Chapter 46) by: (i) increasing glycolysis and gluconeogenesis in the liver (Chapter 43); (ii) reducing glucose transport into storage tissues; (iii) increasing protein catabolism with a consequent release of amino acids from all tissues other than the liver; and (iv) increasing the mobilization of lipids from adipose tissue.

High levels of glucocorticoids also suppress the activity of immune cells to produce an anti-inflammatory effect, and can mimic the actions of aldosterone on the kidney to retain Na^+ and lose K^+ ions. The stress response is appropriate as long as the stress is relieved promptly. Unfortunately, modern life places many of us in positions in which stress is prolonged. This can lead to chronic hypertension, gastric ulceration, immunosuppression and depression (Figure 52.4). Glucocorticoid derivatives, such as **dexamethasone**, are widely used as anti-inflammatory agents in conditions such as arthritis and asthma. Chronically high levels of glucocorticoids eventually cause weakening of the skin, muscle wasting, reduction in bone strength, increased rates of infection due to immunosuppression, and can damage nerve cells in the **hippocampus** that are part of a feedback circuit controlling responses to stress (Figure 52.4). Thus, the long-term therapeutic use of steroids must be very carefully monitored, especially in the young where normal growth may be affected.

Diseases of the adrenal cortex include **Cushing's syndrome**, which results from the excessive release of glucocorticoids and has a range of symptoms similar to those described above, and **Addison's disease**, which is the result of adrenocortical hypoactivity and is characterized by symptoms of hypoglycaemia, weight loss and skin pigmentation.

53 Endocrine control of reproduction

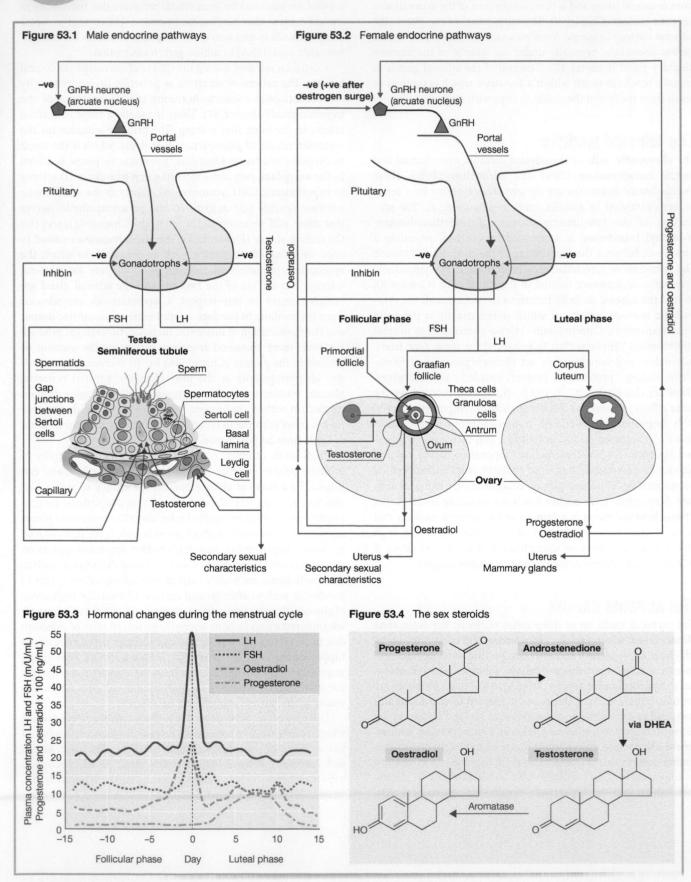

Figure 53.1 Male endocrine pathways

GnRH neurone (arcuate nucleus)
−ve
GnRH
Portal vessels
Pituitary
−ve
Gonadotrophs
−ve
Inhibin
FSH   LH
Testosterone

Testes
Seminiferous tubule
Spermatids
Sperm
Gap junctions between Sertoli cells
Spermatocytes
Sertoli cell
Basal lamina
Leydig cell
Capillary
Testosterone

Secondary sexual characteristics

Figure 53.2 Female endocrine pathways

−ve (+ve after oestrogen surge)
GnRH neurone (arcuate nucleus)
GnRH
Portal vessels
Pituitary
−ve
Gonadotrophs
−ve
Inhibin
Oestradiol
Progesterone and oestradiol

Follicular phase
FSH   LH
Primordial follicle
Graafian follicle
Theca cells
Granulosa cells
Antrum
Testosterone
Ovum

Luteal phase
Corpus luteum

Ovary

Oestradiol
Uterus
Secondary sexual characteristics

Progesterone Oestradiol
Uterus
Mammary glands

Figure 53.3 Hormonal changes during the menstrual cycle

Plasma concentration LH and FSH (m/U/mL)
Progesterone and oestradiol × 100 (ng/mL)

LH
FSH
Oestradiol
Progesterone

55
50
45
40
35
30
25
20
15
10
5
0
−15   −10   −5   0   5   10   15
Follicular phase   Day   Luteal phase

Figure 53.4 The sex steroids

Progesterone   Androstenedione
via DHEA
Oestradiol   Testosterone
Aromatase

Reproductive function in males and females is controlled by common hormonal systems based on the hypothalamic control of the pituitary **gonadotrophins**, individually known as **luteinizing hormone (LH)** and **follicle-stimulating hormone (FSH)**. These glycoproteins are released from the **gonadotrophs** of the anterior pituitary gland under the influence of **gonadotrophin-releasing hormone (GnRH;** Chapter 47) (Figures 53.1 and 53.2). Failure of GnRH release is one cause of infertility. It is released in pulses at intervals of 1–3 h in both males and females, a pattern that is accurately reflected in plasma levels of LH. The pulsatile pattern of GnRH secretion is essential for normal reproductive activity, as continuous exposure of gonadotrophs to the hormone leads to a rapid desensitization of the gonadotrophs and a reduction in the release of gonadotrophins. The releasing hormone acts through receptors coupled to G_q (Chapter 3) to stimulate the release and manufacture of the gonadotrophins.

Actions of gonadotrophins

The gonadotrophins produce their effects via interactions with guanosine triphosphate-binding protein (G-protein)-coupled receptors that activate the intracellular production of cyclic adenosine monophosphate (cAMP) (Chapter 7). In the male, LH acts on the **Leydig cells** of the testes to stimulate the production of the steroid **testosterone**, which acts in concert with FSH on **Sertoli cells** of the **seminiferous tubules** to support **spermatogenesis** (Figure 53.1). Sperm are generated in a two-stage meiosis from spermatocytes via spermatids. Spermatogenesis proceeds most efficiently at a temperature of 34 °C, which is why the testes are located outside the body cavity. A normal adult male produces some 2×10^8 sperm per day, a process that carries on from puberty until the end of life. Sertoli cells also produce **inhibin**, a peptide feedback signal that specifically inhibits the release of FSH from the anterior pituitary.

The situation in females varies over time according to the **menstrual cycle** (Figures 53.2 and 53.3), which lasts for around 28 days but is also ultimately driven by the activity of the hypothalamic GnRH neurones. After puberty, the ovaries contain about 400 000 **primordial follicles**, each of which contains an **ovum** (or **oocyte**) in an arrested state of meiosis. All follicles are present at birth and no new gametes are formed after this time. Small groups of follicles begin to mature spontaneously throughout reproductive life, but only those for which development coincides with the appropriate phase of the cycle reach the stage of ovulation. In the first part of the cycle (the **follicular phase**), LH acts on **theca interna cells** in developing follicles to stimulate the production of testosterone, which is converted to **oestrogens** (mainly **oestradiol**; Figure 53.2) by **aromatase** enzymes in follicular **granulosa cells** under the influence of FSH. Granulosa cells also produce inhibin, which suppresses FSH release. In the follicular phase, oestrogens promote the growth of the uterine endometrial lining and the release of watery secretions at the cervix that enhance the transit of sperm into the uterus. Oestrogens also stimulate the production of LH receptors in granulosa cells. During this time, the actions of FSH and oestrogens stimulate maturing follicles within the ovary, only the largest of which will normally undergo **ovulation**. The remainder wither away by the process of **atresia**. Ovulation occurs at about day 14 of the cycle (Figure 53.3). It is initiated by a large increase in the release of oestradiol from the granulosa cells, stimulated by their newly developed LH receptors. Normally, oestrogens act as a negative feedback signal, inhibiting LH release (Figure 53.2), but the large amounts secreted by the mature follicle *stimulate* LH release, i.e. the system switches from negative to *positive* feedback. This leads to a massive increase in the release of LH, which causes the wall of the most developed follicle to rupture and releases the ovum into the nearest **oviduct** to await fertilization (Chapter 55). Following ovulation, the granulosa cells undergo **hypertrophy** (growth) and the ruptured follicle develops into the **corpus luteum**, and the cycle enters the **luteal phase**. The corpus luteum produces **progesterone** (Figure 53.2), as well as oestrogens, in response to stimulation by LH. Progesterone prepares the reproductive tract for pregnancy, stimulating further growth of the uterine endometrium and altering the nature of cervical secretions to discourage the entry of sperm into the uterus. If fertilization does not occur, the corpus luteum undergoes **luteolysis** after roughly 14 days, a process that results from the reduced ability of LH to support the corpus luteum. In the absence of progesterone and oestradiol, the endometrial lining degenerates and is shed in the process of **menstruation**, followed by the onset of a new cycle. After 30–40 years of menstrual activity, the exhaustion of ovarian follicles causes the female system to enter the **menopause**, after which reproduction is no longer possible. Circulating levels of sex steroids are greatly reduced, leading to drying of the secretory glands in the reproductive tract and other symptoms, including circulatory changes that cause hot flushes. The most pernicious outcome of the menopause is **osteoporosis** (Chapter 51).

All sex steroids exert their effects by interacting with intracellular receptors that bind to deoxyribonucleic acid (DNA) response elements, and thus induce changes in gene expression (Chapter 8). Some of the actions of testosterone are actually mediated by its conversion to the more active **dihydrotestosterone**, produced within the target cells by the action of the enzyme **5-α-reductase**.

Hormonal contraceptives

Human fertility control currently rests firmly on the use by women of hormonal contraceptives. These agents can contain a mixture of synthetic oestrogens and progestogens (analogues of progesterone), or progestogens only, and are administered as daily tablets, depot injections that last for several months, or as long-term (5 years) uterine implants. They probably have multiple sites of action, affecting negative feedback signals to suppress gonadotrophins, the consistency of cervical mucus to prevent sperm penetration, and the sensitivity of the uterine lining to prevent implantation of the embryo.

54 Sexual differentiation and function

Figure 54.1 Male

Bladder
Corpora cavernosum
Corpus spongiosum
Urethra
Glans penis
Seminiferous tubules

Seminal vesicle
Prostate gland
Bulbourethral gland
Bulbocavernosus muscle
Vas deferens
Epididymis
Scrotum
Testis

Figure 54.2 Female

Oviduct
Bladder
Vagina
Clitoris
Labia

Ovary
Uterus
Cervix
Anus

Oviduct
Ovary
Ovarian ligament

Uterus
Cervix
Vagina

Sexual differentiation

Gender is determined by the presence of X and Y chromosomes in the genome. Two X chromosomes provide the female genotype, whereas X and Y chromosomes together give a genetic male. Undifferentiated gonads are apparent after about 4–6 weeks of gestation, and both **Müllerian ducts**, which eventually form the uterus and Fallopian tubes, and **Wolffian ducts**, which form the vas deferens, epididymis and seminal vesicles, are present. The early gonads secrete steroids just as they do in the adult, and these hormones determine the sexual phenotype. In the absence of the *Sry* gene on the Y chromosome and thus testosterone, the Müllerian ducts continue to differentiate whilst the Wolffian ducts regress. The development of reproductive

organs and brain connectivity therefore defaults to a female pattern which is dependent on the secretion of oestrogens.

The *Sry* gene is thought to be responsible for the establishment of testicular development and **Leydig cells** which secrete testosterone. Testosterone stimulates the development of the male genitalia (Figure 54.1) and the organization of neuronal systems in the brain that are involved in sexual function and behaviour. Notably, there is marked growth in the **sexually dimorphic nucleus** of the medial preoptic area of the hypothalamus and in the spinal nucleus that controls the **bulbocavernosus** muscle which is involved in ejaculation. Curiously, testosterone has to be converted to oestrogen by brain aromatases to have these effects. The fetal testis also secretes **anti-Müllerian hormone** (AMH)

Physiology at a Glance, Fourth Edition. Edited by Jeremy P.T. Ward and Roger W.A. Linden.

which causes regression of Müllerian ducts and thus prevents the uterus and Fallopian tube from developing.

Puberty

Although active before birth, the gonadotrophic axis quickly becomes quiescent after parturition and remains so until the onset of puberty at 8–14 years. The trigger for this remains obscure, but may result from endogenous activation of brain pattern generating circuits that stimulate **gonadotrophin-releasing hormone** (GnRH) neurones. **Body mass**, signalled via circulating levels of leptin (Chapter 46) and insulin-like growth factor-1 (IGF-1) (Chapter 49), are important permissive factors in females and undernutrition is associated with failure of the menstrual cycle. Puberty begins when GnRH stimulates cyclic release of **luteinizing hormone** (LH) and **follicle-stimulating hormone** (FSH) from the anterior pituitary (Chapter 53), first at night and then throughout the day. LH stimulates release of testosterone from Leydig cells in males and follicular oestrogens in females, and FSH the onset of spermatogenesis in males and follicle growth in females; they therefore act **synergistically**. This is accompanied by the many physical changes associated with the final growth into an adult (Table 54.1). The appearance of secondary sexual characteristics in the male is thought to be largely stimulated by the testosterone metabolite, dihydrotestosterone. In females, the onset of the cyclic release of LH and thus oestrogens gives rise to the beginning of menstruation (**menarche**) and the development of the mature female body pattern (Table 54.1). The end of puberty marks the onset of full sexual maturity and the conclusion of somatic growth (Chapter 50). Figures 54.1 and 54.2 shows the mature male and female reproductive tracts.

Table 54.1 Primary and secondary sexual characteristics that develop during puberty

Females (mostly stimulated by oestrogens)	Males (stimulated by [dihydro] testosterone)
Growth and maturation of ovaries	Growth and maturation of testes, including descent into scrotum
Growth of external genitalia	Growth of external genitalia and pubic hair
Growth of breasts	Increased size of larynx, leading to deeper voice
Keratinization of vaginal mucosa, enlargement of uterus	Increased muscle mass and strength
Deposition of fat around hips and thighs	Thickened skin
Growth of pubic hair (*stimulated by adrenal androgens*)	Increased and thickened body hair
	Increased bone mass (*also requires oestrogen*)

Sexual function

Sexual attraction and behaviour in humans are the highly complex result of physiological factors, combined with societal and other psychological influences. The overall level of **libido** (sexual motivation) is set by the hypothalamus under the influence of higher centres and the hormonal environment. In males, sexual arousal arises from physical stimulation of the genitalia (a spinal reflex) or from psychological stimuli (by pathways descending from the hypothalamus via the brain stem) that activate sacral parasympathetic nerves (Chapter 8). The penis becomes erect as the result of the dilation of blood vessels entering the **corpora cavernosum** (the main erectile tissue) and **corpus spongiosum** (Figure 54.1). The enhanced flow of blood into the cavernous spaces increases tissue pressure and restricts venous drainage, causing a further build-up of pressure to make the penis fully erect. The parasympathetic nerves cause vasodilatation by the release of acetylcholine, vasoactive intestinal peptide and, primarily, **nitric oxide** (**NO**; Chapter 24). NO increases the manufacture of **cyclic guanosine monophosphate** (**cGMP**) in blood vessel smooth muscle cells to cause them to relax. Sildenafil (Viagra) inhibits the breakdown of cGMP and thus enhances erectile function. The female sexual response sometimes involves erection of the clitoris, but the main manifestations are relaxation of the smooth muscles of the vagina and an increase in mucous secretions that act as a lubricant. Again, these actions are brought about by the activation of parasympathetic nerves. The combined effects of the male and female sexual responses facilitate entry of the penis into the vagina (**intromission**). Frictional forces stimulate mechanoreceptors in the glans penis and the clitoris that eventually lead to reflex activation of the sympathetic nerves that causes **orgasm**. In the male, this involves peristaltic contractions of the epididymis to pump sperm into the urethra, where they are mixed with the secretions of the **bulbourethral gland**, the **seminal vesicle** and the **prostate gland** to form semen. The secretions provide, respectively, lubrication, energy (in the form of the sugar **fructose**) and an alkaline barrier against the acid conditions normally prevalent in the vagina. They also include high levels of **prostaglandins**, the arachidonic acid-derived local hormones that stimulate the motility of sperm and of the female tract. Further peristaltic contractions of the urethra, in combination with the action of the bulbocavernosus muscle, emit the semen bolus into the upper end of the vagina (**ejaculation**). The female orgasm, which may involve the release of pituitary **oxytocin** elicited by mechanical stimulation of the cervix (Chapter 55), results in rhythmic contractions of the vaginal and uterine muscles that promote the flow of semen into the uterus. Sperm move by means of their own motility and by the beating of cilia on the walls of the uterus, but only a few hundred sperm of the millions released in a single ejaculate will complete the 6-h journey from the vagina to the oviducts.

55 Fertilization, pregnancy and parturition

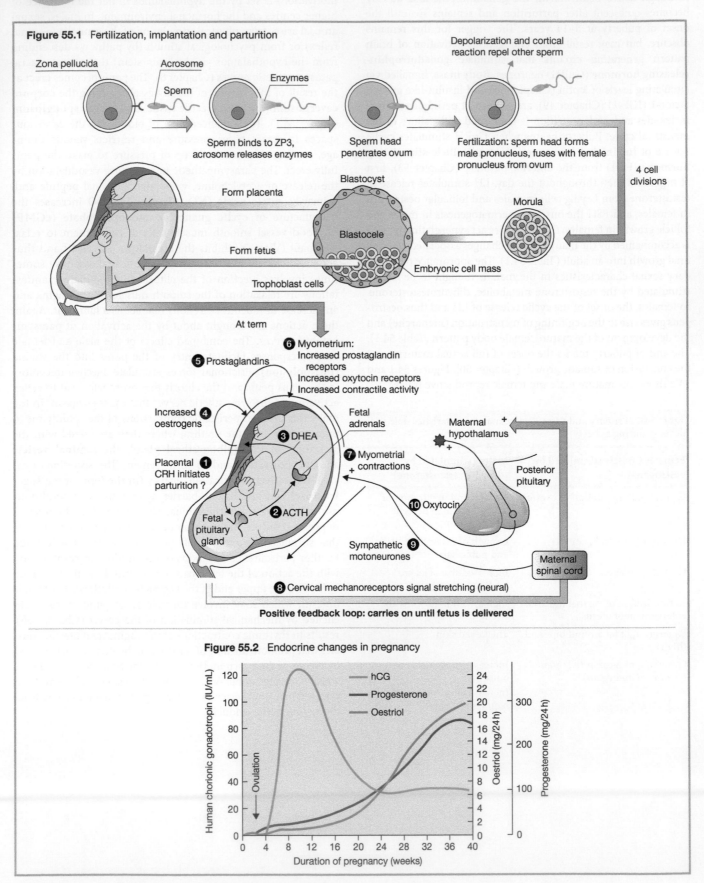

Figure 55.1 Fertilization, implantation and parturition

Zona pellucida

Acrosome

Sperm

Sperm binds to ZP3, acrosome releases enzymes

Enzymes

Sperm head penetrates ovum

Depolarization and cortical reaction repel other sperm

Fertilization: sperm head forms male pronucleus, fuses with female pronucleus from ovum

4 cell divisions

Blastocyst

Form placenta

Blastocele

Form fetus

Morula

Embryonic cell mass

Trophoblast cells

At term

⑥ Myometrium:
Increased prostaglandin receptors
Increased oxytocin receptors
Increased contractile activity

⑤ Prostaglandins

Increased ④ oestrogens

Fetal adrenals

③ DHEA

Placental ① CRH initiates parturition ?

⑦ Myometrial contractions

Maternal hypothalamus

Posterior pituitary

Fetal pituitary gland

② ACTH

⑩ Oxytocin

Sympathetic ⑨ motoneurones

Maternal spinal cord

⑧ Cervical mechanoreceptors signal stretching (neural)

Positive feedback loop: carries on until fetus is delivered

Figure 55.2 Endocrine changes in pregnancy

hCG
Progesterone
Oestriol

Ovulation

Human chorionic gonadotropin (IU/mL)

Oestriol (mg/24 h)

Progesterone (mg/24 h)

Duration of pregnancy (weeks)

Physiology at a Glance, Fourth Edition. Edited by Jeremy P.T. Ward and Roger W.A. Linden.

Fertilization

The unfertilized ovum can survive for up to 24h after ovulation, and sperm remain viable in the uterus for up to 5 days after ejaculation. The environment of the female tract triggers the **capacitation** of sperm. This is a prerequisite for fertilization that involves remodelling of the lipids and glycoproteins of the sperm plasma membrane, coupled with increased metabolism and motility. The ovum is surrounded by the **zona pellucida**, an acellular membrane bearing the glycoprotein **ZP3** that acts as a sperm receptor. Fertilization occurs in the oviduct, when a single capacitated sperm binds to ZP3 and undergoes the **acrosome reaction**. The acrosome is a body containing proteolytic enzymes that is attached to the sperm head (Figure 55.1). When a sperm binds to ZP3, the acrosomal enzymes are released to digest a pathway for the sperm to penetrate the ovum, within which the contents of the sperm head, including its genetic material, are deposited. This event leads to a chain of reactions that denies access to further sperm penetration. The ovum first undergoes electrical depolarization and then discharges granules that impair further sperm binding at the zona pellucida (the **cortical reaction**). In this way, fertilization is normally restricted to one sperm per ovum. Some 2–3h after penetrating the ovum, the sperm head forms the **male pronucleus** which joins with the **female pronucleus** from the ovum (Figure 55.1). Fusion of the pronuclei combines the parental genetic material from the gametes to form the **zygote**.

Pregnancy

The zygote is propelled by cilia and muscular contractions of the Fallopian tube into the uterus, where it implants in the endometrium. During this journey, the zygote undergoes a number of cell divisions to form the **morula**, a solid ball of 16 cells that 'hatches' from the zona pellucida and develops into the **blastocyst**, in which embryonic cells are surrounded by **trophoblasts** (Figure 55.1). The trophoblasts are responsible for implantation, digesting away the uterine endometrial wall to form a space for the embryo, opening up a pathway to the maternal circulation (via the **spiral arteries** of the uterus) and forming the fetal portion of the **placenta**. The tissue engineering activities of trophoblasts are mediated by epidermal growth factor (EGF) (Chapter 49) and interleukin-1β. Implantation is complete within 7–10 days of fertilization, at which time the embryo and early placenta begin to secrete **human chorionic gonadotrophin** (**hCG**). The appearance of hCG in the plasma and urine is one of the earliest signs of successful conception, and its detection forms the basis of pregnancy testing kits. hCG is a glycoprotein similar to LH that stimulates progesterone secretion from the corpus luteum. Progesterone levels rise steadily throughout pregnancy and fall sharply at term (Figure 55.2). This steroid ensures that the smooth muscle of the uterus remains quiescent during gestation (essential for a successful pregnancy), stimulates mammary gland development and prepares the maternal brain for motherhood. The placenta also secretes **chorionic somatomammotrophin**, a growth hormone-like protein that mobilizes metabolic fuels (Chapter 46) and promotes mammary gland growth, and oestrogen (mainly **oestriol**) that stimulates uterine expansion to accommodate the growing fetus. Fetal development occurs within a fluid-filled sac, known as the **amniotic membrane**, which provides a protective buffer against physical trauma. Pregnancy makes many physiological demands on the mother. The ventilation rate, cardiac output and plasma volume increase to supply fetal–maternal oxygen and water demands; the gastrointestinal absorption of minerals is enhanced; and the renal glomerular filtration rate (Chapter 35) rises to cope with fetal waste production.

Parturition

After some 40 weeks of gestation, the fetus is ready for life outside the uterus. The signal that initiates parturition in humans is still not fully understood, and there seems to be a difference between primates and other mammals. In primates, the primary signal is thought to arise from the **fetoplacental unit** (i.e. the fetus plus the placenta), with *placental* (rather than hypothalamic) production of corticotrophin-releasing hormone (CRH) (Figure 55.1, ❶). CRH stimulates release of adrenocorticotropic hormone (ACTH) from the fetal pituitary (❷) which increases dehydroepiandrosterone (DHEA) production from the fetal adrenal cortex (❸) (Chapters 47 and 52). As the placental aromatase enzymes are not rate limiting, an increase in DHEA, a precursor of oestrogen (Chapter 53), automatically increases oestrogen production (❹). Whatever the initiating signal might be, the end result is an increase in the synthesis of prostaglandins E and F by fetal and uterine tissues (❺), with concomitant increases in prostaglandin receptors in the uterine smooth muscle. The prostaglandins stimulate the production of uterine receptors for **oxytocin** and change the pattern of activity in the uterine myometrium from slow, gentle contractions to regular, deep contractions that eventually move the fetus into the cervix (❻❼). The cervix, which is softened by prior release of the prostaglandins, dilates as the fetus is forced downwards. At this time, the amniotic membrane ruptures. Stretching of the cervix activates mechanoreceptors (❽) that stimulate a spinal sympathetic reflex which causes myometrial contraction (❾) and secretion of **oxytocin** from the posterior pituitary gland (❿) (Chapter 47; Figure 55.1). Oxytocin is a powerful stimulant of uterine smooth muscle that causes further contraction of the myometrium and pushes the fetus further into the cervix, resulting in further stimulation of mechanoreceptors and leading to the release of more oxytocin, i.e. this is a positive feedback system. The spinal reflex, aided by waves of oxytocin, generates large, regular contractions of the uterus that eventually expel the fetus and placenta through the vagina, completing the birth process. Oxytocin continues to be useful, as it limits maternal bleeding by causing vasoconstriction. In the fetus, oxytocin closes the **ductus arteriosus**, a blood vessel that shunts blood away from the pulmonary circulation *in utero*, but which would obviously hamper postpartum life should it remain open.

56 Lactation

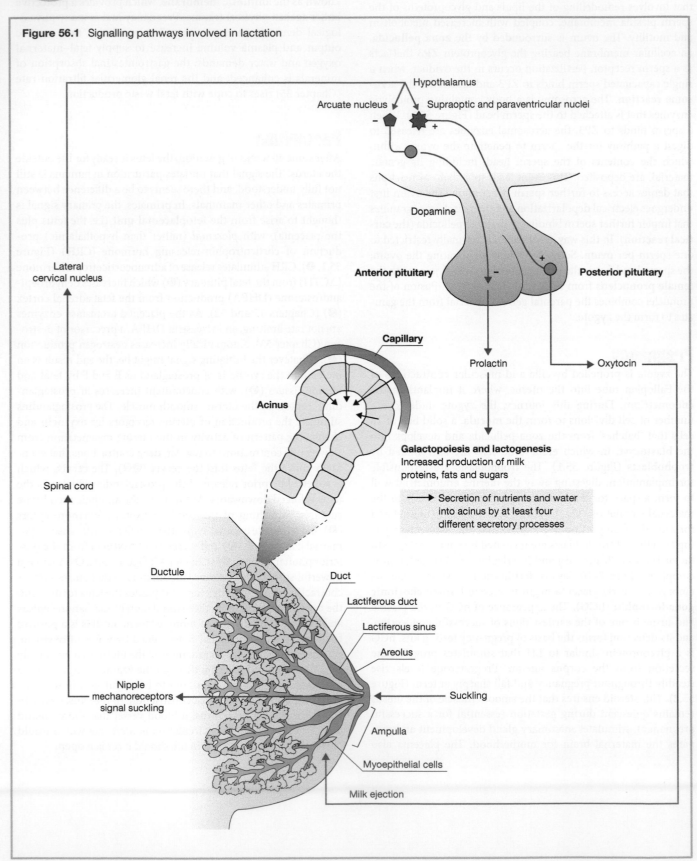

Figure 56.1 Signalling pathways involved in lactation

Hypothalamus

Arcuate nucleus — Supraoptic and paraventricular nuclei

Dopamine

Anterior pituitary **Posterior pituitary**

Lateral cervical nucleus

Capillary

Acinus

Prolactin Oxytocin

Galactopoiesis and lactogenesis
Increased production of milk proteins, fats and sugars

Spinal cord

→ Secretion of nutrients and water into acinus by at least four different secretory processes

Ductule Duct

Lactiferous duct

Lactiferous sinus

Areolus

Nipple mechanoreceptors signal suckling Suckling

Ampulla

Myoepithelial cells

Milk ejection

ilk, which sustains mammalian infants through the first few months of life, is produced by the mammary glands (Figure 56.1) under the influence of the pituitary protein hormone **prolactin** (Chapter 47). The glands comprise several lobules that are composed of **acini** (also called **alveoli**), similar in structure to the salivary glands and the exocrine pancreas (Chapters 40 and 43). The lobules empty into **lactiferous ducts**. As the ducts approach the **areola** (nipple), they open out to form **lactiferous sinuses** before narrowing again to emerge at the **ampulla** on the nipple. The ducts and sinuses are organized so that milk collects within them rather than flowing freely to the ampulla. They are lined by **myoepithelial cells** that contract to expel milk from the breast. Progesterone, oestrogen, prolactin, cortisol and growth hormone are all required to complete development of the mammary glands, which occurs during the late stages of pregnancy; for the rest of adult life the glandular tissue is rather small. Milk is formed by intense activity of the epithelial cells lining the acinus. The acinar secrete fats (triglycerides), proteins (principally **casein**, α-lactalbumin and lactoglobulin B) and sugars (mostly **lactose**) to produce an isotonic liquid that is roughly 4% fat, 1% protein and 7% sugar, with almost 100 additional trace nutrients, including many ions (including Ca^{2+}), some immunoglobulins (antibodies) in the form of IgA (Chapter 11) and growth factors, such as insulin-like growth factor-1 (IGF-1) and epidermal growth factor (EGF) (Chapter 49). **Colostrum**, the first secretion of the mammary glands after birth, is particularly rich in protein, but has a lower sugar concentration than mature milk. It also contains high levels of **antibodies** (Chapter 11) that provide the infant with basic immunological protection in the first days of life. At least four secretory processes are synchronized in the epithelial cells, **exocytosis**, **lipid synthesis** and secretion, **transmembrane secretion** of ions and water, and **transcytosis** of extra-alveolar proteins such as hormones, albumin and immunoglobulins from the interstitial spaces.

Hormonal control

Plasma prolactin levels rise steadily during pregnancy, but the lactogenic effects of the hormone are inhibited by the presence of progesterone and oestrogen, so that its main role during gestation is to promote mammary growth. Note however that progesterone and oestrogen are also essential during late pregnancy to stimulate duct and alveoli growth respectively, and without this pre-exposure the mammary glands will not respond to prolactin after birth. The loss of these placental steroids at term (Chapter 55) allows prolactin to exert its full effects on milk production, provided that cortisol and insulin are also present. **Placental lactogens**, which are similar to prolactin and are thought to bind to the same receptor, may contribute to mammary gland development during pregnancy, though their function in humans is not fully understood. Prolactin acts through a receptor linked to a Janus kinase–signal transduction and activation

of transcription (JAK–STAT) system (Chapter 50) that activates the genes producing milk proteins and the synthetic enzymes for lactose and triglycerides. The production of nutrients is termed **galactopoiesis**. Prolactin also increases blood flow to the gland, and stimulates the delivery of nutrients into milk by exocytosis (proteins) or specific membrane transport systems (sugars, fats, antibodies); these actions are referred to as **lactogenesis**.

Prolactin is an unusual anterior pituitary hormone in that it is released **constitutively** (i.e. without a stimulus) from pituitary lactotrophs, and the primary control from the hypothalamus is inhibitory via **dopamine**, although other hypophysiotropic hormones may also be involved (Chapter 47; Figure 56.1). After birth, the main stimulus that maintains prolactin release is **suckling**. Milk production thus continues for as long as the infant continues to feed from the mother. Prolactin inhibits luteinizing hormone (LH) release from the pituitary and maintains the mother in a low state of fertility until the infant is weaned. This is a useful mechanism for spacing births, but is not 100% effective in humans. Prolactin-secreting tumours of the pituitary render the patient infertile, but this can be overcome by the administration of the dopamine agonist bromocriptine, which inhibits prolactin release long enough for ovulation to occur. Prolactin is released in several conditions other than around birth: sleep, stress, eating and exercise are all associated with elevated plasma prolactin, although the exact function of this release is not yet known.

Milk let down reflex

Prolactin stimulates milk production, but another hormone is required to eject milk from the acini onto the surface of the nipple. Stimulation of areolar mechanoreceptors by suckling infants activates a neural pathway that ascends to the **paraventricular** and **supraoptic nuclei** of the hypothalamus via the lateral cervical nucleus of the brain stem. This pathway excites magnocellular neurones (Chapter 47) to secrete pulses of oxytocin into the blood at 2–10-min intervals. It is not certain how the suckling stimulus, which is continuous, is translated into episodic activity in oxytocin-releasing cells. The oxytocin pulses seem to arise from the simultaneous activation of all oxytocin neurones in both nuclei. The hormone is a potent stimulant of myoepithelial cells, which pump milk from the lactiferous sinuses out through the nipple and into the mouth of the infant. Milk let down encourages further suckling by the recipient, which leads to more oxytocin release, and so makes up another positive feedback system that operates until the infant is sated. This **milk ejection reflex** (Figure 56.1) is also stimulated in response to the crying of infants as a result of psychological **conditioning**. However, the reflex is strongly inhibited by maternal stress, which is one of the most common causes of failure of lactation in new mothers. In animals, the release of oxytocin in the brain has been shown to facilitate maternal behaviour, but works only after pre-exposure to progesterone and oestrogens.

The sensory and motor systems

Part 8

Chapters

57 Introduction to sensory systems

Figure 57.1 Receptor, generator and action potentials

Stimulus (stretch to skin)

Large stretch (**B**)

Small stretch (**A**)

Intensity (mm)

Depolarization

Receptor potential (amplitude-coded signal)

Threshold

Voltage (mV)

Generator potential (generates action potentials)

Action potentials (frequency-coded signals)

Time

Ruffini-type ending

B

A

Figure 57.2 Spatial spread of excitation

(A) In the absence of lateral inhibition

Stimulus

Mechanoreceptors

First synaptic level

Second synaptic level

(B) In the presence of lateral inhibition

Stimulus

First synaptic level

Second synaptic level

NB. All synapses are excitatory except for those marked with * which are inhibitory. For clarity not all inhibitory neurones are shown in the above diagram.

Sensation and perception

The brain obtains its information about the external and internal environment and about the body's relation to the external environment by sensory experience emanating from sensory receptors (sense organs). There are a number of **common steps in sensory reception**: (i) a **physical stimulus** (i.e. touch, pressure, heat, cold, light, etc.); (ii) a **transduction process** (i.e. the translation of the stimulus into a code of action potentials); and (iii) a **response** (i.e. taking a mental note or triggering a motor reaction).

The **specialized nerve ending** (**sensory receptor**), **afferent axon** and its **cell body**, together with the central synaptic connections in the spinal cord or brain stem, are known as **primary afferents**.

Information is transmitted to the brain in the form of action potentials. These action potentials carry this information in the form of **frequency-coded signals** and can signal the following information:

1 The **modality (specificity)** of the system. Such modalities include the 'five special senses': sight, hearing, balance, taste and smell. However, it is easy to list others. The skin itself not only senses pressure and touch, but also cold and warmth, vibration and pain (**somatosensation**). In addition, the body senses both the **external environment** and the **internal environment** (its own state). Examples are the sense of equilibrium (**balance**) and a knowledge of the relative positions of the limbs (**proprioception**). Other modalities that are related to information about the state of the body, and that are not directly apparent, are the senses that assess P_{CO_2} and P_{O_2}, blood pressure, and lung and stomach stretch receptors, the so-called **interoceptors**. Each modality can often be subdivided into further divisions of **quality**, i.e. in the case of taste (sweet, sour, salt, bitter and umami), light (red, green and blue) and hearing (tonal pitches).

2 The **intensity (quantity)** of the stimulus (Figure 57.1). The quantity of a sensory impression corresponds to the strength of the stimulus. As the stimulus strength increases, so does the amplitude of the receptor potential (**amplitude-coded signal**) and, when this eventually reaches a **threshold**, it causes action potentials that increase in their frequency of firing as the receptor potential rises (**temporal** or **frequency coding**). Another way in which the strength of the signal is coded is by increasing the number of afferent fibres that are activated (**spatial** or **recruitment coding**).

3 The **duration** of the stimulus. Many receptors will continue to fire impulses as long as the stimulus is applied; others will signal when a stimulus is applied and when a stimulus is removed. However, in most cases, even if a stimulus persists (e.g. constant touch to the skin), the sensation/perception of it wanes. This involves a process called **adaptation. Adaptation** occurs at all stages of the transformation of the stimulus: in the transduction process, in the conductance mechanism of the receptor potential, in the synaptic transmission from a secondary sensory cell and in the generation of the action potential. It can also be a function of the central nervous system (CNS) itself once the action potentials reach that far.

4 The **localization** and **resolution (acuity)** of the stimulus. The sensory system detects the location of a stimulus, and its fine detail. Both depend on the spacing of receptors (better localization and acuity occur with greater receptor density). The **receptive field** of a sensory neurone itself (sometimes called the **receptor field**) is the area of sensory surface from which that neurone receives an input. Receptor neurones converge onto second-order neurones (usually in the CNS), and then to third- and higher-order neurones. These transitions are made in relay nuclei. The receptor field of the primary receptor is usually a small excitatory area. The receptive field of the second- or higher-order neurone is larger and more complex (because of both convergence and divergence, and excitatory and inhibitory pathways).

The net result is **sensation** and, when interpreted at a conscious level in the light of experience, this becomes **perception**.

Sensory pathways

The coded signals from each of the sensory receptors are relayed to the CNS by peripheral and cranial nerves. Each modality is associated with specific nerves and pathways, e.g. gustatory information is transmitted via facial and glossopharyngeal nerves, and the somatosensory system is transmitted via the dorsal column–medial lemniscal system for the larger afferent fibres (Aα and Aβ) and the anterolateral system (anterior and lateral spinothalamic tracts) for the smaller afferent fibres (Aδ and C). Each sensory system has its unique pathway into and through the CNS to eventually provide an input into the thalamus. The thalamus, in turn, provides an input to the cortex. Each sensory system projects to a specific area of the primary sensory cortex which is primarily concerned with the analysis of the sensory information, and these neurones, in turn, project to the secondary sensory cortex in which more complex processing occurs. There are further projections to associated areas, such as the posterior parietal, prefrontal and temporal cortices, which can again project to the limbic and motor systems. The latter systems are involved in the processing of the sensory information, leading to responses such as complex behavioural and motor responses.

Lateral inhibition. Figure 57.2 shows a neural network comprising two mechanoreceptors in the skin and their associated neurones at the next two synaptic levels. The two receptors are each excited equally by a stimulus applied between them. The **divergent** and **convergent connections** seem to impose an avalanche-like spread of excitation at progressively higher levels of the CNS. Pinpoint stimulation appears to lead to an enlarged, less precise and more diffuse representation at each successive synaptic level (**Ⓐ**). However, this situation is encountered only under pathological conditions (e.g. strychnine poisoning, which blocks inhibiting synapses in the CNS). Inhibition normally prevents the spread of excitation by a phenomenon called **lateral inhibition (Ⓑ)**. At each synaptic relay, each excitatory neurone exerts an inhibitory effect by exciting **inhibitory interneurones**. The neurone with the greatest input (the one in the middle) imposes the strongest inhibition on those on either side of it. Lateral inhibition has been shown to exist at all levels of sensory systems: in the dorsal horn of the spinal cord, in the dorsal column nuclei, in the thalamus and in the cortex, as well as in the visual system. The result is an increased spatial sharpening in the CNS of the representation of the distant peripheral stimulus on moving through the synaptic levels.

Descending inhibition. In practically all sensory systems, higher centres can also exert inhibitory effects on all those at lower levels. Such **central inhibition** can act at a point as far peripheral as the receptor or at the afferent ending in the spinal cord. Like lateral inhibition, descending inhibition can be considered to function as a means of **regulating the sensitivity of the afferent transmission channels**.

The types of synaptic mechanism described above indicate that there is great flexibility in the sensory pathways, and that they are not as hard-wired as many pathway diagrams suggest.

58 Sensory receptors

Figure 58.1 Receptors in hairy and non-hairy skin

Hairy skin

Non-hairy skin

Horny layer
Merkel's discs
Meissners endings
Ruffini-type endings
Hair follicle receptor
Free nerve endings
Eccrine gland
Pacinian corpuscles

Epidermis
Dermis
Subcutaneous tissue

Figure 58.2 Classification of cutaneous mechanoreceptors

	Hairy skin	Non-hairy skin
Slowly adapting (type SAI and SAII) Response Stimulus	Merkel's disc Ruffini-type endings Intensity detectors	Merkel's disc Intensity detectors
Moderately rapidly adapting (type RAI) Response Stimulus	Hair follicle receptors Velocity detectors	Meissner endings Velocity detectors
Very rapidly adapting (type RAII) Response Stimulus	Pacinian corpuscles Acceleration/ vibration detectors	Pacinian corpuscles Acceleration/ vibration detectors

Figure 58.3 Qualities of pain

Pain

Somatic

Visceral

Superficial (from skin)

Deep (from muscle, bone and connective tissues)

(from visceral organs) Such as kidney and gallbladder (stones) and stomach (ulcers)

Initial (fast or first). Sharp, localized pain possibly via Aδ fibres

Delayed (slow or second). Diffuse spatially, less localized and dies out slowly possibly via C fibres

Dull in nature. Poorly localized. Tendency to radiate into surroundings

Dull in nature. Poorly localized. Diffuse in character. Often resembles deep pain

Gives rise to protective reflexes Elicits very few autonomic reflex responses

Associated with unpleasant feelings. Elicits autonomic reflexes of nausea, heavy sweating and lowered blood pressure

The **sensory receptor** is a specialized cell. In mammals, receptors fall into five groups: **mechanoreceptors**, **thermoreceptors**, **nociceptors**, **chemoreceptors** (Chapter 59) and **photoreceptors** (Chapter 60). There is further specialization within these groups. Each receptor responds to one stimulus type; this property is called the **specificity of the receptor**. The stimulus that is effective in eliciting a response is called the **adequate stimulus**.

Transduction processes. Some receptors consist of a nerve fibre alone (e.g. free nerve endings), others consist of a specialized accessory structure (e.g. olfactory receptors, Pacinian corpuscles), and others are more complex and consist of a specialized receptor cell which synapses with a neurone, in other words a secondary sensory cell (e.g. gustatory receptors and Merkel's discs).

Mechanoreceptors. These are found all over the body. Those in the skin have three main qualities: pressure, touch and vibration (or acceleration) (Figures 58.1 and 58.2). When the responses to constant stimuli are studied in the various receptors, the receptors can be divided into three types on the basis of their adaptive properties: **slowly adapting receptors** that continue to fire action potentials even when the pressure is maintained for a long period (e.g. **Ruffini's endings**, **tactile discs**, **Merkel's discs**); **moderately rapidly adapting receptors** that fire for about 50–500 ms after the onset of the stimulus, even when the pressure is maintained (e.g. **hair follicle receptors**, **Meissner's corpuscles**); and **very rapidly adapting receptors** that fire only one or two impulses (e.g. **Pacinian corpuscles**) (Figure 58.2). These three types of receptor are examples of receptors in the skin that detect **intensity**, **velocity** and **vibration** (or **acceleration**), respectively.

Free nerve endings. Each skin nerve, in addition to the large myelinated afferents, contains a large number (over 50% of the fibres) of **smaller myelinated and unmyelinated (Aδ and C) axons**. Some of the C fibres are, of course, efferent postganglionic sympathetic fibres. However, a large number of the remaining fibres are afferents that terminate in **free nerve endings** and not in corpuscular structures (Figure 58.1). Many of these are **thermoreceptors** or **nociceptors**.

Thermoreceptors. Thermoreceptors mediate the sensations of **cold** and **warmth**. In the skin of humans, there are **specific cold and warm points** at which only the sensation of cold or warmth can be elicited. These are specific cold and warmth receptors; however, they share the following characteristics: (i) **maintain discharge** at constant skin temperature, with the discharge rate proportional to the skin temperature (static response); (ii) have **small receptive fields** (1 mm^2 or less), each afferent fibre supplying only one or a few warm or cold points; and (iii) serve not only as **sensors for the conscious sensation of temperature**, but also participate (together with temperature sensors in the hypothalamus and spinal cord) in the **thermoregulation** of the body.

Nociceptors and pain. Pain differs from the other sensory modalities with regard to the kind of information it conveys. It informs us of a threat to our bodies when it is activated by noxious (tissue-damaging) stimuli. **Nociception** is defined as the **reception, conduction and central processing of noxious signals**. This term is used to make a clear distinction between these 'objective' neuronal processes and the 'subjective' sensation of **pain**, which is defined as an **unpleasant sensory and emotional experience associated with actual or potential damage, or described in terms of such damage**.

Nociceptors are found in the skin, visceral organs and muscle (cardiac and skeletal), and are associated with blood vessels. The **qualities of pain** are divided into **somatic** and **visceral**. If somatic pain is derived from the skin, it is called **superficial pain**, and, if from muscle, bone joints or connective tissue, it is called **deep pain**. If superficial pain is produced by piercing the skin with a needle, the subject feels a sharp pain; this easily localized sensation fades away rapidly when the needle is removed. This sharp, localized **initial pain** (also called **first** or **fast** pain) is often followed, particularly at high stimulus intensities, by **delayed pain** (also called **second** or **slow** pain), which has a dull (or burning) character with a delay of about 1 s. This delayed pain is more diffuse spatially, dies out slowly and is not so easily localized. **Deep pain** is dull in nature, poorly localized and has a tendency to radiate into the surroundings.

The responses of the body in terms of both the distress and suffering and the autonomic and motor responses to pain depend on the quality of pain (Figure 58.3). **Delayed pain** and **deep pain** are accompanied by a **feeling of unpleasantness**, and often elicit autonomic reflexes of **nausea**, **heavy sweating** and **lowered blood pressure**. **Initial pain** gives rise, by contrast, to **protective reflexes**, i.e. flexor withdrawal reflex. **Visceral pain** (pain from organs such as the kidney, stomach and gallbladder) tends to be dull and diffuse in character and resembles deep pain.

Histologically, the nociceptors are **free nerve endings** attached to either **Aδ fibres** or **C fibres**. It has been proposed that, in the case of superficial pain, the transmission of **initial (fast)** pain is via Aδ fibres, whereas **delayed (slow)** pain is signalled by the smaller C fibres. The time difference between initial (fast) pain and delayed (slow) pain appears to be explained by the difference in the conduction velocities of the fibres concerned.

Inhibitory influences. Like all other sensory inputs, the nociceptive afferent influx is exposed to inhibitory influences at the receptor, on its way to and through the spinal cord and in the higher levels of the central nervous system. Many of the modern treatments elicit or enhance these inhibitory processes, pharmacologically using drugs, physically using cold or warm wrappings, short-wave radiation, massage and exercise, and by the electrical stimulation of certain structures, including peripheral nerves. **Acupuncture** and **transcutaneous electrical nerve stimulation** (TENS) may possibly depend on the activation and maintenance of inhibitory processes. Naturally occurring **endorphins**, **enkephalins** and **dynorphins** are thought to contribute to these processes. These are endogenous, pain-controlling opiates produced by the body that attach to the specific opiate receptors, so as to inhibit the sensation of pain without affecting the other sensory modalities.

59 Special senses: taste and smell

Figure 59.1 Section through taste bud

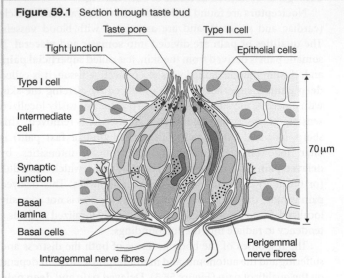

- Taste pore
- Tight junction
- Type I cell
- Intermediate cell
- Synaptic junction
- Basal lamina
- Basal cells
- Intragemmal nerve fibres
- Type II cell
- Epithelial cells
- 70 μm
- Perigemmal nerve fibres

Figure 59.3 Gustatory papillae

Type of papillae	Location	Number of papillae on tongue	Average number of taste buds per papillae	Innervation of taste buds
Fungiform papillae	Anterior two-thirds of tongue	200 (scattered all over dorsal surface)	3 on dorsal surface (range 0–21)	Chorda tympani (facial nerve)
Foliate papillae	Posterior–lateral sides of tongue	2 (one on either side of tongue arranged in 20 parallel folds/rugae)	600 (few in rostral/lateral rugae)	Chorda tympani (facial nerve) anteriorly and glosso-pharyngeal nerve posteriorly
Circum-vallate papillae	Dorsal surface anterior to the sulcus terminalis	Between 8 and 12 (arranged in a V-shaped formation)	250 in sulcus	Glosso-pharyngeal nerve

Figure 59.5 The olfactory organ

- Olfactory bulb
- Olfactory epithelium
- Innervated by trigeminal nerve
- Innervated by glossopharyngeal nerve
- Innervated by vagus nerve

Figure 59.2 Structure and position of lingual gustatory papillae

- Lateral rugae
- Taste bud
- 1 mm
- Taste bud
- von Ebner glands
- Taste bud
- Foliate papilla
- Circumvallate papilla
- Fungiform papilla

Figure 59.4 Transduction mechanisms in gustatory receptors

Salt | Sour | Sweet | Bitter | Umami (amino acids)

Na⁺ — Na^+ H⁺ — H^+ *TRPM5 channel   *TRPM5 channel   *TRPM5 channel

- Apical
- Ca^{2+} stores
- Basolateral
- Ca^{2+} influx
- Transmitter vesicles
- Nerve fibre

**Depolarization → Opening of Ca^{2+} channels → Ca^{2+} influx → Release of transmitter substance → Action potentials in nerve fibre

G-Protein activation → Phospho-lipase C (PLC) → Inositol 1,4,5-trisphosphate (IP_3) → Intracellular Ca^{2+} release

IP_3 and Intracellular Ca^{2+} release causes the opening of TRPM5 channels*, allowing Na⁺ and K⁺ influx → Depolarization**

- Cribriform plate
- Olfactory nerve
- Basal (stem) cells
- Olfactory receptor cells
- Supporting cells
- Mucous layer
- Olfactory epithelium

The so-called special senses comprise the sensations of **taste**, **smell**, **vision**, **hearing** and **balance**. The receptors involved in taste and smell are **chemoreceptors**, those in vision are **photoreceptors**, and those in hearing and balance are **mechanoreceptors**.

The sensations of **taste** and **smell** are two modalities of sense that are very closely related. What the layperson calls 'taste' is really a combination of taste and smell, and probably a number of other modalities. Taken together, a better term would be **flavour**. The modalities of flavour are **taste** (**gustation**), **smell** (**olfaction**), **touch** (**texture**), **temperature** (**thermoreception**) and **common chemical sense** (**chemoreception**).

Gustation

Taste buds (the **gustatory end organs**) (Figure 59.1) are found in the tongue, soft palate, pharynx, larynx and epiglottis, and are unevenly distributed around these regions. Those in the tongue are associated with three of the four types of papillae (**fungiform**, **foliate** and **circumvallate**) (Figure 59.2). Those associated with the other oral tissues are found on the smooth epithelial surfaces. The different papillae occupy specific areas of the tongue. Their associated taste buds are innervated by either the **glossopharyngeal** (**IX**) **nerve** (posterior one-third of the tongue) or the **chorda tympani branch** of the **facial** (**VII**) **nerve** (anterior two-thirds of the tongue). In humans, the number of taste buds varies considerably: on average in the range 2000–5000, but can be as low as 500 or as high as 20 000 (Figure 59.3). Each taste bud is made up of 50–150 **neuroepithelial cells** arranged in a compact, pear-shaped structure (**intragemmal cells**). There is general agreement that there are four types of intragemmal cells: **basal**, **type I** (**dark cells**), **intermediate** and **type II** (**light cells**). Each taste bud comprises a dynamic system in which there is a rapid turnover of cells within each bud. The **lifespan** of an individual receptor cell is about **10 days**. There is a small opening in the surface, the **taste pore**, where the cells have access to the gustatory stimuli (Figure 59.1).

Since Aristotle (384–322 BC), people have tried to categorize taste into **primary** or **basic qualities of taste**. The four qualities that have stood the test of time are **sweet**, **sour**, **salt** and **bitter**, with a fifth categorized by the taste of monosodium glutamate (**umami**). The mechanisms involved in the process of transduction of the signals that eventually produce these basic sensations of taste are complex. In common with many other receptor cells, gustatory receptor cells use **specifically localized ion channel and receptor sites** for transduction. Unlike many other receptor cells, there is **no single membrane transduction event** and the different basic tastes utilize **different ionic mechanisms** (Figure 59.4). **Salt taste** involves Na^+ ions entering the receptor cells via amiloride-sensitive Na^+ channels and **sour taste** involves H^+ ions entering the receptor cell via an acid sensing (PKD2L1) channel. **Sweet, bitter and umami (amino acid) tastes** involve specific taste receptors on the membrane surface and the activation of G-proteins which in turn activate phospholipase C (PLC) and release of inositol 1,4,5-trisphosphate (IP_3) and intracellular Ca^{2+} (Chapter 7). All of these mechanisms lead to depolarization, opening of Ca^{2+} channels in the cell membrane, Ca^{2+} influx, the release of a transmitter substance and activation of the peripheral nerve fibre. Most gustatory stimuli are water soluble and non-volatile and are either already dissolved or are dissolved in saliva during mastication.

The **common chemical sense** has been defined as the sensation caused by the stimulation of **epithelial** or **mucosal free nerve endings** by chemicals. Evidence suggests that these are **polymodal nociceptors** and that, in the mouth, the major contributor to this sense is the **trigeminal** (**V**) **nerve**. The trigeminal innervates almost all regions of the mouth, including the floor of the mouth, the tongue, the hard and soft palate, and the mucosa of the lips and cheek. These nerve endings are stimulated by a number of different chemicals, such as menthol, peppermint, and capsaicin and piperine (found in chilli peppers and black peppers, respectively).

Olfaction

The human olfactory organ, the **olfactory epithelium** or **mucosa**, is a sheet of cells, 100–200-μm thick, situated high in the back of the nasal cavity and on the thin bony partition (the **central septum**) of the nasal passage. The olfactory system responds to airborne, volatile molecules that gain access to the olfactory epithelium with the in-and-out air flow through and behind the nose. The odour molecules are distributed over the receptor sheet in an irregular pattern by the turbulence of the air flow set up by the turbinate bones (Figure 59.5).

The olfactory epithelium contains specialized, elongated nerve cells (**olfactory receptors**) (Figure 59.5). These cells have very thin fibres that run upwards in bundles through perforations in the skull (the **cribriform plate**) above the roof of the nasal cavity. These bundles of nerves constitute the **olfactory** (**I**) **nerve**. They extend only a very short distance, ending in the **olfactory bulbs**, a pair of swellings underneath the frontal lobes. The other end of each olfactory receptor, pointing down into the nasal cavity, is extended into a long process, ending in a knob carrying several hairs (**cilia**) between 20 and 200 μm in length. These cilia are bathed in a thin (35-μm thick) layer of **mucus**, secreted by specialized cells in the olfactory epithelium, in which the molecules of odorous substances dissolve. The molecules diffuse through the surface layer of mucus and stimulate the olfactory receptors. **Hydrophilic** (water-soluble) molecules dissolve readily in the mucus, but the diffusion of less soluble molecules is assisted by 'odour-binding proteins' in the mucus, which are also thought to assist in removing odour molecules from the receptor cells. The mucus layer moves across the surface of the **olfactory mucosa** at 10–60 mm/min towards the **nasopharynx**. This flow of mucus also assists in the removal of odours after they have been sensed. In the membrane of the cilia are **olfactory receptor proteins**, which interact with the smelly molecules, and initiate a cascade reaction inside the cell that leads to a change in the rate of impulses.

Humans are able to **distinguish 10 000 or more different odours**. Individual olfactory receptor neurones fire off spontaneously at between 3 and 60 impulses per second. When stimulated with particular odours, they increase their firing frequency. Each **receptor cell** responds, although not equally, to many different types of odour.

60 Special senses: vision

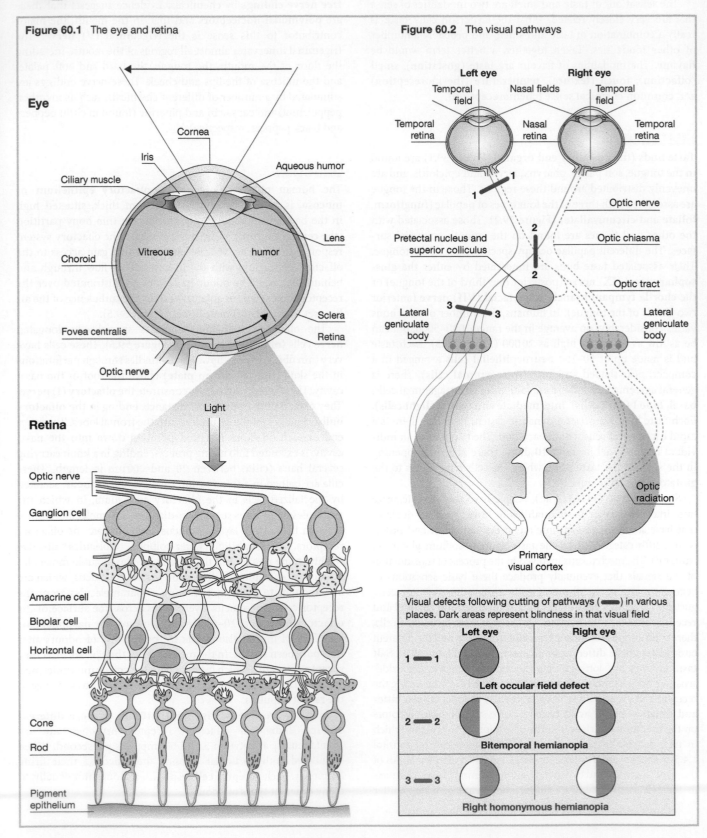

Figure 60.1 The eye and retina

Eye

- Cornea
- Iris
- Ciliary muscle
- Aqueous humor
- Lens
- humor
- Vitreous
- Choroid
- Sclera
- Retina
- Fovea centralis
- Optic nerve

Light

Retina

- Optic nerve
- Ganglion cell
- Amacrine cell
- Bipolar cell
- Horizontal cell
- Cone
- Rod
- Pigment epithelium

Figure 60.2 The visual pathways

Left eye | Right eye

- Temporal field
- Nasal fields
- Temporal field
- Temporal retina
- Nasal retina
- Temporal retina
- Optic nerve
- Optic chiasma
- Pretectal nucleus and superior colliculus
- Optic tract
- Lateral geniculate body
- Lateral geniculate body
- Optic radiation
- Primary visual cortex

Visual defects following cutting of pathways (▬▬) in various places. Dark areas represent blindness in that visual field

	Left eye	Right eye
1 ▬ 1		
Left occular field defect		
2 ▬ 2		
Bitemporal hemianopia		
3 ▬ 3		
Right homonymous hemianopia		

Physiology at a Glance, Fourth Edition. Edited by Jeremy P.T. Ward and Roger W.A. Linden.

ision in humans involves the detection of a very narrow band of light ranging from about **400 to 750 nm** in wavelength. The shortest wavelengths are perceived as blue and the longest as red. The eye contains **photoreceptors** that detect light, but, before the light hits the receptors responsible for this detection, it has to be focused onto the retina (200 μm thick) by the cornea and the lens (Figure 60.1).

The photoreceptors can be divided into two distinct types called **rods** and **cones**. **Rods** respond to **dim light** and **cones** respond in **brighter conditions and can distinguish red, green or blue light.** The rods and cones are found in the deepest part of the retina, and light has to travel through a number of cellular layers to reach these photoreceptors. Each photoreceptor contains molecules of the **visual pigments** (rods: **rhodopsin**; cones: **erythrolabe** [**red**], **chlorolabe** [**green**] and **cyanolabe** [**blue**]); these absorb light and trigger receptor potentials which, unlike other receptor systems, lead to a **hyperpolarization** of the cell. In the dark, the photoreceptors are depolarized and release the neurotransmitter glutamate which *inhibits* activity of **bipolar interneurons**. Light causes the photoreceptors to hyperpolarize, reducing glutamate release and thus increasing activity of bipolar cells. The response is graded according to light intensity.

The layers between the retina surface and the receptor cells contain a number of excitable cells, called **bipolar, horizontal, amacrine** and **ganglion cells**. The vertical bipolar interneurones lie between the receptor cells and the **ganglion cells**, which transmit impulses to the rest of the central nervous system (CNS) via axons in the **optic nerve**. In addition, this complex structure also contains two groups of interneurones (**horizontal** and **amacrine cells**) that function by exerting their influence in a horizontal manner, by causing lateral inhibition on surrounding synaptic connections between receptor cells and bipolar cells, and bipolar cells and ganglion cells, respectively (Figure 60.1).

Each eye contains approximately **126 million photoreceptors (120 million rods and 6 million cones)** but only **1.5 million ganglion cells**. This means that there is a substantial amount of convergence of receptor and bipolar cells onto ganglion cells, but this is not uniform across the retina. At the periphery, there is a large amount of convergence, but, in the region of greatest visual clarity (the **fovea centralis**), there is a 1:1:1 connectivity between a single cone receptor cell, a single bipolar cell and a single ganglion cell. The fovea region has a very high density of cones and very few rods, whereas there is a more even distribution of rods and cones in the other regions of the retina.

Each ganglion cell responds to changes in light intensity over a limited area of the retina, rather than to a stationary light stimulus. This limited area is called the **receptive field** of the cell and corresponds to the group of photoreceptors that has synaptic connections with that particular ganglion cell. Ganglion cells are usually spontaneously active. Approximately half of the ganglion cells in the retina respond with a decrease in firing of their impulses when the periphery of their receptive field is stimulated by light, and increase their firing rate when the centre of the receptive field is lit up (the **ON-centre cells**); the other half increase their firing rate when the periphery is illuminated and decrease their firing rate when the central receptors are stimulated (the **OFF-centre cells**). This allows the output of the retina to signal the relative brightness and darkness of each area being stimulated within the visual field.

The ganglion cells are further subdivided into two main groups: P cells and M cells. P cells receive the central parts of their receptive fields from one or possibly two (but never all three) types of colour-specific cone, whereas M cells receive inputs from all types of cone. M cells are therefore not colour selective, but sensitive to contrast and movement of images on the retina. The division of P and M cells appears to be maintained throughout the visual pathway and they are involved in visual perception.

The optic nerves from the two eyes join at the base of the skull at a structure called the **optic chiasma** (Figure 60.2). Approximately half of each of the optic nerve fibres cross over to the contralateral side; the other half remain on the ipsilateral side and are joined by axons crossing from the other side. The axons of the ganglion cells from the **temporal region** of the retina of the left eye and the **nasal region** of the retina of the right eye proceed into the left optic tract, whereas the axons from the ganglion cells in the **nasal part** of the left eye and the **temporal part** of the right eye form the right optic tract. The neurones that make up the **optic tract** connect to the first relay stations in the pathway: the **lateral geniculate bodies**, the **superior colliculus** and the **pretectal nucleus** of the **brain stem**. Those fibres that synapse in the superior colliculus and the pretectal nucleus are involved in visual reflexes and orientating responses. A small number of fibres also branch off at this point to synapse in the **suprachiasmatic nucleus**, which is concerned with the body clock and circadian rhythms within the body. However, the bulk of the neurones reach the **lateral geniculate nucleus** in the **thalamus**. Each nucleus contains six cellular layers and the information from the two eyes remains separate, each group of fibres synapsing in three of the layers. The **M ganglion cells** terminate in the lower two layers (called **magnocellular** because the cells are relatively large in these layers). Cells in the magnocellular layers are sensitive to contrast and motion, but not colour. The **P ganglion cells** synapse in the upper four layers of the lateral geniculate nucleus (two for each eye), called the **parvocellular** layers. These layers contain relatively small cells which transmit information about colour and fine detail. The fibres from the lateral geniculate nucleus fan backwards and upwards in a bundle (called the **optic radiation**) through the **parietal** and **temporal lobes** to an area of the cerebral cortex called the **primary visual cortex**. Each cortical cell receives inputs from a limited number of cells in the lateral geniculate nucleus, and therefore has its own receptive field or patch of retina to which it responds.

61 Special senses: hearing and balance

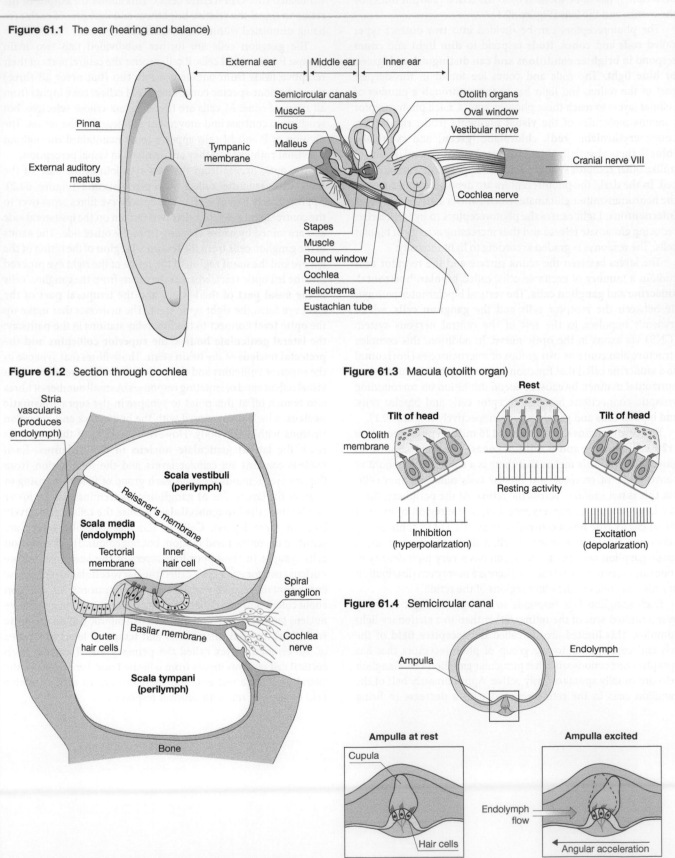

Figure 61.1 The ear (hearing and balance)

External ear | Middle ear | Inner ear

Semicircular canals
Muscle
Incus
Malleus

Pinna

Tympanic membrane

External auditory meatus

Otolith organs
Oval window
Vestibular nerve

Cranial nerve VIII

Cochlea nerve

Stapes
Muscle
Round window
Cochlea
Helicotrema
Eustachian tube

Figure 61.2 Section through cochlea

Stria vascularis (produces endolymph)

Scala vestibuli (perilymph)

Reissner's membrane

Scala media (endolymph)

Tectorial membrane

Inner hair cell

Spiral ganglion

Outer hair cells

Basilar membrane

Cochlea nerve

Scala tympani (perilymph)

Bone

Figure 61.3 Macula (otolith organ)

Rest

Tilt of head

Otolith membrane

Resting activity

Tilt of head

Inhibition (hyperpolarization)

Excitation (depolarization)

Figure 61.4 Semicircular canal

Endolymph

Ampulla

Ampulla at rest

Cupula

Hair cells

Ampulla excited

Endolymph flow

Angular acceleration

Physiology at a Glance, Fourth Edition. Edited by Jeremy P.T. Ward and Roger W.A. Linden.
© 2017 John Wiley & Sons, Ltd. Published 2017 by John Wiley & Sons, Ltd. Companion website: www.ataglanceseries.com/physiology

Hearing

The young healthy human can detect sound wave frequencies of between **40 Hz** and **20 kHz**, but the upper frequency limit declines with age. When sound waves reach the ear, they pass down the **external auditory meatus (the external ear)** to the **tympanic membrane** that vibrates at a frequency and strength determined by the magnitude and pitch of the sound. The vibration of the membrane causes three ear **ossicles (malleus, incus** and **stapes)** in the **middle ear** (an air-filled cavity) to move, which, in turn, displaces fluid within the **cochlea (the inner ear)** as the foot of the stapes moves the **oval window** at the base of the cochlea. This mechanical link prevents the incoming sound energy from being reflected back, and the ossicles improve the efficiency with which the sound energy is transferred from the air to the fluid. Small muscles are attached to the ossicles and contract reflexly in response to loud sounds, thereby dampening the vibration and attenuating the transmission of the sound (Figure 61.1).

The inner ear includes the **cochlea** and also the **vestibular organs** responsible for balance (see later). The receptors involved in both hearing and balance are specialized mechanoreceptors called **hair cells**. Projecting from the apical surface of the hair cell is a bundle of over 100 small hair-like structures called **stereocilia** and a larger stereocilium called the **kinocilium**. Deflection of the stereocilia towards the kinocilium leads to a potential change in the cell (depolarization), the release of a transmitter substance from the base of the hair cell, and activation of the nerve fibres that convey impulses to the higher centres of the brain.

The cochlea comprises a coiled tube of about 3 cm in length (Figure 61.2), with three tubular canals running parallel to one another (**scala vestibuli, scala media** and **scala tympani**).

The scala vestibuli and the scala tympani contain **perilymph** (which is similar to extracellular fluid in composition), and the scala media contains **endolymph** (similar in composition to intracellular fluid). The scala vestibuli and scala tympani are joined at the tip of the coil (the **helicotrema**); at the base of the scala vestibuli is the **oval window** and at the base of the scala tympani is the **round window**, separating the fluid of the inner ear from the air in the middle ear.

The scala media lies between the two perilymph-filled canals; the boundary between it and the scala vestibuli is called **Reissner's membrane**, and the boundary between it and the scala tympani is called the **basilar membrane**. On top of the basilar membrane sits the **organ of Corti** in which the hair cells are situated. There are around 15 000 hair cells distributed in rows along the basilar membrane. There are two types of hair cell: the **inner hair cells** which form a single row and the more numerous **outer hair cells** arranged in three rows. The hair cells are ideally placed to detect small amounts of movement of the basilar membrane. Because of the changing width of the basilar membrane, high-frequency sounds maximally displace the membrane at the base of the cochlea and low-frequency sounds maximally displace the membrane at the apical end of the cochlea.

The auditory signals are relayed through a complex series of nuclei in the brain stem and the thalamus, eventually reaching the **primary auditory cortex** in the temporal lobe of the cerebral cortex.

Balance

The system associated with balance is called the **vestibular system** and is not only involved with balance, but also postural reflexes and eye movements.

As mentioned earlier, the receptors involved in the vestibular system are hair cells. These hair cells are found in the inner ear in close proximity to the cochlea in two **otolith organs** called the **utricle** and **saccule**, and in a structure called the **ampulla** found in the three semicircular canals. The otolith organs are primarily involved in the detection of **linear motion** and **static head position**, and the semicircular canals in the detection of **rotational movements of the head**.

The four otolith organs (two on each side) each contain a structure called the **macula** which comprises a number of hair cells (Figure 61.3). With the head erect, the macula in each utricle is orientated horizontally and that in each saccule is orientated vertically. The base of each macula contains hair cells whose stereocilia project into a gelatinous mass called the **otolith membrane**. When the head is tilted, the force of gravity displaces the otolith membrane, thereby bending the stereocilia. The nerve fibres innervating the hair cells are spontaneously active: displacement in one direction increases firing and displacement in the opposite direction decreases firing of the neurones. The **utricle** sends signals representing **forwards and backwards movements** and the **saccule** conveys information about **vertical movements**.

The semicircular canals each contain an organ called the **ampulla** (Figure 61.4). They respond to **rotational movement of the head**, and the plane of each canal is perpendicular to the other two, so that, between all six (three on each side), they provide information relating to the rotational acceleration of the head during movement around any axis. Each canal contains endolymph and the ampulla comprises hair cells in which the stereocilia project into a gelatinous mass, with the same specific gravity as the endolymph, called the **cupula**. During acceleration in the plane of a particular canal, the endolymph tends to remain stationary because of inertia. The movement displaces the stereocilia and stimulation of the associated nerve fibres occurs. Again, movement in one direction increases firing of the nerves and movement in the opposite direction causes a decrease in firing. Vestibular afferent fibres from the auditory (VIII) nerve have their cell bodies in the **vestibular ganglion** and terminate in one of **four vestibular nuclei in the medulla**. These nuclei also receive inputs from neck muscle receptors and the visual system. They then project to a number of areas of the central nervous system, including the **spinal cord, thalamus, cerebellum** and **oculomotor nuclei**, where they are involved in posture, gait and eye movements. They also project to the **primary somatosensory cortex** and to the **posterior parietal cortex**.

62 Motor control and the cerebellum

Figure 62.1 Major ascending sensory inputs and descending motor outputs

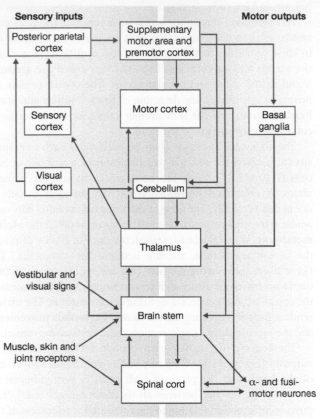

In addition there are looped pathways linking the thalamus, cerebellum, premotor cortex, supplementary motor area, basal ganglia and motor cortex. These have been omitted for the sake of clarity. See Figure 62.2

Figure 62.3 Motor homunculus

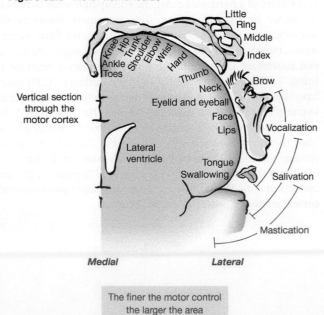

Figure 62.2 Diagram of looped pathways within the motor system

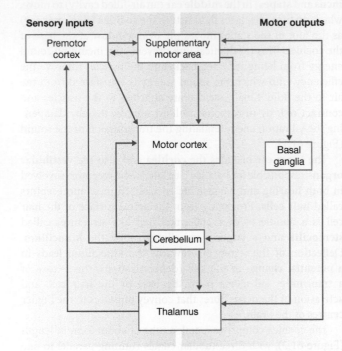

Figure 62.4 Anatomical positions of principal spinal and supraspinal motor and sensory centres

Motor control

Motor control is defined as the control of movements by the body. These movements can be both influenced and guided by the many sensory inputs that are received, or can be triggered by sensory events. They can also be triggered by the need to move using internal mechanisms. The major division of the body into sensory and motor functions is artificial, because almost all motor areas in the central nervous system (CNS) receive sensory inputs.

The organization and physiology of motor systems have been represented as a number of **hierarchical structures**, but these must be viewed with caution, as they are again artificial and, by necessity, oversimplified.

Figure 62.1 shows the major ascending sensory inputs and descending motor outputs, and Figure 62.2 shows the main looped pathways within the CNS.

Voluntary movements can be summarized as follows. Exactly where the idea of a movement is initiated is unknown, but it is thought to be in the areas of the cortex other than the primary sensory or primary motor cortices (the **association cortex**) and possibly the **basal ganglia**. At this stage, sensory information relating to the intended movement is analysed in the **posterior parietal cortex**. This sensory information mainly comes from the **visual** and **sensory cortex**.

The posterior parietal cortex activates the **supplementary motor area** and the **premotor cortex**. This excitation also causes the **basal ganglia loop** and the **cerebrocerebellar loop** to be excited and to lead to a degree of amplitude setting and coordination of the activity. The supplementary motor area and the premotor cortex then initiate activity in the **motor cortex**. In addition, the premotor cortex initiates, via the **anterior corticospinal tract** and the connections to the brain stem **ventromedial pathways**, any postural adjustments needed for the movement.

The motor cortex, via the lateral **corticospinal** and **corticorubrospinal tracts**, then initiates the activity of the muscles. This activity is due to the excitation of both α- and **fusi-motor neurones**. During this movement, there is continuous feedback from **receptors** in the **joints**, **muscles** and **skin**, which can lead to fine adjustments via local **spinal** and **brain stem reflexes**. Furthermore, there is often **visual feedback** which can modulate the motor outputs at the cortical and cerebellar levels. Modulations of the activity at all levels continue throughout the voluntary movement.

Figure 62.4 shows the anatomical sites of the principal motor and sensory centres, and Figure 62.3 shows the relative size of the areas in the motor cortex represented by the different parts of the body (the motor homunculus).

The term **upper motor neurones** refers to those neurones that are wholly in the CNS motor pathways. These descending motor pathways are divided into the **pyramidal tracts**, which originate in the cerebral cortex, and the **extrapyramidal tracts**, which originate in the brain stem. The **pyramidal tracts** descend through the **internal capsule** and terminate in the brain stem. One small group of fibres (the **corticobulbar tract**) terminates on cranial motor nuclei and is involved in controlling eye, facial and masticatory muscles. Another larger group of fibres (the **corticospinal tract**) descends directly from the cortex to the grey matter of the spinal cord but, as it passes through the brain stem,

it divides into two. Approximately **85%** of the fibres cross over the midline (**decussate**) and descend as the **lateral corticospinal tract**, terminating directly onto the α- and fusi-motor neurones. Some of the fibres do not terminate directly onto the motor neurones but excite interneurones instead. These interneurones can be either excitatory or inhibitory in nature.

The other **15%** of corticospinal neurones, the **anterior corticospinal tract**, do not decussate and remain ipsilateral, eventually terminating in the upper thoracic spinal cord, and project bilaterally onto the motor neurones and interneurones that innervate the muscles of the upper trunk and neck.

The **extrapyramidal tract** neurones project to the spinal cord, where they synapse mainly onto interneurones. There are two groups: the **ventromedial** pathways, which terminate in the motor pools of the axial and proximal limb muscles, and the **dorsolateral** pathways, which terminate in the motor pools of the distal limb muscles. The **ventromedial pathways** comprise the **vestibulospinal tract**, which receives neurones from the vestibular system and is involved in the reflex control of balance, the **tectospinal tract**, which is involved in the coordination of eye and body movements, and the **reticulospinal tract**, which is concerned with regulating the excitability of extensor muscle reflexes. The **dorsolateral pathways** comprise mainly the **rubrospinal tract**, which originates in the **red nucleus** in the **midbrain** and projects to similar motor neurone pools as those served by the corticospinal tracts, and are involved with the **reflex control** of **flexor muscles**.

The cerebellum

The cerebellum is anatomically distinct from the rest of the brain and is connected to the brain stem by thick strands of afferent and efferent fibres through **three (cerebellar) peduncles**. Its primary function is the coordination and learning of movements, and it is made up of three functional and anatomical structures: the **spinocerebellum**, which is involved in the control of musculature and posture; the **cerebrocerebellum**, which is involved in the coordination and planning of limb movement; and the **vestibulocerebellum**, which is involved with posture and the control of eye movements. The **spinocerebellum** receives both sensory inputs from the spinal cord and motor inputs from the cerebral cortex. It regulates ongoing movements of axial and distal muscles, by comparison of the descending inputs with the ascending sensory feedback, and regulates muscle tone. The **cerebrocerebellum** receives inputs from the cerebral cortex, particularly the premotor cortex, and is primarily involved in the planning and initiation of movements, particularly involving the visual system. The **vestibulocerebellum** receives inputs and sends outputs to the vestibular nuclei in the medulla, and is involved in the regulation of balance, posture and the control of eye movements.

The cerebellum functions by acting as a **comparator**, comparing sensory and motor inputs and achieving coordinated movements that are both smooth and accurate. It can also function as a **timing device** in which it converts descending motor signals into a sequence of coordinated and smooth events. Finally, it can **store motor information** and regularly update it; therefore, given the right sequence of events, it can lead to the initiation of accurate learnt movements.

63 Proprioception and reflexes

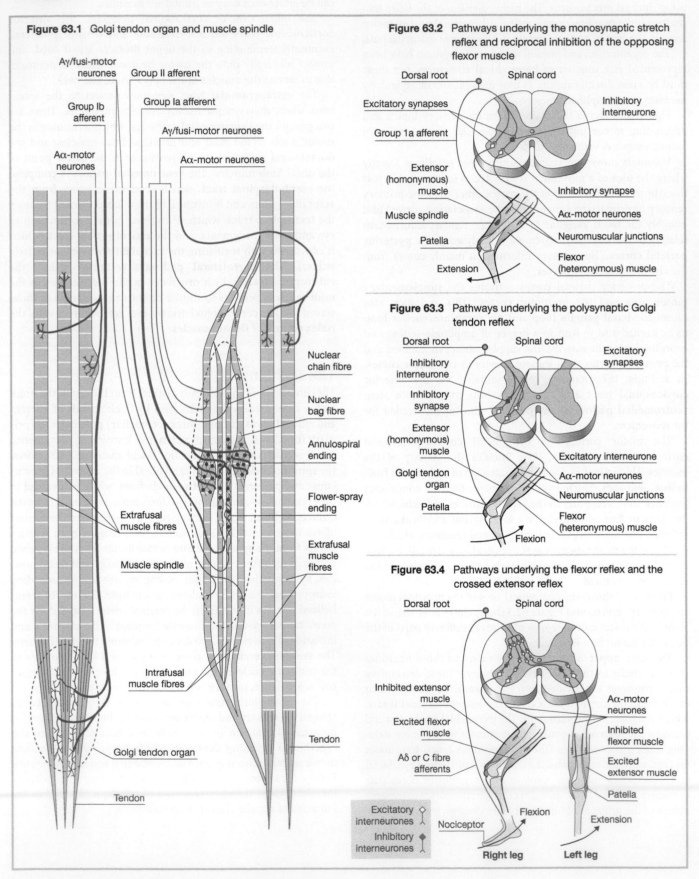

Figure 63.1 Golgi tendon organ and muscle spindle

Aγ/fusi-motor neurones
Group II afferent
Group Ib afferent
Group Ia afferent
Aγ/fusi-motor neurones
Aα-motor neurones
Aα-motor neurones
Nuclear chain fibre
Nuclear bag fibre
Annulospiral ending
Flower-spray ending
Extrafusal muscle fibres
Extrafusal muscle fibres
Muscle spindle
Intrafusal muscle fibres
Tendon
Golgi tendon organ
Tendon

Figure 63.2 Pathways underlying the monosynaptic stretch reflex and reciprocal inhibition of the oppposing flexor muscle

Dorsal root
Spinal cord
Excitatory synapses
Inhibitory interneurone
Group 1a afferent
Extensor (homonymous) muscle
Inhibitory synapse
Muscle spindle
Aα-motor neurones
Patella
Neuromuscular junctions
Extension
Flexor (heteronymous) muscle

Figure 63.3 Pathways underlying the polysynaptic Golgi tendon reflex

Dorsal root
Spinal cord
Inhibitory interneurone
Excitatory synapses
Inhibitory synapse
Extensor (homonymous) muscle
Excitatory interneurone
Golgi tendon organ
Aα-motor neurones
Patella
Neuromuscular junctions
Flexion
Flexor (heteronymous) muscle

Figure 63.4 Pathways underlying the flexor reflex and the crossed extensor reflex

Dorsal root
Spinal cord
Inhibited extensor muscle
Aα-motor neurones
Excited flexor muscle
Inhibited flexor muscle
Aδ or C fibre afferents
Excited extensor muscle
Patella
Nociceptor
Flexion
Extension

Excitatory interneurones
Inhibitory interneurones

Right leg
Left leg

Physiology at a Glance, Fourth Edition. Edited by Jeremy P.T. Ward and Roger W.A. Linden.

We are aware of the orientation of our limbs with respect to one another, we can perceive the movements of our joints and we can accurately assess the amount of resistance (force) that opposes the movements we make. This ability is called **proprioception**. The three qualities of this modality are **position**, **movement** and **force**. The receptors or **proprioceptors** that mediate this modality are principally found in the joint capsules (**joint receptors**), muscles (**muscle spindles**) and tendons (**Golgi tendon organs**).

The **joint capsule** is compressed or stretched when the joint moves, and **mechanoreceptors** within it signal the position of the joint, as well as the direction and velocity of the movement. Individual receptors respond to the position of the joint, as well as the direction and the velocity of the movement, but not the force. The receptor types found in the joint capsule are **Ruffini-type** (slowly adapting) stretch receptors (Chapter 58).

Each muscle contains a number of small muscle fibres (**intrafusal muscle fibres**: 15–30 μm in diameter and 4–7 mm in length) that are thinner and shorter than the ordinary muscle fibre (**extrafusal muscle fibres**: 50–100 μm in diameter and varying in length from a few millimetres to many centimetres). Several intrafusal fibres are grouped together and encased in a connective tissue capsule, called the **muscle spindle**, a specialized receptor that responds to the stretch of a muscle (Figure 63.1). Muscle spindles lie in **parallel** to the extrafusal muscle fibres and are elongated when the muscle is stretched. The primary sensory innervation of the muscle spindle consists of afferent fibres which wind themselves around the centre of the intrafusal muscle fibres (**annulospiral ending**). These are large myelinated fibres (group Ia afferents). These endings are called **primary sensory endings** and, when excited, they evoke a **monosynaptic stretch reflex** involving an excitation of the **homonymous** α-motor neurones and reciprocal inhibition of the **heteronymous** α-motor neurones (Figure 63.2). Many muscle spindles also have a **secondary sensory innervation** (group II afferent). They are thinner and end in **flower-spray endings** (they are not involved in the monosynaptic stretch reflex).

The intrafusal muscle fibres possess a motor innervation, the Aγ- or fusi-motor neurones. They are smaller in diameter than those innervating the extrafusal muscle fibres, the Aα-motor neurones.

Stretching the muscle, thereby extending both the extrafusal and intrafusal muscle fibres, can excite the muscle spindle. However, there is a second way to excite the primary muscle spindle ending – by contraction of the intrafusal muscle fibre brought about by excitation of the fusi- or γ-motor neurone. This does not change the overall length or tension of the entire muscle, as it is too weak; however, it is sufficient to stretch the central portion of the intrafusal fibres, inducing excitation in the primary sensory ending.

Contraction of the extrafusal fibres can be triggered or at least facilitated by the muscle spindle, either by stretch of the whole muscle or by activation of the fusi- or γ-motor neurones. They can complement each other or have a mutually cancelling effect. The threshold of the stretch reflex can also be varied by intrafusal activity.

The **Golgi tendon organs** are stretch receptors found in the muscle tendons (Figure 63.1). Each receptor is associated with the tendon fascicle of about 10 extrafusal muscle fibres, is surrounded by a capsule of connective tissue and is innervated by large myelinated afferent fibres (group Ib fibres). They are in **series** with the extrafusal muscle fibres and respond to tension in the muscle. They can respond both when the muscle contracts and when the muscle is stretched, unlike the muscle spindle which responds predominantly during stretching of the muscle. Golgi tendon organs protect against overloading and provide a protective reflex. In a functional sense, the segmental connections of the Ib fibres are a mirror image of the Ia fibres. A marked increase in muscle tension, whether resulting from stretch, contraction or a combination of the two, will result in **inhibitory** connections with the **homonymous** motor neurones and **excitatory** connections with the **heteronymous** motor neurones. However, none of these connections is monosynaptic; all involve at least two synapses (Figure 63.3).

The properties of the joint receptors make it very likely that they are primarily responsible for mediating the sense of position and movement. The most likely detectors of force sensation are the muscle spindles and Golgi tendon organs. Other receptors also contribute to the sense of force, as well as movement and position, such as mechanoreceptors in the skin.

Polysynaptic motor reflexes. Many receptors in the body, other than those found in muscle, can trigger motor reflexes. Experiments on animals, in which the spinal cord has been severed, have shown that many of these reflexes are restricted to the spinal cord. They are always polysynaptic. The most prominent examples of these reflexes are the flexor reflex and the crossed extensor reflex (Figure 63.4). If a pinprick is made to a toe, the stimulated limb is pulled away. The **flexor reflex** is a flexion of the knee and hip joints. It is a protective reflex, pulling the limb from the site of the noxious stimulus. The delay and the magnitude of the response are very much dependent on the stimulus intensity. The higher the intensity, the shorter the latency and the quicker the response. It can also be observed that the flexion of one limb is always accompanied by the extension of the limb on the other side of the body. In other words, there is an ipsilateral flexor reflex and a contralateral extensor reflex. This contralateral extensor reflex is called the **crossed extensor reflex**. These reflexes are not only enhanced in spinal animals, but also in newborn and premature babies, as during the days just after birth the higher levels of the brain are not fully developed.

Glossary

acini (plural), acinar (adj.) cluster of cells looking like a many-lobed berry

adrenergic relating to adrenaline, noradrenaline

adrenoceptors (α or β) adrenergic receptors for noradrenaline, adrenaline

adventitia outermost connective tissue layer of, e.g. blood vessel or organ

afferent conducting towards, e.g. nerves to the brain, arterioles to the glomerulus

anabolic process or hormone that acts to build up tissues or energy stores; consumes energy

anaerobic metabolic process that does not require oxygen

angiogenesis generation of new blood vessels

anorexigenic suppresses appetite

antidromic conducting in the opposite direction to normal, e.g. in an axon towards the soma

antigen anything that is recognized as foreign by an immunoglobulin

antiporters transporters that exchange molecules across a membrane, e.g. Na^+-K^+ ATPase

anti-pyretic drug that reduces fever

apnoea cessation of breathing

apoptosis programmed cell death (different from necrosis)

atresia narrowing or absence of an orifice or passage in the body

autocoids (*autacoid*) locally acting chemical signalling substance

basal lamina layer of extracellular matrix secreted by cells on which they sit

basement membrane thin membrane an epithelium from underlying tissue (includes basal laminar)

basolateral base and sides of a polarized cell (normally epithelial) away from lumen

catabolic metabolism/breakdown of molecules to release energy

chemoreceptors detect and respond to chemicals, e.g. H^+ (pH), O_2

chemotaxis movement of cell induced by a chemical gradient

cholinergic relating to acetylcholine releasing nerves

clonal expansion division of a single cell into multiple exact copies of itself (a clone)

colloidal osmotic pressure see oncotic pressure

compliance "stretchiness"

crystalloid osmotic pressure due to electrolytes, e.g. Na^+ and Cl^-

cytokine signalling molecule secreted by cells of the immune system that affects other cells

cytosol (cytoplasm) intracellular fluid

diapedesis movement of leucocytes across capillary walls into tissues

dorsolateral of the back and sides

efferent conducting away from, e.g. from the central nervous system

eicosanoid local hormone derived from arachidonic acid, e.g. prostaglandins, leukotrienes

electrolyte any charged ion (e.g. Na^+)

endocytosis import of substances into cells by engulfing in a section of membrane to form a vesicle

enteric of the intestines

epitope amino acid sequence on a protein recognized by an immunoglobulin

exocytosis export of substances from cells via secretory vesicles

extracellular matrix assembly of non-cellular molecules (e.g. collagen) secreted by cells that provide them with both structural support and affect their function

gating process that causes an ion channel open or shut

glabrous hairless (skin)

glycosylation covalent addition of sugar moieties to specific amino acids on a protein

hydrophilic water loving, substance that dissolves easily in water

hydrophobic water hating, substance that does not dissolve easily in water (e.g. lipids, oils)

hypertonic of a greater osmolality than (usually) plasma or interstitial fluid

hypertrophy grows larger than normal

inotropic affects contractility of heart

interstitial fluid fluid between cells

intima (*tunica intima*) innermost layer of organ or blood vessel; endothelium

isometric no change in length while force changes

isotonic no change in force while length changes

lamina propria layer of connective tissue beneath epithelia; part of mucosa

ligand something that binds to a specific receptor or location on a molecule

lipophilic lipid soluble

mitogen substance that causes mitosis and cell division

mucosa (*mucous membrane*) inner lining of lines body cavities and tubes, consists of epithelium and laminar propria

myocardium cardiac muscle

oligopeptide peptide with 20 or less amino acids

oncogenes gene with a potential to cause cancer

oncotic pressure osmotic pressure exerted by proteins across a protein-impermeable but water- and electrolyte-permeable membrane

orexigenic appetite stimulant

orthodromic conducting in a normal direction, e.g. in an axon away from the soma

osmolality (osmotic pressure) reflects number of diffusible particles/molecules in fluid

paracellular transfer of fluid or solute through junctions between cells

partial pressure the part of barometric pressure due to a single component of the gas mixture

phagocytes (phagocytosis) cell that ingests bacteria or debris, e.g. macrophage

phosphorylate transfer of a phosphate group onto a molecule

pinocytosis ingestion of fluid into a cell in small vesicles budded from cell membrane (a form of endocytosis)

plasma membrane (plasmalemma) cell membrane

polar having a charge, e.g. Na^+

polarized cell a cell (normally epithelial) with different properties on top and bottom

proprioception position sensing

pyrogens a substance that induces fever (pyro, Greek for fire)

refractory resistant to a stimulus

sarcolemma membrane (plasmalemma) of a muscle cell

sarcoplasm cytosol (cytoplasm) of a muscle cell

Physiology at a Glance, Fourth Edition. Edited by Jeremy P.T. Ward and Roger W.A. Linden.
© 2017 John Wiley & Sons Ltd. Published 2017 by John Wiley & Sons, Ltd. Companion website: www.ataglanceseries.com/physiology

semi-permeable membrane one that has different permeabilities to different molecules, e.g. cell membrane

serosa (serous membrane) fluid-secreting epithelial membrane, e.g. pleura, peritoneum

stenosis narrowing

syncope fainting

synergistic more than additive

tonic continuous, normally active

transcellular transport transport through a cell, most commonly across epithelia, e.g. glucose reabsorption in renal proximal convoluted tubule

transudation passage of fluid through an epithelium by hydrostatic or osmotic pressure

ultrafiltration filtration across a membrane that only allows small molecules to pass (e.g. glomerulus)

Appendix I: Comparison of the properties of skeletal, cardiac and smooth muscle

Characteristic	Skeletal muscle	Cardiac muscle	Smooth muscle
Cell shape and size	Long cylindrical cells up to 30 cm long and 100 μm wide	Irregular, branched, rod-shaped cells up to 100 μm long and 20 μm wide	Spindle-shaped cells up to 400 μm long and 10 μm wide
Nuclei	Multinucleated	Mostly single nuclei	Single nuclei
Presence of actin and myosin filaments	Yes	Yes	Yes
Striated (presence of sarcomeres)	Yes	Yes	No
Myogenic activity	No	Yes	Yes
Initiation of contraction	Extrinsic (somatic, neural)	Intrinsic (muscle origin) but influenced by extrinsic autonomic (sympathetic and parasympathetic)	Can be intrinsic via plexus of nerves or extrinsic via autonomic (sympathetic and/or parasympathetic), hormones or stretch
Basic muscle tone	Neural activity	None	Both intrinsic and extrinsic factors
Speed of contraction	Fast	Slow	Very slow
Type of contraction	Phasic	Rhythmic	Tonic with some phasic
Electronic coupling between cells (gap junctions)	No	Yes	A few in multiunit and many in unitary
Influence of hormones on contraction	Small	Large	Large
Effect of nerve stimulation	Excitatory	Excitatory or inhibitory	Excitatory or inhibitory
Spontaneous electrical activity	No	Yes	Unitary (yes), multiunit (no)
Extent of innervation	Each cell innervated	Variable	Unitary (sparse), multiunit (almost every cell)
Site of calcium regulation of contraction	Troponin thin filament	Troponin thin filament	Myosin thick filament
Mechanism of excitation–contraction coupling	Via action potentials and T-system	Via action potentials and T-system	Via action potentials, calcium channels and/or second messengers
Source of activating calcium	Sarcoplasmic reticulum	Sarcoplasmic reticulum and some extracellular	Sarcoplasmic reticulum and some extracellular

Physiology at a Glance, Fourth Edition. Edited by Jeremy P.T. Ward and Roger W.A. Linden.
© 2017 John Wiley & Sons, Ltd. Published 2017 by John Wiley & Sons, Ltd. Companion website: www.ataglanceseries.com/physiology

Appendix II: Normal physiological values

Blood fluid volumes	
Blood volume	70 mL/kg body weight
Plasma volume	40 mL/kg body weight
Total body fluid volume	60% body weight (males) 50% body weight (females)
Intracellular fluid volume	65% of total body fluid volume
Extracellular fluid volume	34% of total body fluid volume
Blood cells	
Haematocrit	45% (range 40–50) males 40% (range 36–46) females
Haemoglobin concentration	150 g/L (range 130–170) males 140 g/L (range 120–150) females
Red cell (erythrocyte) count	5×10^{12}/L (range 4.5–6.5) males 4.5×10^{12}/L (range 3.8–5.6) females
Reticulocyte count	2% of erythrocyte count
Erythrocyte sedimentation rate (ESR)	<5 mm/h (males) <7 mm/h (females)
White cells count	7×10^9/L (range 4–11)
Neutrophils	3.5×10^9/L
Lymphocytes	2×10^9/L
Eosinophils	0.2×10^9/L
Monocytes	0.5×10^9/L
Basophils	$<0.1 \times 10^9$/L
Platelet count	2.5×10^{11}/L (range 1.4–4.0)
Plasma	
Plasma protein concentration	60 g/L
Plasma oncotic (colloid osmotic) pressure	25 mmHg
Plasma osmolality	290 mosmol/kg H_2O
Na^+	140 mmol/L
K^+	4 mmol/L
Ca^{2+}	1 mmol/L (free)
Cl^-	108 mmol/L
HCO_3^-	25–30 mmol/L
Cardiovascular function	
Cardiac output, rest	5 L/min
Cardiac output, exercise	>20 L/min
Heart rate, rest	70/min
Heart rate, exercise	180/min
Resting stroke volume	70 mL

Physiology at a Glance, Fourth Edition. Edited by Jeremy P.T. Ward and Roger W.A. Linden.
© 2017 John Wiley & Sons, Ltd. Published 2017 by John Wiley & Sons, Ltd. Companion website: www.ataglanceseries.com/physiology

Systemic arterial blood pressure	110 mmHg (systolic)
	80 mmHg (diastolic)
Pulmonary arterial pressure	25 mmHg (systolic)
	15 mmHg (diastolic)
Central venous pressure	5 cmH$_2$O (range 3–8)
Mean arterial pressure	90 mmHg
Mean blood pressure at start of arterioles	65 mmHg
Capillary pressure	25–35 mmHg (arterial side)
	15 mmHg (venous side)
End diastolic volume (EDV)	130 mL (range 120–140)
End diastolic pressure	<10 mmHg

Percentage of cardiac output to various organs at rest

Brain	14%
Heart	4%
Liver and digestive system	27%
Kidney	20%
Skeletal muscle	21%
Skin	5%
Bone and other tissues	9%

Respiratory function

Static lung compliance	1.5 L/kPa
Intrapleural pressure (quiet breathing)	−4 cmH$_2$O (expiration)
	−9 cmH$_2$O (inspiration)
Tidal volume	500 ml
Respiratory rate (rest)	12/min
Respiratory minute volume	6 L/min
Dead space	150 mL
Alveolar ventilation rate	5 L/min
FEV$_1$/FVC	80% (range 75–90)
Vital capacity (VC)	5.5 L
Inspiratory reserve volume (IRV)	3.3 L
Expiratory reserve volume (ERV)	1.7 L
Total lung capacity (TLC)	7.3 L
Functional reserve capacity (FRC)	3.5 L
Residual volume (RV)	1.8 L

Blood gases and acid–base balance

Systemic arterial pH	7.36 (range 7.3–7.42)
Systemic arterial Po$_2$	13 kPa (98 mmHg)
Systemic arterial Pco$_2$	5.3 kPa (40 mmHg)
Base excess	−2 to +2 mmol/L
Mixed venous blood Po$_2$ (resting)	5.3 kPa (40 mmHg)
Mixed venous blood Pco$_2$ (resting)	6.1 kPa (46 mmHg)
Alveolar Po$_2$	13.3 kPa (100 mmHg)
Alveolar Pco$_2$	5.3 kPa (40 mmHg)
Capillary Po$_2$	5.3 kPa or less (40 mmHg or less)
Capillary Pco$_2$	6.1 kPa or more (46 mmHg or more)

Renal function	
Renal blood flow	1.2 L/min
Renal plasma flow	600 mL/min
Glomerular filtration rate	125 mL/min
Average urine output	1 mL/min
Renal glucose threshold	11 mmol/L
Gastrointestinal function	
Fluid inputs into the digestive system (total = 9 L/day)	
Food and drink	2.0 L
Saliva	1.5 L
Bile (liver)	0.5 L
Gastric secretions	2.0 L
Pancreatic secretions	1.5 L
Intestinal secretions	1.5 L
Fluid removed from the digestive system (total = 9 L/day)	
Absorption from small intestine	7.5 L
Absorption from large intestine	1.4 L
Excreted in faeces	0.1 L
Nervous system	
Equilibrium potential for Na^+	+65 mV
Equilibrium potential for K^+	−90 mV
Resting membrane potential in excitable cells	−70 mV (range −60 to −90)
Resting membrane potential in non-excitable cells	−10 mV
Blood glucose levels	
Normal	
Fasting pre-prandial	4.0–5.9 mmol/L
Post-prandial (2 h after meal)	<7.8 mmol/L
Diabetic fasting pre-prandial	
Pre-diabetes or impaired glucose glycaemia	6.0–6.9 mmol/L
Diagnosis of diabetes	>6.9 mmol/L
HbA_{1C} (glycated haemoglobin), a measure of the average plasma glucose concentration	
Normal	20–41 mmol/L (4–5.9%)
Diabetic patients	>47 mmol/L (>6.5%)

Index

Note:

Glossary (page 142-143) has not been indexed.

Page numbers in *italics* refer to pages on which figures &/or tables appear.

Physiology at a Glance, Fourth Edition. Edited by Jeremy P.T. Ward and Roger W.A. Linden.
© 2017 John Wiley & Sons, Ltd. Published 2017 by John Wiley & Sons, Ltd. Companion website: www.ataglanceseries.com/physiology